Medications and Their Effects on Sleep and Wake

Editors

JOHAN VERBRAECKEN
JAN HEDNER

SLEEP MEDICINE CLINICS

www.sleep.theclinics.com

Consulting Editor
TEOFILO LEE-CHIONG Jr

June 2018 • Volume 13 • Number 2

ELSEVIER

1600 John F. Kennedy Boulevard • Suite 1800 • Philadelphia, Pennsylvania, 19103-2899

http://www.theclinics.com

SLEEP MEDICINE CLINICS Volume 13, Number 2
June 2018, ISSN 1556-407X, ISBN-13: 978-0-323-58417-3

Editor: Colleen Dietzler
Developmental Editor: Donald Mumford

Sleep Medicine Clinics (ISSN 1556-407X) is published quarterly by Elsevier Inc., 360 Park Avenue South, New York, NY 10010-1710. Months of issue are March, June, September and December. Business and Editorial Offices: 1600 John F. Kennedy Blvd., Ste. 1800, Philadelphia, PA 19103-2899. Customer Service Office: 3251 Riverport Lane, Maryland Heights, MO 63043. Periodicals postage paid at New York, NY and additional mailing offices. Subscription prices are $203.00 per year (US individuals), $100.00 (US students), $486.00 (US institutions), $245.00 (Canadian and international individuals), $135.00 (Canadian and international students), $540.00 (Canadian institutions) and $540.00 (International institutions). Foreign air speed delivery is included in all *Clinics* subscription prices. All prices are subject to change without notice. **POSTMASTER:** Send change of address to *Sleep Medicine Clinics*, Elsevier Health Sciences Division, Subscription Customer Service, 3251 Riverport Lane, Maryland Heights, MO 63043. Customer Service: **Tel: 1-800-654-2452 (U.S. and Canada); 314-447-8871 (outside U.S. and Canada). Fax: 314-447-8029. E-mail: journalscustomerservice-usa@elsevier.com (for print support); journalsonline support-usa@elsevier.com (for online support).**

Reprints. For copies of 100 or more of articles in this publication, please contact the Commercial Reprints Department, Elsevier Inc., 360 Park Avenue South, New York, NY 10010-1710. Tel.: 212-633-3874; Fax: 212-633-3820; E-mail: reprints@elsevier.com.

Sleep Medicine Clinics is covered in *MEDLINE/PubMed (Index Medicus).*

PROGRAM OBJECTIVE
The goal of *Sleep Clinics of North America* is to keep practicing physicians up to date with current clinical practice by providing timely articles reviewing the state of the art in patient care.

TARGET AUDIENCE
All practicing physicians and other healthcare professionals.

LEARNING OBJECTIVES
Upon completion of this activity, participants will be able to:
1. Review drug therapy used in parasomicas, hypersomnias, insomnia, obstructive sleep apnea, and circadian sleep-wake rhythm disturbances.
2. Discuss pharmacologic treatment of sleep disorders in pregnancy, as well as pharmacological and non-pharmacological treatment of restless legs syndrome.
3. Recognize drug-induced sleep disordered breathing and ventilatory impairment, as well as drug-induced insomnia and excessive sleepiness.

ACCREDITATION
The Elsevier Office of Continuing Medical Education (EOCME) is accredited by the Accreditation Council for Continuing Medical Education (ACCME) to provide continuing medical education for physicians.

The EOCME designates this enduring material for a maximum of 15 *AMA PRA Category 1 Credit*(s)™. Physicians should claim only the credit commensurate with the extent of their participation in the activity.

All other healthcare professionals requesting continuing education credit for this enduring material will be issued a certificate of participation.

DISCLOSURE OF CONFLICTS OF INTEREST
The EOCME assesses conflict of interest with its instructors, faculty, planners, and other individuals who are in a position to control the content of CME activities. All relevant conflicts of interest that are identified are thoroughly vetted by EOCME for fair balance, scientific objectivity, and patient care recommendations. EOCME is committed to providing its learners with CME activities that promote improvements or quality in healthcare and not a specific proprietary business or a commercial interest.

The planning committee, staff, authors and editors listed below have identified no financial relationships or relationships to products or devices they or their spouse/life partner have with commercial interest related to the content of this CME activity:
Galia V. Anguelova, MD, MSc; Michelle Cao, DO; Joseph Daniel; Sylvie Dujardin, MD; Nicholas-Tiberio Economou, MD, PhD; Jonathan S. Emens, MD; Luigi Ferini-Strambi, MD, PhD; Priya Gopalan, MD; Jonathan P. Hintze, MD; Sebastian C. Holst, PhD; Shahrokh Javaheri, MD; Alison Kemp; Arthur G.Y. Kurvers, MD; Hans-Peter Landolt, PhD; Teofilo Lee-Chiong Jr; Raffaele Manni, MD; Laura P. McLafferty, MD; Lino Nobili, MD, PhD; Dirk Pevernagie, MD, PhD; Katie Pfaff; Angelique Pijpers, MD, PhD; Roselyne M. Rijsman, MD, PhD; Meredith Spada, MD; Paschalis Steiropoulos, MD, PhD, FCCP; Michele Terzaghi, MD; Ann Van Gastel, MD; Johan Verbraecken, MD, PhD; Monique H.M. Vlak, MD, PhD; Ding Zou, MD, PhD.

The planning committee, staff, authors and editors listed below have identified financial relationships or relationships to products or devices they or their spouse/life partner have with commercial interest related to the content of this CME activity:
Helen J. Burgess, PhD: is a consultant/advisor for Natrol, LLC.
Jack D. Edinger, PhD: has received research support from Merck Sharpe & Dohme Corp. and Koninklijke Philips NV.
Ludger Grote, MD, PhD: has participated in a speaker's bureau for Koninklijke Philips NV and AstraZeneca; recevies roayalties and/or holds patents with Johnson & Johnson Consumer, Inc.; has participated in a speaker's burea and received research support from Itamar Medical Ltd and ResMed.
Jan Hedner, MD, PhD: has participated in a speaker's bureau for AstraZeneca, Itamar Medical Ltd., and Koninklijke Philips NV.
Gert Jan Lammers, MD, PhD: has been a consultant/advisor for UCB SA, Jazz Pharmaceuticals, Inc., and Bioprojet.
Paola Proserpio, MD: has been employed by Sapio UFE.

UNAPPROVED/OFF-LABEL USE DISCLOSURE
The EOCME requires CME faculty to disclose to the participants:
1. When products or procedures being discussed are off-label, unlabelled, experimental, and/or investigational (not US Food and Drug Administration [FDA] approved); and
2. Any limitations on the information presented, such as data that are preliminary or that represent ongoing research, interim analyses, and/or unsupported opinions. Faculty may discuss information about pharmaceutical agents that is outside of FDA-approved labelling. This information is intended solely for CME and is not intended to promote off-label use of these medications. If you have any questions, contact the medical affairs department of the manufacturer for the most recent pre-scribing information.

TO ENROLL

To enroll in the *Sleep Medicines Clinic* Continuing Medical Education program, call customer service at 1-800-654-2452 or sign up online at http://www.theclinics.com/home/cme. The CME program is available to subscribers for an additional annual fee of USD $140.

METHOD OF PARTICIPATION

In order to claim credit, participants must complete the following:

1. Complete enrolment as indicated above.
2. Read the activity.
3. Complete the CME Test and Evaluation. Participants must achieve a score of 70% on the test. All CME Tests and Evaluations must be completed online.

CME INQUIRIES/SPECIAL NEEDS

For all CME inquiries or special needs, please contact elsevierCME@elsevier.com.

SLEEP MEDICINE CLINICS

FORTHCOMING ISSUES

September 2018
Sleep Disorders in Women's Health
Kathryn Lee and Fiona Baker, *Editors*

December 2018
Dental Sleep Medicine
Jamison R. Spencer, *Editor*

March 2019
Prevention, Screening and Treatments for Obstructive Sleep Apnea: Beyond Positive Airway Pressure (PAP)
Song Tar Toh, *Editor*

RECENT ISSUES

March 2018
Sleep in Older Adults
Cathy A. Alessi and Jennifer L. Martin, *Editors*

December 2017
Advanced PAP Therapies and Non-invasive Ventilation
Lee K. Brown and Shahrokh Javaheri, *Editors*

September 2017
Hypersomnolence
Ahmed S. BaHammam, *Editor*

ISSUES OF RELATED INTEREST

Otolaryngologic Clinics, Vol. 49, No. 6 (December 2016)
Obstructive Sleep Apnea
Mark A. D'Agostino, *Editor*

THE CLINICS ARE AVAILABLE ONLINE!
Access your subscription at:
www.theclinics.com

Contributors

CONSULTING EDITOR

TEOFILO LEE-CHIONG Jr, MD
Professor of Medicine, National Jewish Health,
University of Colorado Denver, Denver,
Colorado; Chief Medical Liaison, Philips
Respironics, Pennsylvania, USA

EDITORS

JOHAN VERBRAECKEN, MD, PhD
Medical Coordinator, Professor,
Multidisciplinary Sleep Disorders Centre,
Antwerp University Hospital and University
of Antwerp, Antwerp, Belgium

JAN HEDNER, MD, PhD
Medical Director, Professor, Department of
Internal Medicine and Clinical Nutrition, Center
for Sleep and Vigilance Disorders, Sahlgrenska
Academy, University of Gothenburg,
Gothenburg, Sweden

AUTHORS

GALIA V. ANGUELOVA, MD, MSc
Center for Sleep and Wake Disorders,
Haaglanden Medical Center, The Hague, The
Netherlands

HELEN J. BURGESS, PhD
Biological Rhythms Research Laboratory,
Department of Behavioral Sciences, Rush
University Medical Center, Chicago, Illinois,
USA

MICHELLE CAO, DO
Clinical Associate Professor, Division of Sleep
Medicine, Stanford University School of
Medicine, Redwood City, California, USA

SYLVIE DUJARDIN, MD
Sleep Medicine Center Kempenhaeghe,
Heeze, The Netherlands

NICHOLAS-TIBERIO ECONOMOU, MD, PhD
Sleep Study Unit, Department of Psychiatry,
University of Athens, Enypnion Sleep-Epilepsy
Center, Bioclinic Hospital Athens, Athens,
Greece

JACK D. EDINGER, PhD
Professor, Department of Medicine, National
Jewish Health, Denver, Colorado, USA

JONATHAN S. EMENS, MD
Departments of Psychiatry and Medicine,
Oregon Health & Science University, VA
Portland Health Care System, Portland,
Oregon, USA

LUIGI FERINI-STRAMBI, MD, PhD
Division of Neuroscience, University
Vita-Salute San Raffaele, Milan, Italy

PRIYA GOPALAN, MD
Assistant Professor of Psychiatry, Western
Psychiatric Institute and Clinic, University of
Pittsburgh Medical Center, Pittsburgh,
Pennsylvania, USA

LUDGER GROTE, MD, PhD
Professor, Sleep Disorders Center, Pulmonary
Medicine, Sahlgrenska University Hospital,
Gothenburg, Sweden

SEBASTIAN C. HOLST, PhD
Neurobiology Research Unit, Copenhagen
University Hospital, Rigshospitalet,
Copenhagen, Denmark

JAN HEDNER, MD, PhD
Medical Director, Professor,
Department of Internal Medicine and
Clinical Nutrition, Center for Sleep and
Vigilance Disorders, Sahlgrenska Academy,
University of Gothenburg, Gothenburg,
Sweden

JONATHAN P. HINTZE, MD
Clinical Assistant Professor, Division of
Pediatric Sleep Medicine, University of South
Carolina School of Medicine Greenville,
Greenville Health System, Greenville, South
Carolina, USA

SHAHROKH JAVAHERI, MD
Sleep Physician, Bethesda North
Hospital, Emeritus Professor of Medicine,
University of Cincinnati College of
Medicine, Cincinnati, Ohio, USA;
Adjunct Professor of Medicine,
Division of Pulmonary, Critical
Care and Sleep Medicine, The Ohio
State University, Columbus, Ohio,
USA

ARTHUR G.Y. KURVERS, MD
Center for Sleep and Wake Disorders,
Haaglanden Medical Center, The Hague,
The Netherlands

GERT JAN LAMMERS, MD, PhD
Neurologist, Clinical Neurophysiologist
and Somnologist, Staff Member,
Department of Neurology, Leiden
University Medical Center, Leiden,
The Netherlands; Medical Director,
Sleep-Wake Centers of SEIN,
The Netherlands

HANS-PETER LANDOLT, PhD
Institute of Pharmacology and
Toxicology, University of Zürich,
Zürich Center for Interdisciplinary Sleep
Research (ZiS), University of Zürich, Zürich,
Switzerland

RAFFAELE MANNI, MD
Unit of Sleep Medicine and Epilepsy,
C. Mondino National Neurological Institute,
Pavia, Italy

LAURA P. McLAFFERTY, MD
Assistant Professor, Department of
Psychiatry and Human Behavior, Thomas
Jefferson University, Philadelphia,
Pennsylvania, USA

LINO NOBILI, MD, PhD
Department of Neuroscience, Centre of Sleep
Medicine, Centre for Epilepsy Surgery,
Niguarda Hospital, Milan, Italy; Department of
Neuroscience (DINOGMI), University of Genoa,
Genoa, Italy

DIRK PEVERNAGIE, MD, PhD
Sleep Medicine Center Kempenhaeghe,
Heeze, The Netherlands; Departments of
Internal Medicine and Paediatrics, Faculty of
Medicine and Health Sciences, Ghent
University, Ghent, Belgium

ANGELIQUE PIJPERS, MD, PhD
Sleep Medicine Center Kempenhaeghe,
Heeze, The Netherlands

PAOLA PROSERPIO, MD
Department of Neuroscience, Centre of Sleep
Medicine, Centre for Epilepsy Surgery,
Niguarda Hospital, Milan, Italy

ROSELYNE M. RIJSMAN, MD, PhD
Center for Sleep and Wake Disorders,
Haaglanden Medical Center, The Hague,
The Netherlands

MEREDITH SPADA, MD
Child and Adolescent Psychiatry Fellow,
Western Psychiatric Institute and Clinic,
University of Pittsburgh Medical Center,
Pittsburgh, Pennsylvania, USA

**PASCHALIS STEIROPOULOS, MD, PhD,
FCCP**
Sleep Unit, Department of Pulmonology
Medical School, Democritus University of
Thrace, University Campus, Alexandroupolis,
Greece

MICHELE TERZAGHI, MD
Unit of Sleep Medicine and Epilepsy,
C. Mondino National Neurological Institute,
Pavia, Italy

ANN VAN GASTEL, MD
Multidisciplinary Sleep Disorders
Centre and University Department
of Psychiatry, Antwerp University
Hospital, Faculty of Medicine and
Health Sciences, Collaborative Antwerp
Psychiatric Research Institute (CAPRI),

University of Antwerp (UA), Antwerp,
Belgium

MONIQUE H.M. VLAK, MD, PhD
Center for Sleep and Wake Disorders,
Haaglanden Medical Center, The Hague,
The Netherlands

DING ZOU, MD, PhD
Department of Internal Medicine and Clinical
Nutrition, Center for Sleep and Vigilance
Disorders, Sahlgrenska Academy, University of
Gothenburg, Gothenburg, Sweden

Contents

Preface: Medications and Their Effects on Sleep and Wake   xv

Johan Verbraecken and Jan Hedner

Sleep-Wake Neurochemistry   137

Sebastian C. Holst and Hans-Peter Landolt

> The regulated alternations between wakefulness and sleep states reflect complex behavioral processes, orchestrated by distinct neurochemical changes in brain parenchyma. No single neurotransmitter or neuromodulator controls the sleep-wake states in isolation. Rather, fine-tuned interactions within organized neuronal circuits regulate waking and sleep states and drive their transitions. Structural or functional dysregulation and medications interfering with these ensembles can lead to sleep-wake disorders and exert wanted or unwanted pharmacologic actions on sleep-wake states. Knowledge of the neurochemical bases of sleep-wake states, which are discussed in this article, provides the conceptual framework for understanding pharmacologic effects on sleep and wake.

Drug-Induced Insomnia and Excessive Sleepiness   147

Ann Van Gastel

> Psychotropic and nonpsychotropic drugs, which may induce or aggravate insomnia and/or daytime sleepiness, are discussed. These central nervous system effects are possible from the interactions of a drug with any of the many neurotransmitters or receptors that are involved in sleep and wakefulness. Multiple interactions between disease, sleep, comorbid sleep disorders, and direct or indirect influences of pharmacologic agents are possible. Awareness of these effects is important to adapt treatment and reach optimal results for every patient. Besides the importance for health and quality of life, effects on sleep or waking function can be a potential source of noncompliance.

Drug-Induced Sleep-Disordered Breathing and Ventilatory Impairment   161

Ludger Grote

> This article describes current knowledge about drug entities that have the potential to induce, aggravate, or modify sleep-disordered breathing. The drug effects on sleep-disordered breathing may vary by patient age, gender, and comorbidity. In general, the clinical relevance of drug-induced sleep-disordered breathing is increasing in sleep medicine and the evidence in the field is growing in parallel.

Prescription Drugs Used in Insomnia   169

Sylvie Dujardin, Angelique Pijpers, and Dirk Pevernagie

> This article reviews the effects on sleep of prescription drugs that are commonly prescribed for chronic insomnia in adults. The following groups are discussed: benzodiazepines and their receptor agonists, the dual orexin receptor antagonist suvorexant, melatonin and its receptor agonists, sedating antidepressants, and antipsychotics. Together with the neurobiologic and pharmacologic properties of these drugs, clinical effects are described, including subjective and objective effects

on sleep duration, continuity, and architecture. Medical prescription information is given when available. Recently published American and European guidelines for the treatment of insomnia serve as reference frame.

Drugs Used in Narcolepsy and Other Hypersomnias 183
Gert Jan Lammers

Narcolepsy and idiopathic hypersomnia cannot be cured; all available treatments are symptomatic. It is of paramount importance for patients, and their relatives, to be informed about the consequences of these chronic diseases and to become ready to accept the consequences of the diagnosis before starting any treatment. This facilitates the implementation of behavioral modifications and the proper use of medication to decrease the disease burden. A supportive social environment (eg, family members, friends, employer, colleagues, and patient support groups) is instrumental. Current treatment options are discussed with a focus on pharmacologic treatment, including future directions.

Drugs Used in Parasomnia 191
Paola Proserpio, Michele Terzaghi, Raffaele Manni, and Lino Nobili

Patient education and behavioral management represent the first treatment approaches to the patient with parasomnia, especially in case of disorders of arousal (DOA). A pharmacologic treatment of DOA may be useful when episodes are frequent and persist despite resolution of predisposing factors, are associated with a high risk of injury, or cause significant impairment, such as excessive sleepiness. Approved drugs for DOA are still lacking. The most commonly used medications are benzodiazepines and antidepressants. The pharmacologic treatment of rapid eye movement sleep behavior disorder is symptomatic, and the most commonly used drugs are clonazepam and melatonin.

Drug Therapy in Obstructive Sleep Apnea 203
Jan Hedner and Ding Zou

There are several reasons to develop a pharmacologic remedy in obstructive sleep apnea (OSA); but so far, there is no generally effective drug available. Previous attempts to find a drug in OSA therapy were serendipity driven in small pilot trials. There is a growing literature on phenotyping pathophysiologic mechanisms of OSA that may be exploited in strategic drug development programs. This article addresses potential pitfalls encountered in previous studies and highlights several drug candidates under development in the field.

Pharmacologic and Nonpharmacologic Treatment of Restless Legs Syndrome 219
Galia V. Anguelova, Monique H.M. Vlak, Arthur G.Y. Kurvers, and Roselyne M. Rijsman

This article provides an updated practical guide for the treatment of primary restless legs syndrome (RLS). Articles that appeared after the American Academy of Neurology guideline search were reviewed according to the same evidence rating schedule. We found limited evidence for nonpharmacologic treatment options. In moderate to severe primary RLS, pharmacologic options may be considered, including iron supplementation, an $\alpha 2\delta$ ligand, a dopamine agonist, a combination of an $\alpha 2\delta$ ligand and a dopamine agonist, or oxycodone/naloxone. This article includes treatment options in case of augmentation.

Drugs Used in Circadian Sleep-Wake Rhythm Disturbances   231

Helen J. Burgess and Jonathan S. Emens

This article focuses on melatonin and other melatonin receptor agonists, and specifically their circadian phase shifting and sleep-enhancing properties. The circadian system and circadian rhythm sleep-wake disorders are briefly reviewed, followed by a summary of the circadian phase shifting, sleep-enhancing properties, and possible safety concerns associated with melatonin and other melatonin receptor agonists. The recommended use of melatonin, including dose and timing, in the latest American Academy of Sleep Medicine Clinical Practice Guidelines for the treatment of intrinsic circadian rhythm disorders is also reviewed. Lastly, the practical aspects of treatment and consideration of clinical treatment outcomes are discussed.

Pharmacologic Treatment of Sleep Disorders in Pregnancy   243

Laura P. McLafferty, Meredith Spada, and Priya Gopalan

Pregnancy often predisposes women to new-onset sleep disturbances, as well as exacerbations of preexisting sleep disorders. The goals of treating perinatal sleep disorders include the promotion of restorative sleep and the benefits it brings to both mother and fetus. The prescribing of any sleep aid in pregnancy must include consideration of the risks and benefits for both the patient and her fetus. Although data on the perinatal use of sleep aids are limited, there may be effects on fetal development, timing and duration of delivery, and postnatal outcomes.

Sleep-Related Drug Therapy in Special Conditions: Children   251

Nicholas-Tiberio Economou, Luigi Ferini-Strambi, and Paschalis Steiropoulos

Sleep disorders in children may lead to neurodevelopmental and neurocognitive deficits; it is important to diagnose and treat them properly. Apart from the existing challenges in diagnosis, another drawback is that few therapies are currently approved. In this article, a comprehensive summary of the most common pediatric sleep disorders, along with the various pharmacologic and nonpharmacologic approaches for their management, is presented. Special attention has been paid to the currently available treatment options for pediatric insomnia, obstructive sleep apnea, parasomnias, narcolepsy, and restless legs syndrome, and comparisons are made with the corresponding treatment options for sleep disorders in adults.

Hypnotic Discontinuation in Chronic Insomnia   263

Jonathan P. Hintze and Jack D. Edinger

Patients with chronic insomnia are commonly prescribed hypnotic medications. The long-term effects of chronic hypnotics are not known and discontinuation is encouraged but often difficult to achieve. A gradual taper is preferred to abrupt cessation to avoid rebound insomnia and withdrawal symptoms. Written information provided to the patient about medication discontinuation may be helpful. Cognitive behavioral therapy or behavioral therapies alone can improve hypnotic discontinuation outcomes. There is limited evidence for adjunct medications to assist in hypnotic cessation for insomnia.

Effects of Chronic Opioid Use on Sleep and Wake   271

Michelle Cao and Shahrokh Javaheri

Chronic use of opioids negatively affects sleep on 2 levels: sleep architecture and breathing. Patients suffer from a variety of daytime sequelae. There may be a bidirectional relationship between poor sleep quality, sleep-disordered breathing, and daytime function. Opioids are a potential cause of incident depression. The best therapeutic option is withdrawal of opioids, which proves difficult. Positive airway pressure devices are considered first-line treatment for sleep-related breathing disorders. New-generation positive pressure servo ventilators are increasingly popular as a treatment option for opioid-induced sleep-disordered breathing. Treatments to improve sleep quality, sleep-related breathing disorders, and quality of life in patients who use opioids for a long term are discussed.

Preface
Medications and Their Effects on Sleep and Wake

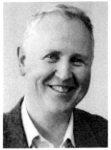

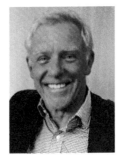

Johan Verbraecken, MD, PhD   Jan Hedner, MD, PhD
Editors

Welcome to this issue of *Sleep Medicine Clinics*, which is dedicated to the topic of medications and their effects on sleep/wake mechanisms. This is a comprehensive overview of current drug therapy in different sleep disorders and of the complex relationship between drugs and sleep-wake.

The number of patients suffering from sleep-related disorders is increasing dramatically, and drug prescription is a common therapeutic measure. Several effective pharmaceuticals have been developed and launched only during the last decade. The sleep disorders addressed in this issue are diverse, but reflect those most relevant with respect to disorders of sleep. Invited authors are experts in their field and represent recognized institutions from all over the world. The introductory article offers a comprehensive overview of the neurochemistry of sleep and wake. Dr Sebastian Holst, Copenhagen University, Denmark, and Prof Hans-Peter Landolt, University of Zürich, Switzerland, are preeminent experts in the area and provide the reader with an up-to-date overview. The following articles in this issue are essentially based on these neurochemistry insights. In another article in this issue, which focused on sleep-related side effects of drugs, Dr Ann Van Gastel, from the Antwerp University Hospital, Belgium, brings two decades of research experience to delineate and discuss this topic. Subsequently, Prof Ludger Grote, from the Gothenburg University, Sweden, addresses sleep-disordered breathing and ventilatory impairment, which occur as a consequence of drug use. The following parts of this issue deal with the potential pharmacologic therapies to consider in the major sleep disorders encountered in clinical sleep medicine. First, we explore the pharmacologic treatment of the most common sleep-related complaint, insomnia. Dr Sylvie Dujardin and colleagues, from the Centre for Sleep Medicine Kempenhaeghe, Heeze, The Netherlands, provide a review of the current pharmacologic management means. Next, Prof Gert Jan Lammers from the University of Leiden and Sleep Centre, SEIN, The Netherlands, provides a cutting-edge update on the current pharmacologic approach in narcolepsy and hypersomnia, and Dr Paola Proserpio and colleagues, from Milan, Pavia, Italy, discuss the current treatment of parasomnias, long considered to be disorders of primarily emotional origin, in their review. Prof Jan Hedner, co-editor, and Dr Ding Zou, from Gothenburg University, Sweden, provide an exhaustive review of what is known about the pharmacologic management of sleep-disordered breathing, and where we might hope to go in the coming decade. Next follows a review of drug therapy in restless legs syndrome by Dr Galia Anguelova and colleagues from The Hague, The Netherlands, and a current update on drugs used in circadian sleep-wake rhythm disorders as well a detailed description of the role of light and melatonin in these disorders by Prof Helen Burgess, from Chicago, Illinois, and Prof Jonathan Emens, from Portland, Oregon.

Before turning to the final two articles, we have addressed special issues that follow with

Sleep Med Clin 13 (2018) xv–xvi
https://doi.org/10.1016/j.jsmc.2018.03.005
1556-407X/18/© 2018 Published by Elsevier Inc.

medication in the specific populations of pregnant women and children. Pregnancy is covered by Prof Laura McLafferty, from Philadelphia and Dr Meredith Spada and Dr Priya Gopalan, from Pittsburgh, Pennsylvania, while the pediatric aspects are summarized by Prof Paschalis Steiropoulos, from Alexandroupolis, and Dr Nicholas-Tiberio Economou, from Athens, Greece, together with Prof Luigi Ferini-Strambi, from Milan, Italy. Finally, we conclude with two articles to remind the reader this topic is not merely one of prescribing drugs but also of their withdrawal. These articles address discontinuation of hypnotic drugs by Dr Jonathan Hintze and Prof Jack Edinger, from Denver, Colorado, and of chronic opioid medication by Prof Michelle Cao from Stanford University, California, and Prof Shahrokh Javaheri, from Cincinnati, Ohio, with respect to their influence on sleep. These areas are arguably some of the most complex, maligned, and infrequently studied topics in the field of sleep medicine. Frequently, there is a need of cognitive behavioral therapy and concerted multidisciplinary efforts to deal with these complex sleep disorders.

In summary, it is our hope that this issue of *Sleep Medicine Clinics* will provide the reader with a better understanding of both the usefulness and the limitations that follow therapeutic drug use in various sleep disorders. Ultimately, we anticipate that the information communicated in this issue will benefit our patients in their quest of better sleep and a better quality of life. We are indebted to the contributing authors of this issue for taking time out of their busy schedules to realize this series. Without them, the project would have been impossible. We also thank Donald Mumford at Elsevier for his tenacious efforts in pushing this project through to its final form.

Johan Verbraecken, MD, PhD
Multidisciplinary Sleep Disorders Centre
Antwerp University Hospital and
University of Antwerp
Wilrijkstraat 10
Edegem, Antwerp 2650, Belgium

Jan Hedner, MD, PhD
Centre for Sleep and Wakefulness Disorders
Sahlgrenska Academy
University of Gothenburg
Medicinaregatan 8B
Gothenburg 41346, Sweden

E-mail addresses:
johan.verbraecken@uza.be (J. Verbraecken)
Jan.hedner@lungall.gu.se (J. Hedner)

Sleep-Wake Neurochemistry

Sebastian C. Holst, PhD[a],*, Hans-Peter Landolt, PhD[b,c]

KEYWORDS

- Neurotransmitters • Neuromodulators • Glutamate • Acetylcholine • Norepinephrine • Dopamine
- GABA • Adenosine

KEY POINTS

- Behavioral states alternate between wakefulness, rapid-eye movement and non-rapid eye movement sleep.
- Waking and sleep states are highly complex processes, elegantly fine-tuned by cerebral neurochemical changes in the neurotransmitters and neuromodulators glutamate, acetylcholine, γ-amino-butyric acid, norepinephrine, dopamine, serotonin, histamine, hypocretin, melanin-concentrating hormone, adenosine, and melatonin.
- No single neurotransmitter or neuromodulator, but rather their complex interactions within organized neuronal ensembles, regulate waking and sleep states and drive their transitions.
- Dysregulation or medications interfering with these neurochemical systems can lead to sleep-wake disorders and functional changes of wakefulness and sleep.
- The neurochemical pathways presented here provide a conceptual framework for the understanding of the effects of currently used medications on wakefulness and sleep.

INTRODUCTION

Based on behavioral and (neuro) physiologic characteristics derived from polysomnographic recordings, the 3 distinct vigilance states of wakefulness, rapid eye movement (REM) sleep, and non-REM (NREM) sleep can be unambiguously defined in mammals. Wakefulness with eyes closed is typically associated with electroencephalographic (EEG) activity in the alpha range (8–12 Hz) and with high-frequency, desynchronized activity greater than 40 Hz. In a normal sleep episode, voluntary muscle control is gradually lost and NREM and REM sleep episodes alternate in a cyclic pattern. In NREM sleep, the EEG shows slow, high-amplitude activity reflecting widespread, synchronous oscillations of neurons exhibiting alternating periods of firing and silence (burst-pause firing pattern).[1] The so-called EEG delta activity (<4.5 Hz) is under tight homeostatic control and exhibits a declining trend in the course of the night, which reflects the dissipation of sleep need and the decline in sleep intensity.[2] The EEG in REM sleep (sometimes called paradoxic sleep) is partly reminiscent of EEG activity in drowsy wakefulness, yet it is characterized by muscle atonia with occasional muscle twitches and rapid eye movements.

Disclosure: The authors' research has been supported by the Swiss National Science Foundation (320030_163439), Zürich Center for Interdisciplinary Sleep Research, Clinical Research Priority Program "Sleep & Health" of the University of Zürich, Zürich Center for Integrative Human Physiology, Neuroscience Center Zürich, and Novartis Foundation (08C42) for Medical-Biological Research (to H.P. Landolt) and the Lundbeck Foundation (R209-2015-3438) (to S.C. Holst).
[a] Neurobiology Research Unit, Copenhagen University Hospital, Rigshospitalet, 28 Juliane Maries Vej 6931, Copenhagen 2100, Denmark; [b] Institute of Pharmacology and Toxicology, University of Zürich, Winterthurerstrasse 190, Zürich 8057, Switzerland; [c] Zürich Center for Interdisciplinary Sleep Research (ZiS), University of Zürich, Zürich, Switzerland
* Corresponding author. Institute of Pharmacology and Toxicology, University of Zürich, Winterthurerstrasse 190, Zürich 8057, Switzerland.
E-mail address: holst@nru.dk

Distinct neurotransmitter nuclei and neuronal pathways modulate and maintain these three behavioral states. First insights were reported by Constantin von Economo[3] (1876–1931) who studied patients with a type of viral encephalitis that was never seen before, encephalitis lethargica. von Economo discovered that the encephalitis was associated with lesions to distinct brain areas in the midbrain and brainstem reticular formation. Lesions of the ventral periaqueductal gray and posterior hypothalamus were associated with severe hypersomnia, whereas lesions of the hypothalamic anterior preoptic area extending into the basal ganglia were associated with insomnia. These findings were the first in a series of fundamental studies eventually leading to the postulation of an ascending reticular activating system (ARAS).[4] The ARAS arises from a network of neuronal clusters in the brainstem, which activates forebrain, thalamus, and cortex, mainly in wakefulness but to some extent also in REM sleep. Today, the ARAS is no longer seen as a loose reticular system but, instead, as consisting of a network of individual nuclei expressing distinct neurotransmitters that promote arousal (**Fig. 1**). The key modulatory neurotransmitters of the ascending activating system include acetylcholine (ACh), several monoamines (norepinephrine [NE], serotonin [5-hydroxy-tryptamine, 5-HT], histamine [His],

dopamine [DA]), and the slow-acting neuropeptide hypocretin (Hcrt; aka orexin). More recently, the fast-acting amino acid glutamate has been proposed to be the main regulator of arousal.[5] Together with GABA (γ-amino-butyric acid), these neurochemicals play important roles in promoting waking and sleep states, which provide a useful conceptual framework to understand the effects of medications on wakefulness and sleep. With the recent advent of powerful optogenetic and chemogenetic tools, experimental in vivo control of neuronal activity by stimulating or inhibiting distinct neuronal ensembles permitted exciting new insights into the causal underpinnings of brain state transitions. A comprehensive summary of these insights are beyond the scope of this article; this has been the topic of excellent recent overviews.[6,7] Nevertheless, some recent progress in current understanding of sleep-wake neurochemistry made by investigating sleep-wake circuits with optogenetic techniques are covered.

THE NEUROCHEMICAL UNDERPINNINGS OF WAKEFULNESS
Acetylcholine

ACh-releasing nuclei in the pedunculopontine (PPT) and laterodorsal tegmental nuclei (LDT) of the pons project primarily to the basal forebrain (BF), as well

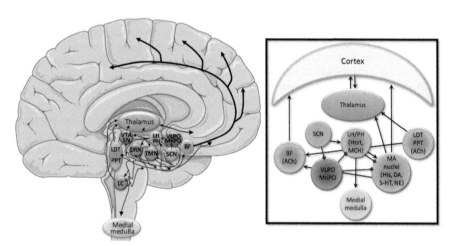

Fig. 1. Anatomical locations of major neurotransmitter nuclei (left) and simplified overview of their major connections relevant for sleep-wake regulation (right). Wakefulness (orange): Cholinergic (Ach) tegmental (LDT or PPT) neurons and monoaminergic (MA) neurons of upper brain stem and hypothalamus innervate thalamus and basal forebrain (BF). The MA neurons have a pronounced role and directly innervate the cerebral cortex. Hypocretin (Hcrt) neurons of lateral or posterior hypothalamus (LH or PH) reinforce the activity of this ascending arousal pathway and directly excite the (BF). NREM sleep (purple): GABA-ergic VLPO and MnPO nuclei, which inhibit the ascending arousal pathways, are active in NREM sleep. REM sleep (cyan): Ach-ergic neurons of LDT or PPT promote REM sleep, during which NE and 5-HT neurons are silent. Entry into REM is inhibited by Hcrt neurons and facilitated by the VLPO. Connections from the SCN are important in regulating the timing of wakefulness and sleep. Black arrows indicate an excitatory connection. Red squares and lines indicate an inhibitory connection. Please refer to main text for full list of abbreviations.

as to the thalamic relay and reticular cells. This pathway is crucial for gating thalamic signaling to the cortex, and is importantly involved in the promotion of both wakefulness and REM sleep. A second cluster of ACh-releasing neurons is located in the BF, which projects widely to the cortex. ACh activates ionotropic nicotinic receptors and metabotropic muscarinic receptors. Nicotinic receptors are expressed in presynaptic and postsynaptic membranes. When they are activated, sodium and calcium ions rapidly enter the cells, leading to membrane depolarization. Muscarinic receptors are part of the superfamily of G-protein-coupled receptors (GPCRs). Five types of muscarinic receptors are currently known. The M_1, M_3, and M_5 receptors are coupled with G_q proteins that activate phospholipase C and adenylyl cyclase. They are expressed in the cortex and striatum, as well as other brain regions. M_2 and M_4 are coupled to $G_{i/o}$ proteins, and their activation inhibits adenylyl cyclase. These receptors are found, among other regions, in the BF, where they act as autoreceptors and are thought to control ACh synthesis and release. The cholinergic neurons in the central nervous system (CNS) are active mainly in wakefulness and REM sleep, and have a firing rate in the theta range.[8] They promote cortical arousal and REM sleep, while reducing NREM sleep.[9–11]

Recent optogenetic studies in mice have improved our understanding of the role of ACh and other wake-promoting neurotransmitters in controlling vigilance states. With this method, selected neurons are genetically modified to express channelrhodopsin-2 (ChR2), a light-activated nonspecific cation channel. When ChR2 is activated by a light pulse, influx of cations such as Ca^{2+} is triggered and the ChR2-expressing cells are activated.[12] Optogenetic activation of the cholinergic PPT or LDT neurons in mice during NREM sleep leads to a rapid transition into REM sleep, yet not into wakefulness.[13] On the other hand, optogenetic stimulation of PPT or LDT neurons during wakefulness is associated with moderate arousal.[13] Interestingly, activation of ChR2-expressing cholinergic neurons of the BF during wakefulness also promotes arousal, whereas activation during NREM sleep leads to transition, at roughly equal amount, into wakefulness and REM sleep.[14] These observations suggest that the cholinergic neurons in the brainstem are more involved in regulating transitions into REM sleep, whereas the cells of the BF are more linked to general arousal.

Another recent study using optogenetics could corroborate that the ACh neurons of the BF contribute to arousal and the promotion of wakefulness.[15] Nevertheless, by also stimulating the glutamatergic and GABA-ergic neurons of the

BF, it was found that the three neuronal cell groups exert similar effects on arousal.[15] Interestingly, activation of BF GABA-ergic neurons substantially enhanced wakefulness. However, when BF glutamatergic and cholinergic neurons were activated, the effects on arousal were minor.[15–18] In conclusion, although ACh neurons of the BF likely modulate wakefulness, it now seems that subgroups of BF GABA-ergic neurons may be more important than cholinergic neurons for the regulation of arousal.

Monoamines

The monoamines promoting arousal and maintaining wakefulness include NE, 5-HT, DA, and His. The primary site of production and release of NE is the locus coeruleus (LC), of 5-HT the raphe nucleus (DRN), of DA the ventral tegmental area (VTA) and substantia nigra (SN), and of His the hypothalamic tuberomammillary nucleus (TMN). With the exception of the dopaminergic cell groups, all these nuclei fire at high rates in wakefulness, lower rates in NREM sleep, and are virtually silent in REM sleep.[19–21] They have widespread CNS projections and innervate cortex, brainstem, ventrolateral preoptic (VLPO) nucleus, thalamus, and the BF, making them ideally located to promote and sustain wakefulness.

Norepinephrine

The LC is an important small cell cluster involved in the regulation of arousal.[20] It is located in the brainstem and consists of roughly 25,000 NE neurons. NE can activate both the α and β families of adrenergic receptors, which are part of the GPCR superfamily. Adrenergic receptors are divided into 3 main types: α_1 (mainly G_q coupled), α_2 (inhibitory autosynaptic and postsynaptic receptors, $G_{i/o}$ coupled), and β receptors (G_s coupled), which are all widely expressed in the CNS.[22] Optogenetic stimulation of the noradrenergic neurons in the LC is associated with immediate transitions from sleep to wakefulness and increased locomotor activity,[23] highlighting the role of the LC in maintaining behavioral arousal. Recent evidence also suggests a role for NE in the sleep-driven macroscopic pathway referred to as the glymphatic system. This system is governed by a flow of cerebrospinal fluid into the brain through perivascular (also known as Virchow–Robin) spaces, which enables the removal of macroscopic waste products from the brain parenchyma in NREM sleep.[24,25] Increased glymphatic function in NREM sleep results from an increased interstitial space volume fraction, which seems to be driven by reduced LC-derived NE-ergic tone.[25] However, the increase in interstitial space that enables glymphatic flow during sleep may not solely be driven by NE. The size of the interstitial space can also be reduced by a wake-promoting cocktail of monoamines, ACh, and Hcrt, and even by altering the concentrations of potassium, calcium, and magnesium ions in the cerebrospinal fluid.[26,27]

Serotonin

The major nuclei releasing 5-HT, the DRN, are located along the midline of the brainstem and reticular formation. Besides 5-HT neurons, the DRN also contains DA-ergic, GABA-ergic, glutamatergic, and neuropeptide-releasing neurons. Moreover, the DRN is innervated by GABA, glutamate, ACh, NE, His, Hcrt, and melanin-concentrating hormone (MCH)-expressing neurons originating from several other brain areas, rendering serotonergic influences on sleep-wake regulation highly complex in nature. Furthermore, the 5-HT receptors are subdivided into 7 distinct families: 5-HT_1 to 5-HT_7 receptors. Similar to the other monoamines, all 5-HT receptors, except the ligand-gated 5-HT_3 ion channel, belong to the GPCR superfamily. The 5-HT_1 and 5-HT_5 receptors are coupled to $G_{i/o}$ protein, the 5-HT_2 receptor is coupled to G_q protein, and the 5-HT_4, 5-HT_6, and 5-HT_7 receptors are coupled to G_s protein. The many 5-HT receptor subtypes and the widespread effects of 5-HT in the CNS have made it challenging to elucidate the distinct roles for 5-HT in sleep-wake regulation.[28] Intriguingly, 5-HT_{1A} and 5-HT_{1B} receptor knockout mice have enhanced amounts of REM sleep,[29,30] whereas mutant mice without 5-HT_{2A} or 5-HT_{2C} receptors show enhanced durations of wakefulness and reduced NREM sleep.[31,32] Overall, the current evidence suggests that 5-HT transmission generally promotes wakefulness, inhibits REM sleep, and can interfere with slow wave sleep.[33] Optogenetic stimulation of DRN 5-HT neurons has been attempted and found to enhance patience in an anticipated-reward paradigm.[34] With respect to sleep-wake regulation, optogenetic activation of DRN 5-HT neurons has not been examined. However, it was recently shown that optogenetic activation of DRN DA neurons promote wakefulness and contribute to the regulation of sleep-wake states.[35]

Histamine

The TMN is a small His-releasing cell cluster found inferior to the hypothalamus. The TMN shows a projection pattern that is similar to the LC and the DRN, including strong reciprocal innervation with the VLPO.[36] Three types of His-ergic GPCRs have so far been classified in the brain: H_1, H_2, and H_3 receptors that are coupled to G_q, G_s, and G_i

proteins. It is well known that antihistamines are sedative, which is a common side effect of early H_1 receptor antagonists (eg, diphenhydramine) in the treatment of allergies. The release of His within the TMN by optogenetic photostimulation activates H_3 autoreceptors and suppresses inhibitory GABA-ergic inputs to TMN.[37] Moreover, His from the TMN enhanced the inhibition of the VLPO. Combined, these observations support a role for His in stabilizing wakefulness.

Dopamine

Psychostimulant and wake-promoting agents typically enhance DA-ergic neurotransmission.[38] However, with respect to sleep-wake regulation, this neurotransmitter has long been thought to be of limited importance because DA-ergic neurotransmission in cats showed only minor alterations across the sleep-wake cycle. By contrast, more recent evidence in rats revealed that extracellular DA levels in the medial prefrontal cortex and parts of the nucleus accumbens (NAc) of the ventral striatum are high in wakefulness and REM sleep, and significantly lower in NREM sleep.[39,40] Thus, similar to the other monoamines, DA may indeed play an important role in regulating wakefulness and sleep. Five types of DA-ergic GPCRs are known. The D_1-like (D_1 and D_5) DA receptors are coupled to G_s protein and are mainly stimulatory. On the contrary, the D_2-like (D_2, D_3, and D_4) DA receptors are coupled to inhibitory G_i protein. Importantly, D_1 and D_2 receptors form functional heteromers with adenosine A_1 and A_{2A} receptors (see later discussion), such that the binding of adenosine results in reduced dopaminergic signaling.

Both distinct subtypes of DA and adenosine receptors are primarily expressed in the NAc, a brain region recently suggested to play a crucial role in sleep-wake regulation.[6] The NAc is innervated by DA projections of the mesolimbic pathway originating in the VTA. By integrating signals from cortex, thalamus, amygdala, and midbrain, the NAc is able to inhibit several other arousal pathways via GABA-ergic interneurons. Experimental inhibition and activation of the NAc, thus, promote wakefulness and sleep.[41–43] Several studies interrogated DA-ergic neurotransmission by optogenetics, in particular with respect to reward and addiction. However, a recent study in rats, elegantly showed that destruction of DA afferents in the SN pars compacta (SNc), projecting via the nigrostriatal pathway to the dorsal striatum, enhanced wakefulness and induced sleep-wake fragmentation.[44] The investigators then optogenetically stimulated the SNc DA neurons, which resulted in increased firing and enhanced sleep,[44] suggesting that the nigrostriatal DA-ergic pathway promotes sleep. Taken together, it is likely that distinct roles for DA in sleep-wake regulation are region-specific and pathway-specific, and probably also dose-dependent.

Neuropeptides

Approximately 100 neuropeptides have been described in the human brain.[45] They typically act via GPCRs, exert long-lasting dynamic modulatory effects at the synapse, and do not cross the blood-brain barrier. These characteristics make them difficult targets for pharmacologic interventions.

Hypocretin

Several neuropeptides, including Hcrt, MCH, galanin, oxytocin, neuropeptide Y, somatostatin, ghrelin, and substance P, play important roles in regulating mood, reward, arousal, and sleep.[46] With respect to sleep-wake regulation, Hcrt and MCH especially deserve mention. These peptides are released from a small cluster of neurons found solely in the lateral hypothalamus (LH). The MCH contributes mainly to the promotion and maintenance of sleep[47] (see later discussion).

The Hcrt-producing neurons project to all previously described nuclei of the arousal pathways, especially to LC, DRN, and TMN. They also release glutamate and play important roles in maintaining arousal and stabilizing the wake state. Similar to the other wake-promoting systems, the Hcrt neurons are mainly active in wakefulness, especially when animals are exploring, and become silent in REM sleep and NREM sleep.[48] The Hcrt binds to 2 subtypes of GPCRs, referred to as Hcrt-1 and Hcrt-2 receptors. Activation of these receptors increases intracellular calcium levels. The loss of Hcrt neurons causes narcolepsy with cataplexy, which is characterized by behavioral state instability, most likely caused by an insufficient inhibition of the circuits regulating REM sleep and NREM sleep.[49,50] Supporting the wake-promoting role of Hcrt, optogenetic activation of Hcrt neurons triggers brief awakenings from both REM sleep and NREM sleep, an effect that is diminished with increasing sleep pressure.[51,52] Combined, these findings suggest that sleep-dependent processes feed back to Hcrt neurons and inhibit their wake-promoting actions.

THE NEUROCHEMICAL UNDERPINNINGS OF SLEEP
Neuropeptides: Melanin-Concentrating Hormone

The MCH expressing neurons in the LH are intermingled with Hcrt neurons and also produce GABA. These neurons innervate many of the Hcrt-target regions, including the LC and the DRN.[53] However, in contrast to Hcrt, the MCH projections are inhibitory and fire at high rates in REM sleep, are less active in NREM sleep, and remain almost silent in wakefulness.[54] Thus, MCH neurons likely promote REM sleep and inhibit wakefulness. Indeed, MCH-deficient mice spend less time in both REM and NREM sleep.[55] On the contrary, when the MCH neurons are optogenetically activated, either REM sleep alone[56,57] or both REM sleep and NREM sleep[58] were found to be enhanced. Although more research is warranted, it seems evident that MCH neurons inhibit wakefulness and functionally oppose Hcrt neurons in regulating the transition between wakefulness and sleep states.[57]

Adenosine

Based on the knowledge that the world's most readily consumed psychostimulant, caffeine, antagonizes adenosine receptors, adenosine and adenosine receptors have long been suggested to be important for sleep-wake regulation.[59–62] Compelling evidence now suggests that the neuromodulator adenosine contributes to the regulation of the increase in sleep pressure during wakefulness and the decrease in sleep propensity during sleep. Four subtypes of G-protein-coupled adenosine receptors have been identified to mediate adenosine's cellular effects: A_1, A_{2A}, A_{2B}, and A_3 receptors. Activation of A_1 and A_3 receptors inhibits adenylyl cyclase by coupling to $G_{i/o}$ protein, whereas A_{2A} and A_{2B} receptors mediate their effects by increased adenylyl cyclase activity through coupling to G_s protein.[63] The A_1 and A_{2A} receptors are strongly expressed in the brain, yet their local expression patterns vary.[64] By contrast, A_{2B} and A_3 receptors are expressed with only low abundance in cerebral structures, and their roles in sleep-wake regulation are not well established. Adenosine has many properties of a presumed endogenous sleep-regulating substance. It has long been known that adenosine, when infused into the intracerebroventricular space, promotes sleep.[65] Moreover, extracellular adenosine levels in the brain of animal models are typically higher in the active phase (dominated by wakefulness) when compared with a phase of rest (dominated by sleep). Similarly, adenosine in the BF is increased by sleep deprivation and normalized by recovery sleep.[66,67] Nevertheless, lesion and pharmacologic studies revealed that accumulation of adenosine in the BF is not necessary for sleep induction, nor are BF cholinergic neurons essential for sleep drive.[68] In conclusion, although adenosine contributes to sleep-wake regulation, a causal role for adenosine in the BF as a single regulator of sleep homeostasis has not been established.

γ-Amino-butyric Acid

Constantin von Economo[3] was the first to describe that lesions to the hypothalamic anterior preoptic area were associated with symptoms of insomnia. Today, it is widely accepted that the VLPO, as well as its neighboring region, the median preoptic area (MnPO), contain high densities of neurons that are active in and even a few minutes before initiation of NREM sleep. The VLPO or MnPO neurons fire less in REM sleep and are almost silent in wakefulness.[69,70] Lesions to the VLPO in cats dramatically reduce sleep.[71] The VLPO neurons are well-positioned to innervate arousal systems of brainstem and hypothalamus, including the DRN, LC, LDT, PPT, SNc, VTA, TMN, and Hcrt-producing neurons in the LH.[5] The VLPO contains GABA-ergic, as well as galanin-ergic projections, both associated with inhibitory transmission on effector targets.[6] Specific activation of GABA-ergic neurons in the VLPO enhance NREM sleep, while reducing wakefulness.[72]

Apart from VLPO or MnPO, novel GABA-ergic structures and pathways that are active in NREM sleep have been discovered in recent years, yet their specific roles in sleep-wake regulation are not yet well established.[6] The actions of GABA are mediated via ligand-gated ion channels referred to as $GABA_A$ and $GABA_C$ receptors, as well as via G_i protein-coupled $GABA_B$ receptors that promote potassium ion conductance on their activation. The pharmacologic properties of GABA receptors are well-investigated, although extremely complex. The $GABA_A$ receptor is the target for the clinically widely used sleep-inducing medications, benzodiazepines and Z-drugs (nonbenzodiazepine structure). This receptor subtype consists of a chloride ion channel composed of 5 subunits assembled from a symphony of α, β, γ, and other less frequent subunit variants.[73] In conclusion, GABA-ergic neurons of the VLPO, together with the MnPO, seem to regulate inhibitory inputs to the ARAS and to promote the transition from wakefulness to sleep and the maintenance of NREM sleep.

Melatonin

The endogenous biological master clock regulating the daily sleep-wake cycle is localized in the suprachiasmatic nucleus (SCN) of the hypothalamus. The SCN is a small neuronal cluster consisting of roughly 20,000 neurons.[74] The SCN functions as an endogenous zeitgeber with a roughly 24-hour periodicity, operating virtually independently of prior sleep and wakefulness. The SCN is primarily entrained by light, which is detected by retinal ganglion cells and transmitted via melanopsin-releasing neurons of the retinohypothalamic tract.[75,76] Nevertheless, other zeitgebers, such as temperature[77] and feeding,[78] also modulate the endogenous clock. The actual timekeeping is maintained by interconnected SCN neurons and transcriptional or translational feedback loops of core and associated clock genes.[74,79]

The SCN has projections to the pineal gland and other hypothalamic nuclei, including the dorsomedial hypothalamic (DMH) nucleus. The DMH seems especially important for the SCN in modulating sleep-wake timing, because abolition of DMH neurons also abolishes sleep-wake timing in experimental animals.[80] The DMH extends strong glutamatergic and GABA-ergic projections to the LH and VLPO, respectively, which allow the SCN to regulate sleep and wakefulness.[81] An important regulator of SCN function is melatonin. Melatonin is often referred to as the hormone of darkness. When compared with the biological day, its concentration is elevated about 10-fold during the biological night in both diurnal and nocturnal species. Melatonin binds to MT_1 (aka MT_{1A}) and MT_2 (MT_{1B}) melatonin receptors, which are GPCRs linked to $G_{i/o}$ protein, inhibiting the production of cyclic adenosine-monophosphate. Melatonin receptors are highly expressed in the SCN. Their signaling cascade activated by melatonin is complex and not yet fully understood.[82] Nevertheless, the US Food and Drug Administration recently approved the MT_1-MT_2 receptor agonist ramelteon for treatment of insomnia. In addition, agomelatine, an MT_1-MT_2 receptor agonist and selective $5-HT_{2B/C}$ receptor antagonist, shifts the phase of the circadian system and may improve sleep. Nevertheless, its usefulness for primary sleep disorders remains debated.[83]

The roles for melatonin in sleep-wake regulation were recently highlighted in a diurnal zebrafish model, in which the synthesis of melatonin was genetically abolished.[84] The mutant fish showed a general loss of circadian rhythmicity and strongly reduced sleep compared with normal fish when kept in constant dark conditions. These findings suggest that melatonin not only modulates circadian but also homeostatic aspects of sleep-wake regulation. Interestingly, melatonin may induce sleep by the production of adenosine. Thus, when adenosine receptors were activated in the fish mutants, their wake-phenotype could be rescued, further strengthening the association of melatonin with sleep-wake homeostasis. Despite the basic importance of these data, the simple nervous system of zebrafish may not be directly comparable to humans, and melatonin may play even more complex roles in mammalian sleep-wake regulation.

SYNOPSIS AND PERSPECTIVES

Clinical observations and research spanning from sleep-wake disordered patients to genetically engineered animal models have consistently identified the ascending arousal pathways, the VLPO, and the SCN as important players in the regulation of wakefulness and sleep see **Fig. 1**. In waking, distinct cell clusters of the brain stem, BF, and hypothalamus activate the thalamus, hypothalamus, cortex, and spinal cord motor neurons. Concurrently, the sleep promoting center of the VLPO is inhibited by the SCN, thereby promoting cortical arousal. In REM sleep, REM-on brain stem nuclei containing ACh, glutamate, and GABA promote activity in BF and cortex and induce muscle atonia and rapid eye movements. On the contrary, MCH-containing hypothalamic neurons suppress REM-off brain centers, including the ventrolateral part of the periaqueductal gray matter (vlPAG), LPT, DRN, and LC. In NREM sleep, GABA and galanin-containing VLPO neurons inhibit arousal nuclei in the brain stem, hypothalamus, and BF. The endogenous sleep regulatory substance adenosine can actively excite sleep active cells of the VLPO.

In NREM sleep, DRN 5-HT-ergic and LC NE-ergic neurons inhibit cholinergic LDT and PPT cells. These DRN and LC neurons become silent in REM sleep, which enables the cholinergic LDT and PPT neurons, in synchrony with GABA-ergic innervation, to generate the REM sleep state.

The pathways previously presented provide a conceptual framework of the neurochemical bases of sleep-wake regulation and the currently available pharmacologic interventions to treat sleep-wake disorders. Powerful new methods to interrogate sleep-wake regulating circuits have recently revealed additional molecular, cellular, and network mechanisms and pathways in sleep-wake regulation, which may lead to an extension of the traditional views of sleep-wake neurochemistry.[6,7] For example, the glutamatergic medial parabrachial nucleus in the dorsal pontine tegmentum regulates arousal[85] and the GABA-ergic parafacial zone in the pontomedullary junction promotes sleep.[86] Furthermore, novel studies in humans and animals using different methodologies further suggest diverse additional brain regions, neuronal structures, and receptors as important regulators of wakefulness and sleep.[87–92] These insights highlight the complexity of the mammalian brain and the sophisticated and fine-tuned regulation of wakefulness and sleep. Future progress is needed to pave the way for the development of novel rational sleep-wake therapeutics.

REFERENCES

1. Steriade M, McCormick D, Sejnowski T. Thalamo-cortical oscillations in the sleeping and aroused brain. Science 1993;262(5134):679–85.
2. Achermann P, Borbély AA. Sleep homeostasis and models of sleep regulation. In: Kryger MH, Roth T, Dement WC, editors. Principles and practice of sleep medicine. 5th edition. St Louis (MO): Saunders; 2011. p. 431–44.
3. von Economo C. Sleep as a problem of localization. J Nerv Ment Dis 1930;71(3):249.
4. Moruzzi G, Magoun HW. Brain stem reticular formation and activation of the EEG. Electroencephalogr Clin Neurophysiol 1949;1(1):455–73.
5. Saper CB, Fuller PM. Wake–sleep circuitry: an overview. Curr Opin Neurobiol 2017;44:186–92.
6. Luppi PH, Fort P. Neuroanatomical and neurochemical bases of vigilance states. Handb Exp Pharmacol 2018. https://doi.org/10.1007/164_2017_84.
7. Tyree SM, de Lecea L. Optogenetic investigation of arousal circuits. Int J Mol Sci 2017;18:e1773.
8. Lee MG. Cholinergic basal forebrain neurons burst with theta during waking and paradoxical sleep. J Neurosci 2005;25(17):4365–9.
9. Baghdoyan HA, Lydic R. M2 muscarinic receptor subtype in the feline medial pontine reticular formation modulates the amount of rapid eye movement sleep. Sleep 1999;22(7):835–47.
10. Nissen C, Power AE, Nofzinger EA, et al. M1 muscarinic acetylcholine receptor agonism alters sleep without affecting memory consolidation. J Cogn Neurosci 2006;18(11):1799–807.
11. Zhang L, Samet J, Caffo B, et al. Cigarette smoking and nocturnal sleep architecture. Am J Epidemiol 2006;164(6):529–37.
12. Boyden ES, Zhang F, Bamberg E, et al. Millisecond-timescale, genetically targeted optical control of neural activity. Nat Neurosci 2005;8(9):1263–8.
13. Van Dort CJ, Zachs DP, Kenny JD, et al. Optogenetic activation of cholinergic neurons in the PPT or LDT induces REM sleep. Proc Natl Acad Sci U S A 2015;112(2):584–9.
14. Han Y, Shi YF, Xi W, et al. Selective activation of cholinergic basal forebrain neurons induces immediate sleep-wake transitions. Curr Biol 2014;24(6):693–8.

15. Xu M, Chung S, Zhang S, et al. Basal forebrain circuit for sleep-wake control. Nat Neurosci 2015; 18(11). https://doi.org/10.1038/nn.4143.

16. Anaclet C, Pedersen NP, Ferrari LL, et al. Basal forebrain control of wakefulness and cortical rhythms. Nat Commun 2015;6. https://doi.org/10.1038/ncomms9744.

17. Chen L, Yin D, Wang TX, et al. Basal Forebrain cholinergic neurons primarily contribute to inhibition of electroencephalogram delta activity, rather than inducing behavioral wakefulness in mice. Neuropsychopharmacology 2016;41(8):2133–46.

18. Kim T, Thankachan S, McKenna JT, et al. Cortically projecting basal forebrain parvalbumin neurons regulate cortical gamma band oscillations. Proc Natl Acad Sci U S A 2015;112(11):3535–40.

19. Jacobs BL, Fornal CA. Activity of serotonergic neurons in behaving animals. Neuropsychopharmacology 1999;21(2 Suppl):9S–15S.

20. Takahashi K, Kayama Y, Lin JS, et al. Locus coeruleus neuronal activity during the sleep-waking cycle in mice. Neuroscience 2010;169(3):1115–26.

21. Takahashi K, Lin J-S, Sakai K. Neuronal activity of histaminergic tuberomammillary neurons during wake-sleep states in the mouse. J Neurosci 2006; 26(40):10292–8.

22. Ramos BP, Arnsten AFT. Adrenergic pharmacology and cognition: focus on the prefrontal cortex. Pharmacol Ther 2007;113(3):523–36.

23. Carter ME, Yizhar O, Chikahisa S, et al. Tuning arousal with optogenetic modulation of locus coeruleus neurons. Nat Neurosci 2010;13(12):1526–35.

24. Iliff JJ, Wang M, Liao Y, et al. A paravascular pathway facilitates CSF flow through the brain parenchyma and the clearance of interstitial solutes, including amyloid β. Sci Transl Med 2012;4(147): 147ra111.

25. Xie L, Kang H, Xu Q, et al. Sleep drives metabolite clearance from the adult brain. Science 2013; 342(6156):373–7.

26. Ding F, O'donnell J, Xu Q, et al. Changes in the composition of brain interstitial ions control the sleep-wake cycle. Science 2016;352(6285): 550–5.

27. Landolt HP, Holst SC. Ionic control of sleep and wakefulness. Science 2016;352(6285):517–8.

28. Landolt H-P, Wehrle R. Antagonism of serotonergic 5-HT2A/2C receptors: mutual improvement of sleep, cognition and mood? Eur J Neurosci 2009;29(9): 1795–809.

29. Boutrel B, Franc B, Hen R, et al. Key role of 5-HT1B receptors in the regulation of paradoxical sleep as evidenced in 5-HT1B knock-out mice. J Neurosci 1999;19(8):3204–12.

30. Boutrel B, Monaca C, Hen R, et al. Involvement of 5-HT1A receptors in homeostatic and stress-induced adaptive regulations of paradoxical sleep:

31. Frank MG, Stryker MP, Tecott LH. Sleep and sleep homeostasis in mice lacking the 5-HT2c receptor. Neuropsychopharmacology 2002;27(5): 869–73.

32. Popa D, Léna C, Fabre V, et al. Contribution of 5-HT2 receptor subtypes to sleep-wakefulness and respiratory control, and functional adaptations in knock-out mice lacking 5-HT2A receptors. J Neurosci 2005;25(49):11231–8.

33. Monti JM. Serotonin control of sleep-wake behavior. Sleep Med Rev 2011;15(4):269–81.

34. Miyazaki KW, Miyazaki K, Tanaka KF, et al. Optogenetic activation of dorsal raphe serotonin neurons enhances patience for future rewards. Curr Biol 2014;24(17):2033–40.

35. Cho JR, Treweek JB, Robinson JE, et al. Dorsal raphe dopamine neurons modulate arousal and promote wakefulness by salient stimuli. Neuron 2017; 94(6):1205–19.e8.

36. Sherin JE, Elmquist JK, Torrealba F, et al. Innervation of histaminergic tuberomammillary neurons by GABAergic and galaninergic neurons in the ventrolateral preoptic nucleus of the rat. J Neurosci 1998;18(12):4705–21.

37. Williams RH, Chee MJS, Kroeger D, et al. Optogenetic-mediated release of histamine reveals distal and autoregulatory mechanisms for controlling arousal. J Neurosci 2014;34(17): 6023–9.

38. Holst SC, Valomon A, Landolt HP. Sleep pharmacogenetics: personalized sleep-wake therapy. Annual review of pharmacology and toxicology 2016;56: 577–603.

39. Dahan L, Astier B, Vautrelle N, et al. Prominent burst firing of dopaminergic neurons in the ventral tegmental area during paradoxical sleep. Neuropsychopharmacology 2007;32(6):1232–41.

40. Léna I, Parrot S, Deschaux O, et al. Variations in extracellular levels of dopamine, noradrenaline, glutamate, and aspartate across the sleep-wake cycle in the medial prefrontal cortex and nucleus accumbens of freely moving rats. J Neurosci Res 2005;81(6):891–9.

41. Holst SC, Landolt HP. Sleep homeostasis, metabolism, and adenosine. Curr Sleep Med Rep 2015; 1(1):27–37.

42. Lazarus M, Huang Z-L, Lu J, et al. How do the basal ganglia regulate sleep wake behavior? Trends Neurosci 2012;35(12):723–32.

43. Monti JM, Monti D. The involvement of dopamine in the modulation of sleep and waking. Sleep Med Rev 2007;11(2):113–33.

44. Qiu MH, Yao QL, Vetrivelan R, et al. Nigrostriatal dopamine acting on globus pallidus regulates sleep. Cereb Cortex 2016;26(4):1430–9.

45. Burbach JPH. Neuropeptides from concept to online database www.neuropeptides.nl. Eur J Pharmacol 2010;626(1):27–48.
46. Richter C, Woods IG, Schier AF. Neuropeptidergic control of sleep and wakefulness. Annu Rev Neurosci 2014;37(1):503–31.
47. Monti JM, Torterolo P, Lagos P. Melanin-concentrating hormone control of sleep-wake behavior. Sleep Med Rev 2013;17(4):293–8.
48. Mileykovskiy BY, Kiyashchenko LI, Siegel JM. Behavioral correlates of activity in identified hypocretin/orexin neurons. Neuron 2005;46(5):787–98.
49. España RA, Scammell TE. Sleep neurobiology from a clinical perspective. Sleep 2011;34(7): 845–58.
50. Mochizuki T, Crocker A, McCormack S, et al. Behavioral state instability in orexin knock-out mice. J Neurosci 2004;24(28):6291–300.
51. Adamantidis AR, Zhang F, Aravanis AM, et al. Neural substrates of awakening probed with optogenetic control of hypocretin neurons. Nature 2007; 450(7168):420–4.
52. Carter ME, Adamantidis A, Ohtsu H, et al. Sleep homeostasis modulates hypocretin-mediated sleep-to-wake transitions. J Neurosci 2009;29(35): 10939–49.
53. Kilduff TS, De Lecea L. Mapping of the mRNAs for the hypocretin/orexin and melanin-concentrating hormone receptors: networks of overlapping peptide systems. J Comp Neurol 2001;435(1):1–5.
54. Konadhode RR, Pelluru D, Shiromani PJ. Neurons containing orexin or melanin concentrating hormone reciprocally regulate wake and sleep. Front Syst Neurosci 2015;8. https://doi.org/10.3389/fnsys. 2014.00244.
55. Willie JT, Sinton CM, Maratos-Flier E, et al. Abnormal response of melanin-concentrating hormone deficient mice to fasting: hyperactivity and rapid eye movement sleep suppression. Neuroscience 2008; 156(4):819–29.
56. Jego S, Glasgow SD, Herrera CG, et al. Optogenetic identification of a rapid eye movement sleep modulatory circuit in the hypothalamus. Nat Neurosci 2013;16(11):1637–43.
57. Tsunematsu T, Ueno T, Tabuchi S, et al. Optogenetic manipulation of activity and temporally controlled cell-specific ablation reveal a role for MCH neurons in sleep/wake regulation. J Neurosci 2014;34(20): 6896–909.
58. Konadhode RR, Pelluru D, Blanco-Centurion C, et al. Optogenetic stimulation of MCH neurons increases sleep. J Neurosci 2013;33(25):10257–63.
59. Bodenmann S, Hohoff C, Freitag C, et al. Polymorphisms of ADORA2A modulate psychomotor vigilance and the effects of caffeine on neurobehavioural performance and sleep EEG after sleep deprivation. Br J Pharmacol 2012;165(6):1904–13.
60. Huang Z-L, Qu W-M, Eguchi N, et al. Adenosine A2A, but not A1, receptors mediate the arousal effect of caffeine. Nat Neurosci 2005;8(7):858–9.
61. Landolt H-P. Sleep homeostasis: a role for adenosine in humans? Biochem Pharmacol 2008;75(11):2070–9.
62. Rétey JV, Adam M, Khatami R, et al. A genetic variation in the adenosine A2A receptor gene (ADORA2A) contributes to individual sensitivity to caffeine effects on sleep. Clin Pharmacol Ther 2007;81(5):692–8.
63. Sebastião AM, Ribeiro JA. Adenosine receptors and the central nervous system. Handb Exp Pharmacol 2009;471–534. https://doi.org/10.1007/978-3-540-89615-9_16.
64. Urry E, Landolt H-P. Adenosine, caffeine, and performance: from cognitive neuroscience of sleep to sleep pharmacogenetics. Curr Top Behav Neurosci 2015;25:331–66.
65. Virus RM, Djuricic-Nedelson M, Radulovacki M, et al. The effects of adenosine and 2'-deoxycoformycin on sleep and wakefulness in rats. Neuropharmacology 1983;22(12 PART 2):1401–4.
66. Porkka-Heiskanen T, Strecker RE, McCarley RW. Brain site-specificity of extracellular adenosine concentration changes during sleep deprivation and spontaneous sleep: an in vivo microdialysis study. Neuroscience 2000;99(3):507–17.
67. Porkka-Heiskanen T, Strecker RE, Thakkar M, et al. Adenosine: a mediator of the sleep-inducing effects of prolonged wakefulness. Science 1997;276(5316): 1265–7.
68. Blanco-Centurion C, Xu M, Murillo-Rodriguez E, et al. Adenosine and sleep homeostasis in the basal forebrain. J Neurosci 2006;26(31):8092–100.
69. Sherin JE, Shiromani PJ, McCarley RW, et al. Activation of ventrolateral preoptic neurons during sleep. Science 1996;271(5246):216–9.
70. Suntsova N, Szymusiak R, Alam MN, et al. Sleep-waking discharge patterns of median preoptic nucleus neurons in rats. J Physiol 2002;543(2): 665–77.
71. McGinty DJ, Sterman MB. Sleep suppression after basal forebrain lesions in the cat. Science 1968; 160(3833):1253–5.
72. Saito YC, Tsujino N, Hasegawa E, et al. GABAergic neurons in the preoptic area send direct inhibitory projections to orexin neurons. Front Neural Circuits 2013;7. https://doi.org/10.3389/fncir.2013.00192.
73. Rudolph U, Möhler H. GABA-based therapeutic approaches: GABAA receptor subtype functions. Curr Opin Pharmacol 2006;6:18–23.
74. Gachon F, Nagoshi E, Brown SA, et al. The mammalian circadian timing system: from gene expression to physiology. Chromosoma 2004;113(3):103–12.
75. Berson DM, Dunn FA, Takao M. Phototransduction by retinal ganglion cells that set the circadian clock. Science 2002;295(5557):1070–3.

76. Gooley JJ, Lu J, Chou TC, et al. Melanopsin in cells of origin of the retinohypothalamic tract. Nat Neurosci 2001;4(12):1165.

77. Blake MJF. Relationship between circadian rhythm of body temperature and introversion-extraversion. Nature 1967;215(5103):896–7.

78. Richter CP. A behavioristic study of the activity of the rat. Comparative Psychological Monographs 1922; 1(2):1–54.

79. Colwell CS. Linking neural activity and molecular oscillations in the SCN. Nat Rev Neurosci 2011;12(10): 553–69.

80. Chou TC, Scammell TE, Gooley JJ, et al. Critical role of dorsomedial hypothalamic nucleus in a wide range of behavioral circadian rhythms. Journal of Neuroscience 2003;23(33):10691–702.

81. Fuller PM, Gooley JJ, Saper CB. Neurobiology of the sleep-wake cycle: sleep architecture, circadian regulation, and regulatory feedback. J Biol Rhythms 2006; 482–93. https://doi.org/10.1177/0748730406294627.

82. Hardeland R, Cardinali DP, Srinivasan V, et al. Melatonin-A pleiotropic, orchestrating regulator molecule. Prog Neurobiol 2011;350–84. https://doi.org/ 10.1016/j.pneurobio.2010.12.004.

83. De Berardis D, Fornaro M, Serroni N, et al. Agomelatine beyond borders: current evidences of its efficacy in disorders other than major depression. Int J Mol Sci 2015;1111–30. https://doi.org/10.3390/ ijms16011111.

84. Gandhi AV, Mosser EA, Oikonomou G, et al. Melatonin is required for the circadian regulation of sleep. Neuron 2015;85(6):1193–9.

85. Fuller P, Sherman D, Pedersen NP, et al. Reassessment of the structural basis of the ascending arousal system. J Comp Neurol 2011;519(5):933–56.

86. Anaclet C, Lin J-S, Vetrivelan R, et al. Identification and characterization of a sleep-active cell group in the rostral medullary brainstem. J Neurosci 2012; 32(50):17970–6.

87. Dang-Vu TT, Schabus M, Desseilles M, et al. Functional neuroimaging insights into the physiology of human sleep. Sleep 2010;33(12):1589–603.

88. Dang-Vu TT, Schabus M, Desseilles M, et al. Spontaneous neural activity during human slow wave sleep. Proc Natl Acad Sci U S A 2008;105(39): 15160–5.

89. Dittrich L, Morairty SR, Warrier DR, et al. Homeostatic sleep pressure is the primary factor for activation of cortical nNOS/NK1 neurons. Neuropsychopharmacology 2015;40(3):632–9.

90. Holst SC, Sousek A, Hefti K, et al. Cerebral mGluR5 availability contributes to elevated sleep need and behavioral adjustment after sleep deprivation. Elife 2017;6. https://doi.org/10.7554/eLife.28751.

91. Maquet P, Degueldre C, Delfiore G, et al. Functional neuroanatomy of human slow wave sleep. J Neurosci 1997;17(8):2807–12.

92. Murphy M, Riedner BA, Huber R, et al. Source modeling sleep slow waves. Proc Natl Acad Sci U S A 2009;106(5):1608–13.

Drug-Induced Insomnia and Excessive Sleepiness

Ann Van Gastel, MD[a,b]

KEYWORDS

- Drugs • Medication • Psychotropic • Nonpsychotropic • Sleep • Insomnia • Sedation • Sleepiness

KEY POINTS

- Undesirable side effects of insomnia and/or sleepiness may occur with many prescribed drugs, psychotropics as well as nonpsychotropics.
- These central nervous system (CNS) effects can be explained by the interactions of a drug with any of the numerous neurotransmitters and receptors that are involved in sleep and wakefulness.
- A close—sometimes bidirectional—relationship between disease and (disturbed) sleep/wakefulness is often present. Drug effects may increase the complexity of this interaction.
- Effects of disease and/or drugs on sleep and wakefulness may create a vicious circle, influencing health and quality of life.
- Direct and indirect effects of drugs on the disease as well as on sleep and wakefulness need to be weighed.

INTRODUCTION

Sleep and waking function are closely connected in a 24-hour rhythm. The central nervous system (CNS) structures involved in the promotion of the waking state include neurons containing serotonin (5-HT), norepinephrine (NE), dopamine (DA), acetylcholine (ACh), histamine (HA), orexin (OX), and glutamate (GLU). Selective activation of either DA receptor D_1 or DA receptor D_2; 5-HT, $5-HT_1$, $5-HT_{2A}$, $5-HT_{2C}$, $5-HT_6$, and $5-HT_7$ receptors; NE α_1 receptor; HA H_1 receptor; ACh m_1 receptor; OX OX_1 and OX_2 receptors; or GLU AMPA, kainite, and N-methyl-D-aspartate receptors increases wake and reduces non–rapid eye movement (REM) and REM sleep.[1] Neurons that constitute the non-REM sleep–inducing system contain γ-aminobutyric acid (GABA) and galanin and inhibit cells involved in the promotion of wake. Somnogens, including adenosine, prostaglandin D_2, nitric oxide, and cytokines, also promote sleep, mainly non-REM sleep, in humans.[2] The REM sleep induction regions include predominantly glutamatergic neurons.[3]

Many drugs have the potential to disrupt sleep and waking function due to their pharmacologic effects at any of the numerous receptors and neurotransmitters involved in sleep-wake regulation. As such, insomnia and/or daytime sleepiness are common side effects of psychotropic as well as nonpsychotropic medication. The lipophilicity, which determines the easiness with which a drug crosses the blood-brain barrier (BBB), and the receptor binding profile determine its possible CNS effects.

Some general considerations have to be taken into account. First, there can be beneficial as well as adverse effects of drugs on sleep and wakefulness (**Table 1**). The effects may be desired when a drug is prescribed with the goal of creating sleep

There are no conflicts of interest. There are no funding sources.
[a] Multidisciplinary Sleep Disorders Centre and University Department of Psychiatry, Antwerp University Hospital, Wilrijkstraat 10, Antwerp 2650, Belgium; [b] Faculty of Medicine and Health Sciences, Collaborative Antwerp Psychiatric Research Institute (CAPRI), University of Antwerp (UA), Campus Drie Eiken, Universiteitsplein 1, Antwerp 2610, Belgium
E-mail address: Ann.Van.Gastel@uza.be

Sleep Med Clin 13 (2018) 147–159
https://doi.org/10.1016/j.jsmc.2018.02.001

Table 1
Drug-induced adverse effects of insomnia or sleepiness with possible mechanism of action

Drug Class or Individual Drug	Induced Sleep-Wake Disturbance	Possible Mechanism of Action
ANTIDEPRESSANTS		
Sedating TCA (eg, amitriptyline and doxepin)	Sleepiness	Antagonism at NE α_1, HA H_1, and ACh receptors
Activating TCA	Insomnia	Inhibition of serotonin and NE reuptake
SSRI	Insomnia	Inhibition of serotonin and NE reuptake
SNRI	Insomnia	Inhibition of serotonin and NE reuptake
Bupropion	Insomnia	Inhibition of NE and DA reuptake
MAOI	Insomnia	Inhibition of MAO enzyme
Atypical sedating AD (eg, trazodone and mirtazapine)	Sleepiness	Antihistaminergic effect, 5-HT_2-receptor antagonism
ANTIPSYCHOTICS		
First generation	Mostly sleepiness, insomnia also reported	Antagonism at NE α_1, HA H_1, ACh, and DA receptors
Second generation, for example, clozapine, olanzapine, and quetiapine	Variable effects Sleepiness	DA-receptor and 5-HT-receptor antagonism; effects at other receptors vary for each agent
ANTIEPILEPTICS	Mostly sleepiness	Decreased neuronal excitation by variable mechanisms
ANTIPARKINSONIAN AGENTS		
DA replacement drugs	Low-dose sleepiness, high-dose insomnia	DA-receptor agonism
ANALGETICS		
NSAIDs		Prostaglandin synthesis inhibition
Opioids	Sleepiness	μ-Opioid and κ-opioid receptor agonism
Triptans	Sleepiness?	5-HT_1-receptor antagonism
ANTIHISTAMINES		
First generation	Sleepiness	Antagonism at HA H_1 receptor
Second generation	None to mild sleepiness	None to little BBB transport
CARDIOVASCULAR DRUGS		
β-Blocking agents	Insomnia	β receptor and 5-HT-receptor antagonism; melatonin suppression
β- and α_1-blocking agent	Insomnia, also sleepiness reported	β and 5-HT receptor antagonism; melatonin suppression; α_1-receptor antagonism
α_1 Antagonists		α_1-receptor antagonism
α_2 Agonist		α_2-receptor stimulation
ANGIOTENSIN-CONVERTING ENZYME INHIBITORS		Interfering dry cough
Angiotensin receptor blockers		?
Loop diuretics	Insomnia	Nocturia
CORTICOSTEROIDS	Insomnia, sleepiness also reported	Multiple effects on HPA axis; effects on cytokines
THEOPHYLLINE	Insomnia?	Adenosine antagonist

(eg, hypnotics) or alertness (eg, stimulants). When the desired effects go on too long, however, they become undesired, for example, hangover effects of hypnotics or insomnia complaints provoked by a stimulant. Second, knowing how a good sleep is necessary for optimal functioning and well-being, drug effects may have far-reaching consequences. Effects on sleep quality or on sleep duration also affect daytime functioning. When a patient presents with daytime sleepiness, it may either be a direct effect of a drug or an indirect effect as the consequence of a disturbed sleep. Third, the mechanisms by which (un)wanted effects occur vary. They may directly affect the CNS (eg, drugs that stimulate the serotonergic system may disrupt sleep) or indirectly (eg, causing or aggravating conditions that disturb sleep like restless legs syndrome [RLS] or periodic limb movement disorder [PLMD]). The effects may be more or less obvious when sleep is interrupted by periods of wakefulness than when sleep architecture as registered by polysomnography is disturbed. Finally, the effects can be present in cases of administration of a drug (eg, sedative effect) or withdrawal of a drug (eg, rebound insomnia).

In this article, several classes of pharmacologic agents and individual drugs are discussed, mainly regarding their effects of inducing or aggravating insomnia and/or daytime somnolence. Due to the overlap of terms used in studies and in clinical practice, the terms, *sedation*, *(daytime) sleepiness*, and *(hyper-)somnolence*, are used interchangeably.

ANTIDEPRESSANTS

Antidepressants (ADs) are mainly used for the treatment of depression. Some ADs are also used in other conditions like anxiety disorders, obsessive-compulsive disorder, eating disorders, and primary headache disorder, or in the treatment of chronic pain. Sedating ADs are used off-label for the treatment of chronic insomnia. ADs may alter sleep patterns both indirectly (ie, by their effect on an underlying depression and the associated sleep abnormalities) and through direct effects on sleep. A close, bidirectional relationship between insomnia and depression is clearly demonstrated.[4]

ADs can be divided into 3 main classes, according to their major action mechanism.[5] The largest group of ADs consists of monoamine reuptake inhibitors. These agents increase the amount of monoamines in the synapse by inhibiting mainly the reuptake of serotonin and/or NE. Monoamine oxidase inhibitors (MAOIs) also increase the level of serotonin and/or NE (and to a lesser extent

DA) by preventing breakdown by the monoamine oxidase (MAO) enzyme. A third diverse group of compounds has complex effects on monoamine mechanisms but shares the ability to block 5-HT$_2$ receptors.

Depending on their acute pharmacologic properties, effects of ADs on sleep and daytime alertness are variable. Acute effects of ADs on sleep not only are reflected in patients' subjective complaints but also can be demonstrated in studies with PSG.[6]

Monoamine Reuptake Inhibitors

The monoamine reuptake inhibitors class of ADs includes tricyclic ADs (TCAs) and the newer, more selective reuptake inhibitors, which also potently inhibit the presynaptic uptake of serotonin and/or NE and/or DA but exert relatively weak effects on other neurotransmitter/receptor systems.

Tricyclic antidepressants
TCAs inhibit the reuptake of both serotonin and NE, but TCAs are nonspecific monoamine reuptake inhibitors. They also have antagonist activities at a variety of neurotransmitter receptors, like NE α_1, HA H$_1$, and ACh receptors, which are associated with many side effects, including sedative effects. TCAs demonstrate wide intraclass variability with respect to effects on nocturnal sleep and daytime sleepiness. Tertiary amine TCAs (eg, amitriptyline and trimipramine) tend to be more sedating, whereas secondary amine TCAs (desipramine and nortriptyline) tend to be more activating.[7] The TCA doxepin is Food and Drug Administration approved for the treatment of maintenance insomnia in very low doses, of 3 mg and 6 mg. These low doses are presumed to promote sleep by antagonizing only the HA-based arousal pathways without any other receptor effects.[8]

Selective serotonin reuptake inhibitors
Selective serotonin reuptake inhibitors (SSRIs), like (es)citalopram, fluoxetine, fluvoxamine, paroxetine, and sertraline, potently inhibit the presynaptic uptake of serotonin while exerting relatively weak effects on other neurotransmitter/receptor systems. Based on data from a Food and Drug Administration study register,[6,7] the highest rates of treatment-emergent insomnia and somnolence with SSRIs were found in patients suffering from obsessive-compulsive disorder treated with high-dose fluvoxamine, 31% and 27%, respectively. The lowest rate of treatment-emergent insomnia complaints (below 2%) was reported with citalopram. The average prevalence of treatment-emergent insomnia in clinical trials with SSRI was 17% compared with 9% of patients randomized

to the placebo arm. The average rate of treatment-emergent somnolence in patients treated with SSRI amounted to 16% compared with 8% of patients receiving placebo.[6,7]

Serotonin-norepinephrine reuptake inhibitors

Venlafaxine and duloxetine are serotonin-NE reuptake inhibitors (SNRIs). They are associated with frequent subjective complaints of insomnia and daytime somnolence as well as vivid dreams.[7] In clinical trials with SNRIs, both treatment-emergent insomnia and somnolence were the most frequent (both equal to 24%) in patients with generalized anxiety disorders treated with venlafaxine. Treatment-emergent insomnia was reported on average in 13% of SNRI-treated patients compared with 7% of the placebo arm. Treatment-emergent somnolence was reported on average in 10% of SNRI-treated patients in comparison to 5% of patients receiving placebo.[7]

Norepinephrine reuptake inhibitor

Reboxetine is the only available NE reuptake inhibitor (NRI). There is a dearth of studies reporting the incidence of side effects of insomnia/hypersomnolence with reboxetine.[9]

Norepinephrine-dopamine reuptake inhibitor

Bupropion is the only representative exerting NE and DA reuptake inhibitor (NDRI). Besides its approval as an AD, it is also registered in the United States as an aid for smoking cessation and seasonal affective disorder.

Bupropion is associated with reports of insomnia in patients treated for depression and seasonal affective disorder, with rates ranging from 11% to 20% depending on the dose, formulation, and condition treated.[7] Bupropion is one of the few ADs that shortens REM latency and increases total REM sleep time.[10] This finding is in contrast to most other ADs, which are prominent suppressants of REM sleep.[11]

Monoamine Oxidase Inhibitors

Drugs belonging to this class of ADs act as MAOIs. They deactivate MAO irreversibly (eg, phenelzine and tranylcypromine) or reversibly (moclobemide). Treatment with MAOIs is associated with frequent complaints of insomnia.[7]

5-HT$_2$ Antagonists

This class of ADs constitutes a diverse group of drugs (mirtazapine, mianserine, trazodone, and agomelatine), which share the ability to block 5-HT$_2$ receptors.

In clinical studies with mirtazapine, 54% of patients reported hypersomnolence compared with 18% of patients in the placebo arm. Mirtazapine produces predominantly antihistaminergic effects at lower doses (<30 mg/d) compared with increasingly predominant noradrenergic effects at higher doses.[6]

In clinical studies with trazodone, the reported prevalence of treatment-emergent insomnia complaints in patients with major depressive disorder was very low (below 2%), but the rate of treatment-emergent somnolence was very high: 46% in patients treated with trazodone compared with 19% of patients receiving placebo. It is common knowledge in clinical practice that trazodone's use as an AD is often limited by its tendency to produce daytime somnolence. In that respect, it is often used, at low doses, as a sleep aid although this effect has not been well studied.[7]

Agomelatine is a nonsedative AD drug exerting agonistic action at melatonergic M$_1$ and M$_2$ receptors and antagonistic action at serotonergic 5-HT$_{2c}$ receptors.

In summary, ADs are associated with different insomnia and somnolence rates, with class-specific or drug-specific effects depending on their mechanisms of action. Some ADs may deteriorate sleep quality mainly due to activation of serotonergic 5-HT$_2$ receptors and increased noradrenergic and dopaminergic neurotransmission. Among them, most prominent are SNRIs, NRIs, NDRIs, MAOIs, SSRIs, and activating TCAs. On the contrary, ADs with antihistaminergic action, like sedating TCAs, mirtazapine, and mianserine, or strong antagonistic action at serotonergic 5-HT$_2$ receptors, like trazodone, quickly improve sleep.[6]

In a meta-analysis of occurring insomnia and somnolence with 14 newer, more selective acting ADs during the treatment of major depression, the highest incidence of insomnia was found for bupropion and desvenlafaxine. Agomelatin was the only AD with a lower likelihood of inducing insomnia than placebo. Fluvoxamine and mirtazapine showed the highest frequency of somnolence. Bupropion induced somnolence to a lower extent than placebo.[9]

Most ADs with strong serotonergic action can cause or exacerbate restless legs or periodic limb movements and may cause insomnia and/or hypersomnolence indirectly through these effects.

Withdrawal effects that occur after long-term treatment with most ADs include insomnia, nightmares, and excessive dreaming related to REM rebound.[12]

ANTIPSYCHOTICS

Antipsychotics (APs) are mainly used for the treatment of psychotic disorders and schizophrenia.

APs are divided into typical, or first-generation, APs (FGAs) and the newer atypical, or second-generation, APs (SGAs).[13] Some of the newer atypical APs are also approved for the treatment of bipolar disorder or as an adjunctive treatment of major depression. APs have direct effects on sleep as well as the ability to promote sleep by attenuating symptoms that interfere with sleep, such as psychosis and agitation.

AP effects are mainly exerted by DA receptor antagonism. Many FGAs also exert effects on various monoamines as well as on HA, ACh, and/or NE α_1 receptors. These effects may increase the likelihood of somnolence.[7] FGAs are associated with side effects of extrapyramidal symptoms (EPs) at clinically AP effective dosages. The SGAs—also described as serotonin-DA antagonists—differ from FGAs by their higher ratio interactions with serotonin receptor subtypes, notably the 5-HT$_{2A}$ subtype, as well as with other neurotransmitter systems. All SGAs have different chemical structures, receptor affinities, and side-effect profiles, which are hypothesized to account for the distinct tolerability profiles associated with each of them. SGAs cause fewer EPs but have the propensity to cause weight gain, lipid elevations, and diabetes.[13]

First-Generation Antipsychotics

Among the FGAs, very high rates of somnolence are reported for chlorpromazine (33%) and thioridazine (35% to 57%) as well as for haloperidol (23%). Insomnia/disturbed sleep is also reported with haloperidol and thioridazine by approximately one-quarter of patients.[14]

Second-Generation Antipsychotics

The highest rate of somnolence, in 52% of patients, is reported for clozapine. Insomnia/disturbed sleep was reported in only 4% of patients.[14] Somnolence was also frequently reported with risperidone (30%) and olanzapine (29%) and moderately frequent with quetiapine and ziprasidone (16%). Although ziprasidone and quetiapine are expected to be sedating given their pharmacologic profiles, they seem less sedating than other drugs, possibly because of their short half-lives. Aripiprazole is least sedating (12%).[14]

In a study comparing somnolence associated with asenapine, olanzapine, risperidone, and haloperidol relative to placebo, only asenapine and olanzapine had significantly higher rates of somnolence relative to placebo.[15]

Objective measures of daytime sleepiness are rare. Both clozapine and olanzapine, however, reduce multiple sleep latency test (MSLT) results

in schizophrenic patients.[16] A placebo-controlled study showed increased Epworth Sleepiness Scale scores with quetiapine but not with lurasidone in patients with acute schizophrenia.[17]

Among the SGAs, insomnia is highest, with aripiprazole reported in approximately one-quarter of patients. Insomnia is also reported with risperidone (17%) and olanzapine (18%) and in 9% of patients with quetiapine and ziprasidone. Suggested possible mechanisms for this reported insomnia include 5-HT$_{1A}$–receptor agonism and RLS symptoms secondary to dopaminergic antagonism. Also, the 5 agents with the highest incidence of EPs—haloperidol, thioridazine, aripiprazole, risperidone, and olanzapine—have the 5 highest rates of sleep disturbance.[14]

In a 14-day randomized controlled trial PSG study evaluating the effects of paliperidone extended release in patients with schizophrenia-related insomnia, an improved sleep architecture and sleep continuity was found.[18] In another trial, single arm, with longer duration, insomnia was the most common adverse event, occurring in 17.9% of patients treated with paliperidone.[19]

A low-dose quetiapine is increasingly used off-label for the treatment of chronic insomnia. Quetiapine exhibits strong H$_1$-receptor antagonism and moderate affinity for 5-HT$_{2A}$ receptors. Antagonism at these sites is believed responsible for quetiapine's sedative effects.[7] In an open-label pilot study,[20] 18 adults with insomnia were treated with quetiapine, 25 mg at bedtime, with dosages increased to 50 mg in 7 patients and 75 mg in 1 patient. There were improvements in subjective and objective sleep parameters after 2 weeks that continued at 6 weeks. Transient morning hangover was a frequently reported adverse effect.

ANTIEPILEPTICS

The mechanism of action of antiepileptic drugs (AEDs) is via facilitation of GABA, sodium and calcium channel inhibition, inhibition of glutaminergic transmission, or other unknown mechanisms.[21] In addition to the treatment of epilepsy, several AEDs are used in other diseases, for example, in bipolar disorders or chronic pain conditions. Topiramate is used for the treatment of sleep-related eating disorder.

Antiepileptic Drugs in the Treatment of Epilepsy

Sleep and epilepsy have reciprocal effects, because sleep is a strong modulator of epileptic activity. Most seizures occur during non-REM sleep; seizures are rare in REM sleep. Poor sleep quality or quantity induces worsened seizure control, which in turn deteriorates sleep. Hence, a vicious circle is established.[22] Sleep disruption may be caused by seizures, anticonvulsants, or a coexisting sleep disorder. Patients with epilepsy are particularly sensitive to the adverse effects of sleep disruption.[23] In addition, most AEDs affect sleep architecture. These effects may be mediated by mechanism of action or may be indirectly due to treatment effects on epileptic phenomena.[24] Moreover, sleep disorders are common in epilepsy, and many of them have a higher prevalence in patients with epilepsy than in the general population. Treatment of them may improve seizure control. In adults with epilepsy, 40% to 55% of patients had insomnia, whereas 28% to 48% of patients with epilepsy reports daytime sleepiness.[22]

Sleepiness is one of the most commonly reported adverse effects of AEDs. In general, drugs acting on GABAergic neurotransmission (benzodiazepines, barbiturates, tiagabine, and vigabatrin) have the highest reported incidence of sleepiness or fatigue, amounting to 15% to 30% or more.[25] Placebo-controlled trials showed no difference between tiagabine and placebo in the incidence of sedation, but open-label long-term studies showed a 25% incidence of sedation with tiagabine.[26] Drugs acting primarily through sodium channel blockade (carbamazepine and phenytoin) show an incidence of sedation of 5% to 10%.[25] Drugs acting via calcium blockade or with multiple mechanisms of action show varying incidence of sedation: rates of 5% to 15% were reported for gabapentin (GBP), lamotrigine, pregabalin (PGB), and zonisamide. For levetiracetam and topiramate, sedation incidence of 15% to 27% was reported.[25]

Insomnia has been reported with lamotrigine.[27]

Compared with healthy controls or untreated patients with epilepsy, patients on phenobarbital, carbamazepine, phenytoin, or valproate have shown increased sleepiness on MSLT or decreased alertness on a maintenance of wakefulness test.[28]

In a review of objective sleep metrics,[24] daytime sleepiness was found not changed by topiramate, lamotrigine, zonisamide, and vigabatrin in patients with epilepsy but was increased by phenobarbital. Daytime sleepiness was unchanged at 1000-mg daily dose for levetiracetam but increased at 2000-mg daily dose. Other studies showed subjective sleepiness with zonisamide[29] and topiramate.[30] The not straightforward results from different studies may be related to several factors. Patients with epilepsy report increased sleepiness, so it is possible that this was attributed to

treatment. Also patients who reported sleepiness subjectively may not have objective sleepiness.[24]

In reports of impaired driving, use of anticonvulsants has been associated with an almost doubled risk of collision rate. Some studies in epileptic patients, however, have commented on the benefit of therapy. Because preventing seizures on the road reduce the incidence of collision, optimal therapy is the key. A large multicenter study discovered higher crash rates in patients not taking their AEDs appropriately compared with medication-adherent patients. This highlights the complex relationships between disease and risks as well as pharmacotherapy and risks. So considering driving ability in epileptic patients, outweighing the decreased risk of collusion against possible sedative effects of AEDs is essential.[31]

Antiepileptic Drugs in the Treatment of Other Disorders

GBP and PGB are newer antiepileptic agents that share some aspects of their mechanism of action. They are presumed to work via the $\alpha_2\delta$ unit of voltage-gated calcium channels, binding to which reduces calcium influx that decreases the release of several excitatory neurotransmitters.[21] GBP and PGB are approved for the treatment of neuropathic pain. Sedation is reported to occur in 15% to 25% of patients using these drugs to treat neuropathic pain.[28] GBP and PGB also are a recognized treatment of RLS/PLMD.[32] PGB is also indicated for the treatment of generalized anxiety disorder.

ANTIPARKINSON DRUGS

The primary treatment of Parkinson disease (PD) is DA replacement. Levodopa and DA agonists (eg, pramipexole, ropinirole, and rotigotine) are the principal drugs used. Adjunctive treatments include, among others, dopamine decarboxylase inhibitors (carbidopa and benserazide), which prevent peripheral conversion of levodopa to DA; catechol-O-methyltransferase inhibitors (entacapone and tolcapone), which prolong the duration of the effect of levodopa; and MAO-B inhibitors (selegiline and rasagiline), which block the breakdown of DA.[33]

Sleep disorders are among the most common nonmotor manifestations in PD. Most frequently reported are insomnia, REM sleep behavior disorder, RLS, sleep-disordered breathing, and excessive daytime sleepiness (EDS).[34] Multiple causes for these sleep-related complaints are possible: abnormalities in sleep-wake regulation caused by the disease; motor symptoms, such as rigidity, tremor, dystonia, and poor bed mobility; other sleep disorders; concurrent medical or psychiatric illness; or the medications used for the treatment. As such, it is difficult to determine whether changes in sleep and waking behavior after drug administration are due to the direct effects of a drug or the indirect effects of a drug on the disease.[25]

It is suggested that low doses of dopaminergic medications tend to improve sleep whereas higher doses are likely to disrupt sleep.[34] An increased risk of insomnia compared with placebo was reported in randomized controlled trials for DA agonists, for DA agonist withdrawal, for selegiline and rasagiline (although some data suggest otherwise for rasagiline), and for entacapone. Higher total levodopa equivalent dose and levodopa equivalent dose contributed by DA agonists have been associated with worse measures of subjective and objective sleep in PD. Benefits on motor symptoms have to be weighed against risks of worsening insomnia due to dopaminergic stimulation. Drug-related improvement in PD symptoms may outweigh the sleep-disrupting effects of the drug, resulting in an improvement in sleep overall. Additionally, sleep dysfunction can be associated with and influence motor and nonmotor symptoms in this patient population.[35]

EDS is also common among patients with PD. EDS is more likely to affect patients with advanced PD.[35] Several studies also support a relationship between dopaminergic therapy and EDS. Levodopa equivalent dose independently predicts subjective sleepiness and subjective sleepiness correlated with use of DA agonists. Sudden-onset sleep episodes are more likely among patients on DA agonists. On the other hand, some studies do not support a relationship between dopaminergic therapy and EDS.[35] No increased EDS compared with placebo was shown for rasagiline. In an open-label study, selegiline in combination with reduction or discontinuation of DA agonists led to reduction or resolution of somnolence in 94% subjects with EDS.

ANALGESICS

In patients with chronic pain, a vicious circle often develops, with pain disrupting sleep and poor sleep further exacerbating pain.[4] Improving sleep quantity and quality in patients with pain may break this vicious circle and as a consequence enhance a patient's overall health and quality of life. So, when using an analgetic, it seems important to know the effects on sleep.[21]

Nonsteroidal Anti-inflammatory Drugs

Nonsteroidal anti-inflammatory drugs (NSAIDs) are among the most commonly used analgesics.

Their therapeutic action is largely due to the inhibition of the 2 isoenzymes of cyclo-oxygenase (COX), COX-1 and COX-2, which are important for the production of prostaglandins. Prostaglandins play a role in regulation of sleep and wakefulness.[36] Prostaglandin D_2 increases proportionately with increased duration of wake and may be involved in sleep initiation.[37] Proposed possible underlying mechanisms of sleep disruption after NSAID intake may relate to the direct and indirect consequences of inhibiting prostaglandin synthesis, including decrease of prostaglandin D_2, reduced melatonin secretion, and modification of body temperature.[38,39]

PSG studies about the influence of NSAIDs on sleep are limited and results are mixed. In healthy patients, acetaminophen does not seem to change sleep structure. For ibuprofen and aspirin, no effects[40] to delayed sleep onset, increased wake after sleep onset, increased stage 2 sleep, decreased slow-wave sleep, and reduced sleep efficiency[39,41] were reported. A study on the effect of tenoxicam on rheumatoid arthritis patients reported improvement in pain but no changes in PSG parameters during 90 days of treatment.[42] A trial on women with dysmenorrhea treated with therapeutic doses of diclofenac reported subjective and objective improvement in sleep, including sleep quality, sleep efficiency, REM sleep, and a reduction of stage 1 sleep.[43]

Opioids

Opioids are used as major analgetics. Their effects are mediated by specific opioid receptors of which 3 major types are described: mu (μ), kappa (κ), and delta (δ).[36] Centrally occurring opioids bind to these receptors to exert control over various biological systems, including pain regulation and the sleep-wake cycle. The effect of opioids on the sleep-wake cycle is believed controlled by opioid receptors, their indirect actions on GABAergic transmission, and other neurotransmitter systems and neuromodulators, such as adenosine. One of the mechanisms by which opioids are said to disrupt sleep is through their effects on the availability of adenosine in sites that are important in REM and non-REM sleep.[44]

Somnolence is a common side effect of opioid medication.[28] It varies with used dose, duration of use, age, and underlying disease.[28] The sedative effects may lead to the impression that they promote sleep. On the contrary, opioids have been shown to decrease both REM sleep and SWS in the postoperative period as well as in chronic opiate use and abuse.[45,46] Increased nocturnal awakenings have also been shown.

Nevertheless, the strong analgesic properties of these drugs permit sleep in people who are otherwise unable to sleep, such as those with chronic pain syndromes or severe RLS.

Triptans

Triptans are used for the treatment of migraine and cluster headache. They exert their therapeutic action via agonist effects at the 5-HT$_1$ receptor.[47]

Reported somnolence is highest with the more lipophilic triptans with active metabolites, such as eletriptan, zolmitriptan, and rizatriptan. Reported somnolence is lowest with less lipophilic triptans without active metabolites, such as sumatriptan, almotriptan, and naratriptan.[48]

Different opinions exist over whether the reported somnolence is the result of the effects of a drug on the serotonergic system (less likely because serotonin is mostly a wake-promoting neurotransmitter) or reflects a symptom of the wider migraine attack.[47] This was illustrated by pooled data from 7 placebo-controlled trials of triptan use in acute migraine. Higher rates of somnolence were shown in responders than nonresponders, whereas similar rates of somnolence were shown in patients who responded to either active treatment or placebo. It is suggested that this must be due, at least to a significant part, to headache relief and unmasking of somnolence as a symptom of the syndrome of a migraine attack, rather than just a side effect of treatment.[49]

H$_1$ ANTIHISTAMINES

HA is widely present throughout the body and the CNS. In most tissues, HA is stored in mast cells, which mediate allergic responses. In the CNS, HA serves as a neurotransmitter promoting wakefulness. Different types of HA receptors have been described. H$_1$ antihistamines are the mainstay in the treatment of allergic disorders.[50]

First-generation H$_1$ antihistamines have a much stronger sedative effects than second-generation H$_1$ antihistamines. The first-generation H$_1$ antagonists (eg, chlorpheniramine, diphenhydramine, and hydroxyzine) are lipophilic molecules that can easily permeate the BBB. The second-generation H$_1$ antihistamines (eg, bilastine, ebastine, and fexofenadine) are more hydrophilic molecules that do not easily enter the CNS and have as such no (or less) effect on wakefulness. Among second-generation H$_1$ antihistamines, cetirizine shows a more noticeable sedative effect than others. Central H$_1$-receptor occupancy varies from almost negligible (eg, fexofenadine) to 30% for cetirizine.[51] According to brain H$_1$-receptor occupancy, antihistamines might objectively be classified into 3 categories of sedating, less sedating, and nonsedating antihistamines.[52] Nonsedating antihistamines should be preferentially used whenever possible, because most are equally efficacious, whereas adverse effects of sedating antihistamines can be serious.[52]

Because of the sedative side effects, H$_1$ antagonists are used off-label for the treatment of insomnia. These agents are varyingly effective and may result in daytime sleepiness.

CARDIOVASCULAR DRUGS
β-Adrenergic Blocking Agents

β-Adrenergic blocking drugs are widespread used for a variety of diseases, cardiovascular as well as noncardiovascular, like migraine, posttraumatic stress disorder, and anxiety disorders. Reported side effects include tiredness, insomnia, and vivid dreams, which may manifest as frank nightmares in some.[53] Several features of β-blocking agents seem to play a role in these CNS side effects. A higher lipophylicity carries a higher risk of entrance in the CNS, but other characteristics like high β$_2$ and/or 5-HT–receptor occupancy also seem important in potentially causing sleep disruption. Taking into account all these pharmacologic features, it is suggested that bisoprolol, atenolol, betaxolol, acebutolol, nebivolol, and nadolol involve the lowest risk for insomnia, and sotalol, timolol, pindolol, and carvedilol carry a moderate risk for insomnia, whereas the highest risk for insomnia is borne by labetalol, metoprolol and propranolol.[25]

β-Blocking agents also inhibit melatonin production by blocking sympathetic signaling to the pineal gland.[54–56] Because the pineal gland is located outside the BBB, both lipophilic (such as propranolol) and hydrophilic (such as atenolol) β-blocking agents suppress melatonin, leading to a reduced circadian signal to initiate sleep, which may help explain the insomnia associated with β-blocker use.[47] An acute study in healthy subjects showed that melatonin supplementation to the β-blocker restores sleep. In a 3-week study of melatonin supplementation in hypertensive patients chronically treated with β-blockers, improved sleep quality was reported.[57]

β-Blockers that have vasodilatating properties through α$_1$ blockade, for example, carvedilol and labetalol, also are associated with fatigue and somnolence.[25]

α$_1$ Antagonists

Prazosin is increasingly used off-label to treat nightmares in patients with posttraumatic stress disorder. Insomnia and hallucinations are listed as some of the rare side effects of prazosin by the manufacturer. Low-dose prazosin was associated with nightmares and sleep disturbances in a case report of an elderly patient without previously diagnosed mental illness or coexisting environmental risk factors for nightmares.[58]

α₂-Adrenergic Agonists

For the central-acting antihypertensives, clonidine and methyldopa, sedation is a common side effect, occurring in 30% to 75% of patients. The severity seems to diminish with time. There are also reports of insomnia and nightmares with these drugs.[25]

Angiotensin-Converting Enzyme Inhibitors

A low incidence of central side effects (eg, captopril and cilazapril) is reported.[25] Indirectly, sleep disturbance can be initiated or aggravated, because angiotensin-converting enzyme inhibitors can precipitate a dry, irritating cough, which may interfere with sleep.[25] Spirapril was associated with insomnia at high doses of 6 mg.[59] Ramipril improved subjective sleep reports in heart failure patients.[60]

Angiotensin Receptor Blockers

In patients receiving losartan, more adverse effects, including insomnia, were reported, compared with controls who were taking angiotensin-converting enzyme inhibitors or calcium channel blockers.[61]

Loop Diuretics

Research of the effects of loop diuretics on sleep is scarce. Diuretic intake, however, is often associated with nocturia, which may result in sleep fragmentation.[62] On the other hand, it was indicated by preliminary work that administration of loop diuretics may improve OSA by reducing peripharyngeal edema.[63]

Statins

Placebo-controlled studies of lovastatin, pravastatin,[64] and simvastatine[65] showed no increased sleep disturbance.

CORTICOSTEROIDS

Corticosteroids, effectors of the hypothalamic-pituitary-adrenal axis (HPA) system, elicit their actions through binding to 2 types of intracellular receptors located in the CNS, the mineralocorticoid receptors and the glucocorticoid receptors. Glucocorticoid receptors are widely distributed in the CNS,[66] including anatomic regions implicated in the control of sleep and waking. Corticosteroids are used in a wide medical array. Adverse drug reactions to corticosteroids are known to be associated with the way of administration, the size of the dose, chemical properties, and the length of time for which a drug is prescribed.[67] Behavioral alterations are commonly associated with elevated levels of cortical steroids. Sleep disturbances are recognized as a prominent symptom among these behavioral alterations.[66]

Knowing the link between chronic insomnia and cortisol,[68,69] an association between corticoid administration and insomnia could be expected. The results of objective studies, however, seem inconsistent. In a large study with the use of high-dose prednisolone versus placebo for optic neuritis, 53% of patients treated with prednisolone for optic neuritis reported sleep disturbance compared with 20% on placebo.[70] Otherwise, clinical trials on intranasal corticosteroids report that the improved nasal congestion is associated with improved quality of life, with better sleep and reduced fatigue.[71] Dexamethasone has been shown to increase alertness[66] as well as increase slow-wave sleep.[67] In clinical studies of children with acute lymphoblastic leukemia treated with corticosteroids, both insomnia and hypersomnia are reported as adverse side effects attributed to dexamethasone.[72] Several mediating mechanisms may explain these apparently contradictory research and clinical findings noted in different studies of the effects of corticosteroids and sleep.

Corticosteroids affect sleep at multiple levels of the nervous system.[66,67,73] On the one hand, corticosteroids can cause a direct increase in alertness. On the other hand, corticosteroids inhibit the release of corticotropin-releasing hormone (CRH) by the HPA axis feedback loop. CRH activates the locus coeruleus–NE system, thereby increasing wakefulness. This indirect CRH inhibition decreases wakefulness and increases slow-wave sleep.[72]

Another potential mechanism for the effects of dexamethasone on sleep involves inflammatory cytokines. Tumor necrosis factor (TNF)-α, interleukin (IL)-1, and IL-6 are important in sleep regulation[74] and they are associated with daytime sleepiness. TNF-α, IL-1, and IL-6 have been identified as mediators of sickness syndrome in human and animal studies and they are believed important factors mediating fatigue.[75]

THEOPHYLLINE

Theophylline, related in chemical structure and pharmacologic action to caffeine, is mainly used in the treatment of asthma and chronic obstructive pulmonary disease. Several mechanisms of action have been suggested to explain the effectiveness of theophylline. Adenosine receptor antagonism is believed responsible for some of the CNS side effects, including insomnia and restlessness.[76]

The effect of theophylline on sleep quality and cognitive performance in patients has been the subject of controversy. Two almost identical studies were undertaken to examine the direct effects of theophylline on sleep quality and cognitive performance, without confounding effects from bronchodilatation, in healthy subjects.[77] In 1 study it was shown that theophylline does not affect sleep quality or cognitive performance in normal adults,[78] whereas, on the contrary, an increased number of arousals and reduced total sleep time were shown in the other study.[79] Dose-dependent increase in MSLT latency and performance was noted with short-term administration of theophylline in healthy persons.[80] Theophylline-associated sleep disturbances were shown in children with cystic fibrosis.[81] A meta-analysis of 12 studies of theophylline, however, did not indicate impairment in cognition or behavior.[82]

Impaired quality of sleep is common among patients with bronchial asthma[83] and chronic obstructive pulmonary disease.[84] Overall, notwithstanding the—in some studies—reported negative effects of theophylline on sleep architecture, the positive effects on sleep of ameliorated respiration at night presumably outweigh the minimal negative effects on sleep architecture.

DISCUSSION

When choosing a pharmacologic agent for a patient, the adverse-effect profile is the most important consideration after the main therapeutic effect.[85] Awareness of possible side effects like disturbed sleep and/or daytime sleepiness is important to adapt treatment and reach optimal results for every patient. Besides the importance for health and quality of life, effects on sleep or waking function can be a potential source of noncompliance. Nevertheless, although direct negative effects on sleep or waking function may show themselves in healthy persons, the resulting effects of drugs in patients may not be straightforward. As described previously, the positive effects of theophylline on nighttime respiration in patients presumably outweigh the negative effects on sleep architecture described in healthy persons. As in many conditions, a close bidirectional relationship between disease and sleep exists; drug effects may lead this vicious circle in both ways. In the bidirectional connection between, for example, sleep and pain, direct negative effects

of opioids on sleep may be present, but indirect effects (ameliorating sleep by reducing pain during the night) may be clinically more important and set an important upward trend for the patient. Vice versa, as, for example, in the bidirectional relationship between insomnia and depression, unwanted drug effects may be further complicating this interaction, for example, aggravating insomnia in an otherwise positive AD response. Disease, sleep disturbances, and medication may also interact for example, in epilepsy, where sleep disruption may be caused by seizures, by anticonvulsants, or by coexisting sleep disorders, any of which may have an adverse impact on daily functioning. Also, benefits gained in reducing 1 sleep problem may be offset by causing or exacerbating another sleep problem.[86] For example, loop diuretics have been associated with decreases in OSA severity. A side effect of diuretic administration, however, is nocturia. Given the entanglement between sleep, health, and quality of life, awareness of effects of drugs on sleep is essential. A vigilant clinician is needed to optimize treatment to the need of the patient.

REFERENCES

1. Monti JM. The effect of second-generation antipsychotic drugs on sleep parameters in patients with unipolar or bipolar disorder. Sleep Med 2016;23: 89–96.
2. Monti JM. The neurotransmitters of sleep and wake, a physiological reviews series. Sleep Med Rev 2013; 17:313–5.
3. Luppi PH, Clément O, Fort P. Paradoxical (REM) sleep genesis by the brainstem is under hypothalamic control. Curr Opin Neurobiol 2013;23:1–7.
4. Sateia MC, Buysse DJ. Insomnia diagnosis and treatment. 1st edition. London: Informa healthcare; 2010.
5. Wilson S, Argyropoulos S. Antidepressants and sleep: a qualitative review of the literature. Drugs 2005;65(7):927–47.
6. Wichniak A, Wierzbicka A, Wałęcka M, et al. Effects of antidepressants on sleep. Curr Psychiatry Rep 2017;19(9):63.
7. Doghramji K, Jangro WC. Adverse effects of psychotropic medications on sleep. Psychiatr Clin North Am 2016;39(3):487–502.
8. Roth T, Rogowski R, Hull S, et al. Efficacy and safety of doxepin 1 mg, 3 mg, and 6 mg in adults with primary insomnia. Sleep 2007;30(11):1555–61.
9. Alberti S, Chiesa A, Andrisano C, et al. Insomnia and somnolence associated with second-generation antidepressants during the treatment of major depression: a meta-analysis. J Clin Psychopharmacol 2015;35(3):296–303.

10. Nofzinger EA, Reynolds CF 3rd, Thase ME, et al. REM sleep enhancement by bupropion in depressed men. Am J Psychiatry 1995;152(2):274–6.

11. Holshoe JM. Antidepressants and sleep: a review. Perspect Psychiatr Care 2009;45(3):191–7.

12. Haddad PM. Antidepressant discontinuation syndromes. Drug Saf 2001;24(3):183–97.

13. Sadock BJ, Sadock VA, Ruiz P. Kaplan and Sadock's synopsis of psychiatry. Behavioral sciences/clinical psychiatry. 11th edition. Philadelphia: Wolters Kluwer; 2015.

14. Krystal AD, Goforth HW, Roth T. Effects of antipsychotic medications on sleep in schizophrenia. Int Clin Psychopharmacol 2008;23(3):150–60.

15. Gao K, Mackle M, Cazorla P, et al. Comparison of somnolence associated with asenapine, olanzapine, risperidone, and haloperidol relative to placebo in patients with schizophrenia or bipolar disorder. Neuropsychiatr Dis Treat 2013;9:1145–57.

16. Kluge M, Himmerich H, Wehmeier PM, et al. Sleep propensity at daytime as assessed by Multiple Sleep Latency Tests (MSLT) in patients with schizophrenia increases with clozapine and olanzapine. Schizophr Res 2012;135(1–3):123–7.

17. Loebel AD, Siu CO, Cucchiaro JB, et al. Daytime sleepiness associated with lurasidone and quetiapine XR: results from a randomized double-blind, placebo-controlled trial in patients with schizophrenia. CNS Spectr 2014;19(2):197–205.

18. Luthringer R, Staner L, Noel N, et al. A double-blind, placebo-controlled, randomized study evaluating the effect of paliperidone extended-release tablets on sleep architecture in patients with schizophrenia. Int Clin Psychopharmacol 2007;22(5):299–308.

19. Üçok A, Saka MC, Bilici M. Effects of paliperidone extended release on functioning level and symptoms of patients with recent onset schizophrenia: an open-label, single-arm, flexible-dose, 12-months follow-up study. Nord J Psychiatry 2015;69(6):426–32.

20. Wiegand MH, Landry F, Brückner T, et al. Quetiapine in primary insomnia: a pilot study. Psychopharmacology (Berl) 2008;196(2):337–8.

21. Bohra MH, Kaushik C, Temple D, et al. Weighing the balance: how analgesics used in chronic pain influence sleep? Br J Pain 2014;8(3):107–18.

22. Jain SV, Kothare SV. Sleep and epilepsy. Semin Pediatr Neurol 2015;22(2):86–92.

23. Bazil CW. Nocturnal seizures and the effects of anticonvulsants on sleep. Curr Neurol Neurosci Rep 2008;8(2):149–54.

24. Jain SV, Glauser TA. Effects of epilepsy treatments on sleep architecture and daytime sleepiness: an evidence-based review of objective sleep metrics. Epilepsia 2014;55(1):26–37.

25. Schweitzer PK, Randazzo AC. Drugs that disturb sleep and wakefulness. In: Kryger MH, Roth T, Dement WC, editors. Principles and practice of sleep medicine. 6th edition. Philadelphia: Elsevier; 2017. p. 480–98.

26. Vossler DG, Morris GL 3rd, Harden CL, et al, Postmarketing Antiepileptic Drug Survey (PADS) Group Study Investigators. Tiagabine in clinical practice: effects on seizure control and behavior. Epilepsy Behav 2013;28(2):211–6.

27. Sadler M. Lamotrigine associated with insomnia. Epilepsia 1999;40(3):322–5.

28. Schweitzer PK. Excessive sleepiness due to medications and drugs. In: Thorpy MJ, Billiard M, editors. Sleepiness: causes, consequences and treatment. United Kingdom: Cambridge University Press; 2011. p. 386–98.

29. Leppik IE. Zonisamide. Epilepsia 1999;40(Suppl. 5):S23–9.

30. Glauser TA. Topiramate. Epilepsia 1999;40(Suppl. 5):S71–80.

31. Hetland A, Carr DB. Medications and impaired driving. Ann Pharmacother 2014;48(4):494–506.

32. Garcia-Borreguero D, Kohnen R, Silber MH, et al. The long-term treatment of restless legs syndrome/Willis-Ekbom disease: evidence-based guidelines and clinical consensus best practice guidance: a report from the International Restless Legs Syndrome Study Group. Sleep Med 2013; 14(7):675–84.

33. Connolly BS, Lang AE. Pharmacological treatment of Parkinson disease: a review. JAMA 2014;311(16):1670–83.

34. Videnovic A, Golombek D. Circadian and sleep disorders in Parkinson's disease. Exp Neurol 2013;243:45–56.

35. Chahine LM, Amara AW, Videnovic A. A systematic review of the literature on disorders of sleep and wakefulness in Parkinson's disease from 2005 to 2015. Sleep Med Rev 2017;35:33–50.

36. Schug SA, Garrett WR, Gillespie G. Opioid and nonopioid analgesics. Best Pract Res Clin Anaesthesiol 2003;17(1):91–110.

37. Datta S, Maclean RR. Neurobiological mechanisms for the regulation of mammalian sleep-wake behavior: reinterpretation of historical evidence and inclusion of contemporary cellular and molecular evidence. Neurosci Biobehav Rev 2007;31(5):775–824.

38. Horne JA. Aspirin and nonfebrile waking oral temperature in healthy men and women: links with SWS changes. Sleep 1989;12:516–21.

39. Murphy PJ, Badia P, Myers BL, et al. Nonsteroidal anti-inflammatory drugs affect normal sleep patterns in humans. Physiol Behav 1994;55(6):1063–6.

40. Gengo F. Effects of ibuprofen on sleep quality as measured using polysomnography and subjective measures in healthy adults. Clin Ther 2006;28(11):1820–6.

41. Horne JA, Percival JE, Traynor JR. Aspirin and human sleep. Electroencephalogr Clin Neurophysiol 1980;49(3–4):409–13.

42. Lavie P, Nahir M, Lorber M, et al. Nonsteroidal anti-inflammatory drug therapy in rheumatoid arthritis patients. Lack of association between clinical improvement and effects on sleep. Arthritis Rheum 1991;34:655–9.

43. Lacovides S, Avidon I, Bentley A, et al. Diclofenac potassium restores objective and subjective measures of sleep quality in women with primary dysmenorrhea. Sleep 2009;32(8):1019–26.

44. Moore JT, Kelz MB. Opiates, sleep, and pain: the adenosinergic link. Anesthesiology 2009;111(6): 1175–6.

45. Cronin AJ, Keifer JC, Davies MF, et al. Postoperative sleep disturbance: influences of opioids and pain in humans. Sleep 2001;24:39–44.

46. Onen SH, Onen F, Courpron P, et al. How pain and analgesics disturb sleep. Clin J Pain 2005;21(5): 422–31.

47. Nesbitt AD. Headache, drugs and sleep. Cephalalgia 2014;34(10):756–66.

48. Dodick DW, Martin V. Triptans and CNS side-effects: pharmacokinetic and metabolic mechanisms. Cephalalgia 2004;24(6):417–24.

49. Goadsby PJ, Dodick DW, Almas M, et al. Treatment-emergent CNS symptoms following triptan therapy are part of the attack. Cephalalgia 2007;27(3):254–62.

50. Hu Y, Sieck DE, Hsu WH. Why are second-generation H1-antihistamines minimally sedating? Eur J Pharmacol 2015;765:100–6.

51. Tashiro M, Sakurada Y, Iwabuchi K, et al. Central effects of fexofenadine and cetirizine: measurement of psychomotor performance, subjective sleepiness, and brain histamine H1-receptor occupancy using 11C-doxepin positron emission tomography. J Clin Pharmacol 2004;44(8):890–900.

52. Yanai K, Yoshikawa T, Yanai A, et al. The clinical pharmacology of non-sedating antihistamines. Pharmacol Ther 2017;178:148–56.

53. Pagel JF, Helfter P. Drug induced nightmares–an etiology based review. Hum Psychopharmacol 2003; 18(1):59–67.

54. Arendt J, Bojkowski C, Franey C, et al. Immunoassay of 6-hydroxymelatonin sulfate in human plasma and urine: abolition of the urinary 24-hour rhythm with atenolol. J Clin Endocrinol Metab 1985;60:1166–73.

55. Nathan PJ, Maguire KP, Burrows GD, et al. The effect of atenolol, a beta1-adrenergic antagonist, on nocturnal plasma melatonin secretion: evidence for a dose-response relationship in humans. J Pineal Res 1997;23:131–5.

56. Stoschitzky K, Sakotnik A, Lercher P, et al. Influence of beta-blockers on melatonin release. Eur J Clin Pharmacol 1999;55(2):111–5.

57. Scheer FA, Morris CJ, Garcia JI, et al. Repeated melatonin supplementation improves sleep in hypertensive patients treated with beta-blockers: a randomized controlled trial. Sleep 2012;35(10): 1395–402.

58. Kosari S, Naunton M. Sleep disturbances and nightmares in a patient treated with prazosin. J Clin Sleep Med 2016;12(4):631–2.

59. Kantola I, Terént A, Honkanen T, et al. Efficacy and safety of spirapril, a new ace-inhibitor, in elderly hypertensive patients. Eur J Clin Pharmacol 1996; 50(3):155–9.

60. Gundersen T, Wiklund I, Swedberg K, et al. Effects of 12 weeks of ramipril treatment on the quality of life in patients with moderate congestive heart failure: results of a placebo-controlled trial. Ramipril Study Group. Cardiovasc Drugs Ther 1995;9(4): 589–94.

61. Samizo K, Kawabe E, Hinotsu S, et al. Comparison of losartan with ACE inhibitors and dihydropyridine calcium channel antagonists: a pilot study of prescription-event monitoring in Japan. Drug Saf 2002;25(11):811–21.

62. Riegel B, Moser DK, Anker SD, et al. State of the science: promoting self-care in persons with heart failure: a scientific statement from the American Heart Association. Circulation 2009;120(12):1141–63.

63. Bucca CB, Brussino L, Battisti A, et al. Diuretics in obstructive sleep apnea with diastolic heart failure. Chest 2007;132(2):440–6.

64. Ehrenberg BL, Lamon-Fava S, Corbett KE, et al. Comparison of the effects of pravastatin and lovastatin on sleep disturbance in hypercholesterolemic subjects. Sleep 1999;22(1):117–21.

65. Keech AC, Armitage JM, Wallendszus KR, et al. Absence of effects of prolonged simvastatin therapy on nocturnal sleep in a large randomized placebo-controlled study. Oxford Cholesterol Study Group. Br J Clin Pharmacol 1996;42(4):483–90.

66. Meixner R, Gerhardstein R, Day R, et al. The alerting effects of dexamethasone. Psychophysiology 2003; 40(2):254–9.

67. Friess E, Tagaya H, Grethe C, et al. Acute cortisol administration promotes sleep intensity in man. Neuropsychopharmacology 2004;29(3):598–604.

68. Vgontzas AN, Bixler EO, Lin HM, et al. Chronic insomnia is associated with nyctohemeral activation of the hypothalamic-pituitary-adrenal axis: clinical implications. J Clin Endocrinol Metab 2001;86(8): 3787–94.

69. Rodenbeck A, Huether G, Rüther E, et al. Interactions between evening and nocturnal cortisol secretion and sleep parameters in patients with severe chronic primary insomnia. Neurosci Lett 2002; 324(2):159–63.

70. Chrousos GA, Kattah JC, Beck RW, et al. Side effects of glucocorticoid treatment. Experience of the

optic neuritis treatment trial. JAMA 1993;269(16): 2110–2.

71. Lunn M, Craig T. Rhinitis and sleep. Sleep Med Rev 2011;15(5):293–9.

72. Rosen G, Harris AK, Liu M, et al. The effects of Dexamethasone on sleep in young children with Acute Lymphoblastic Leukemia. Sleep Med 2015; 16(4):503–9.

73. Steiger A. Sleep and the hypothalamo-pituitary-adrenocortical system. Sleep Med Rev 2002;6: 125–38.

74. Krueger K, Rector D, Churchill L. Sleep and cytokines. Sleep Med Clin 2007;2(2):161–9.

75. Bryant P, Trinder J, Curtis N. Sick and tired: does sleep have a vital role in the immune system? Nat Rev Immunol 2004;4:457–67.

76. Vassallo R, Lipsky JJ. Theophylline: recent advances in the understanding of its mode of action and uses in clinical practice. Mayo Clin Proc 1998; 73(4):346–54.

77. Smith PL, Schwartz AR. The effect of theophylline on sleep in normal subjects. Chest 1993;103(1):5–6.

78. Fitzpatrick MF, Engleman HM, Boellert F, et al. Effect of therapeutic theophylline levels on the sleep quality and daytime cognitive performance of normal subjects. Am Rev Respir Dis 1992;145(6): 1355–8.

79. Kaplan J, Fredrickson PA, Renaux SA, et al. Theophylline effect on sleep in normal subjects. Chest 1993; 103(1):193–5.

80. Roehrs T, Merlotti L, Halpin D, et al. Effects of theophylline on nocturnal sleep and daytime sleepiness/alertness. Chest 1995;108(2):382–7.

81. Avital A, Sanchez I, Holbrow J, et al. Effect of theophylline on lung function tests, sleep quality, and nighttime SaO2 in children with cystic fibrosis. Am Rev Respir Dis 1991;144(6):1245–9.

82. Stein MA, Krasowski M, Leventhal BL, et al. Behavioral and cognitive effects of methylxanthines. A meta-analysis of theophylline and caffeine. Arch Pediatr Adolesc Med 1996;150(3):284–8.

83. Janson C, Gislason T, Boman G, et al. Sleep disturbances in patients with asthma. Respir Med 1990; 84(1):37–42.

84. Mulloy E, McNicholas WT. Theophylline improves gas exchange during rest, exercise, and sleep in severe chronic obstructive pulmonary disease. Am Rev Respir Dis 1993;148(4 Pt 1):1030–6.

85. Novak M, Shapiro CM. Drug-induced sleep disturbances. Focus on nonpsychotropic medications. Drug Saf 1997;16(2):133–49.

86. Jiménez JA, Greenberg BH, Mills PJ. Effects of heart failure and its pharmacological management on sleep. Drug Discov Today Dis Models 2011;8(4): 161–6.

Drug-Induced Sleep-Disordered Breathing and Ventilatory Impairment

Ludger Grote, MD, PhD

KEYWORDS

- Sleep apnea • Hypoventilation • Opiates • Benzodiazepines • Growth hormone • Anabolic steroids
- Baclofen

KEY POINTS

- To assess the risk and severity for drug-induced sleep-disordered breathing (SDB), it is important to consider patients' clinical data and comorbidities.
- Opiates can induce clinically relevant central and obstructive SDB with a very typical breathing pattern.
- Benzodiazepines can induce obstructive and reduce central SDB. The negative effects may be limited in most patients but older age, comorbidities, and known severe sleep apnea are strong contraindications as long as sleep apnea is untreated.
- Additional drug classes with a potential for respiratory impairment during sleep include growth hormone, phosphodiesterase inhibitors, baclofen, and sodium oxybate.
- When sleep apnea is already known and treated, such drug classes can be used with caution.

INTRODUCTION

The interaction between certain drug classes and SDB is of clinical relevance for sleep medicine. Specific patient populations with acute and chronic pain, chronic insomnia, or hormone replacement treatment may face the induction of SDB. In more severe cases, nocturnal hypoventilation and respiratory failure have been reported as adverse effects of commonly used medications. Abuse of pain killers or anabolic steroids constitute another problem that may compromise adequate breathing during sleep. Current classification of sleep disorders characterizes the different subtypes of drug-induced SDB.[1] This article summarizes the current knowledge and suggests problem-solving strategies in certain clinical situations.

Data on the effect size of drug-induced SDB are conflicting. A recent Cochrane analysis studied the effects of 10 different drugs potentially affecting respiration during sleep.[2] A total of 293 subjects with verified sleep apnea, often of mild to moderate degree, from 14 randomized controlled studies were included in the analysis. Drugs investigated were the opiate remifentanil and benzodiazepine-receptor agonists, such as eszopiclone, zolpidem, brotizolam, flurazepam, nitrazepam, ramelteon, and sodium oxybate, used in the treatment of narcolepsy. Within-group comparisons showed only mild deteriorations in overnight oxygenation and apneic events; no systematic increases in the apnea-hypopnea index (AHI) or the Oswestry disability index were observed. Some studies even showed beneficial effects on the AHI (eszopiclone and sodium oxybate). The investigators concluded that there was no current evidence for a systematic deterioration of SDB by the investigated substances.

Sleep Disorders Center, Pulmonary Medicine, Sahlgrenska University Hospital, Bruna Straket 5, Gothenburg 413 45, Sweden
E-mail address: Ludger.grote@lungall.gu.se

Sleep Med Clin 13 (2018) 161–168
https://doi.org/10.1016/j.jsmc.2018.03.003
1556-407X/18/© 2018 Elsevier Inc. All rights reserved.

sleep.theclinics.com

In sharp contrast, data from large pharmacovigilance databases using a case-control design suggest that benzodiazepines (odds ratio [OR] 2.6), opium alkaloids (OR 2.1), sodium oxybate (OR 64.3), and other psychotropic agents may significantly increase the risk for sleep-disordered breathing classified as a severe adverse drug reaction.[3] These studies clearly demonstrate that the population of patients at risk may vary significantly between the randomized controlled trial (RCT) settings and clinical reality. Safe and beneficial administration of those drugs depends greatly on a careful patient selection and treatment follow-up.

OPIATES

Opiate treatment is accompanied by the well-known side effect of respiratory depression, which becomes most clinically relevant during sleep.[4] Both conditions have synergistic effects on breathing by reducing respiratory rate and decreasing tonic respiratory drive. Animal experiments have elegantly shown the dose-response relationship between pharmacologic mu-receptor stimulation by opiates and 2 major effects on breathing during sleep[5]:

1. Reduction of upper airway muscle tone
2. Reduction of respiratory rate and irregular breathing (atactic breathing).

These animal studies showed that the effect of opiates is generated by neurokinin-1 receptor-stimulation of pre-Bötzinger complex respiratory neurons and that the pharmacologic blockage of those receptors was able to reverse the opiate-induced respiratory depression.[5]

In human sleep studies, both effects have been known for longer time and a dose-response relationship between opiate use and obstructive sleep apnea (OSA) has been established.[4,6–8] In addition, frequent central sleep apneas and irregular breathing have been identified in patients using opiate treatment.[9–11] A typical opiate-induced respiratory pattern during sleep is illustrated in **Fig. 1**. The combination of the previously mentioned effects (1) and (2) may lead to significant sleep-related hypoventilation. This risk is particularly present in patients with risk factors for hypoventilation during sleep, including comorbid obesity, respiratory disease (eg, chronic obstructive pulmonary disease [COPD]), neuromuscular disease, preexisting severe obstructive OSA, or in the elderly (**Table 1**).

Given the knowledge previously summarized, several clinical scenarios need to be addressed. First, patients with chronic pain have often typical risk factors for SDB, such as older age or obesity. This increases the likelihood of undiagnosed preexisting sleep apnea in pain patients receiving opiate treatment. Indeed, a strong association has been recognized between SDB, obesity, and pain.[12] One potential mechanism may be linked to nocturnal hypoxia as an enhancer of pain on awakening[12] and pain was reported to be improved after alleviation of nocturnal hypoxia by

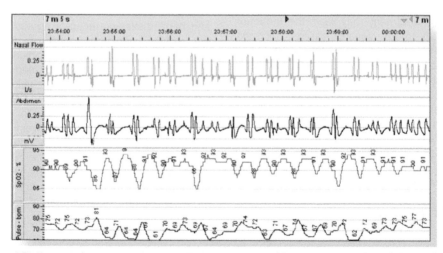

Fig. 1. Opiate-induced central sleep apnea in a 32-year-old man participating in a methadone program. A repetitive lack of flow and effort occurs in the nasal flow and the abdominal effort signals, which indicates repetitive central apneas of short duration. Mild oxygen desaturations can be detected in the oxygen saturation signal (SpO$_2$). Highly characteristic for opiate-induced central sleep apnea are the high variability of apnea length and the irregularity of the respiratory effort.

Table 1
Detrimental effects of certain drug classes on breathing during sleep

Drug Class	OSA	CSA	Sleep-Related Hypoventilation	Patients at Risk
		Type of SDB		
Opiates	Increase in obstructive SDB, more prominent in preexisting OSA and patients with OSA risk factors (eg, obesity)	Frequent (up to 70%) central apneas during NREM sleep, irregular breathing, dose-response relationship, sleep fragmentation CSA often combined with OSA	Known in patients with risk factors for hypoventilation (eg, obesity, respiratory and neuromuscular disease, and preexisting OSA), or in the elderly	Comorbidities such as obesity, moderate to severe OSA, respiratory disease (eg, COPD), neuromuscular disease
BRAs	Aggravation of upper airway obstruction	Beneficial effect has been reported by modification of a pathologic low arousal threshold	In patients with risk factors for sleep-related hypoventilation Case reports, no systematic evaluation Clear contraindication for use in these risk populations	Elderly Severe OSA Impaired respiratory function Neuromuscular disease
Anabolic steroids	Low likelihood for increases in obstructive SDB	Increases in arousal from sleep and light sleep, indirect risk factor for central SDB	No consistent reports	Frequent off-label use outside medical control Risk for combination with other drugs or alcohol
GH	GH substitution in patients without pituitary deficiency may induce obstructive apneas and hypopneas	No consistent reports	No consistent reports	Patients with central obesity Increase in neck size has been documented after GH treatment

(continued on next page)

Table 1
(continued)

Drug Class	Type of SDB			Patients at Risk
	OSA	CSA	Sleep-Related Hypoventilation	
Baclofen	In patients with known OSA, the event frequency was increased after intrathecal baclofen administration in high doses	Central apneas and severe CSA when applied intrathecal with high doses. Pharmacovigilance data indicate increased prevalence of sleep apnea syndromes with baclofen used in alcohol addiction	No consistent reports	Patients with known sleep apnea. Use of high oral and intrathecal doses can aggravate or induce clinically significant sleep apnea (central and obstructive)
Sodium oxybate	Uncontrolled data and pharmacovigilance reports indicate increased risk for OSA. Not verified in 2 RCTs	No consistent reports	No consistent reports	Patient selection important. Increased risk in comorbid SDB, respiratory disease, CNS-depressant drugs. Alcohol aggravates the risk
PDI	Uncontrolled data reported increase in OSA. Not replicated in RCTs	No consistent reports	No consistent reports	

Abbreviations: BRA, benzodiazepine receptor agonist; CNS, central nervous system; CSA, central sleep apnea; GH, growth hormone; NREM, non-rapid eye movement; PDI, phosphodiesterase inhibitor; SDB, sleep-disordered breathing.

continuous positive airway pressure (CPAP) treatment.[13] Therefore, it is recommended to consider the symptoms and clinical findings of OSA before and during chronic opiate treatment. In case of suspected opiate-induced SDB (frequent nocturnal awakenings, nocturnal dyspnea, reported snoring), objective sleep investigation is necessary. Second, perioperative and postoperative use of opiates may be closely monitored to avoid aggravation of respiratory instability and hypoventilation during sleep. The threshold for an objective assessment of breathing and oxygenation during sleep should be low. Third, age per se increases the likelihood for opiate-induced respiratory depression during sleep. Prolonged elimination half-lives and modified receptor sensitivity to opiate treatment have been described.[4] Risk for opiate-induced respiratory depression is 3 to 8 times higher in patients from the seventh to the ninth decade compared with younger age. Careful consideration of opiate treatment (dose and use) and follow-up of daytime and nighttime respiratory status is necessary to avoid patient harm in the elderly. Fourth, patients with substance abuse may be enrolled in methadone programs. Methadone is known to induce similar effects on respiration as other opiates. However, development of tolerance to the respiratory depression has been reported in patients receiving methadone over several months.[4] Because methadone dosage may be readjusted during long-term treatment, respiratory symptoms need to be monitored closely to avoid adverse respiratory events.

BENZODIAZEPINE RECEPTOR AGONISTS

Data suggest that benzodiazepine receptor agonists (BRAs) reduce muscle tone in the upper airway, as well as reduce the chemoreceptor response to hypoxia.[14] In part, longer obstructive breathing events with prolonged hypoxemic episodes have been documented. On the other hand, a certain OSA phenotype with a low arousal threshold has been recently identified.[15] Elevation of the arousal threshold by BRA treatment had beneficial effects with a reduction of the total AHI by approximately 40%.[16] The effect was mainly attributed to the reduction of central and mixed apneas.

Specific concerns have been raised for the use of BRA hypnotics in patients with severe OSA, obesity, and/or COPD. Two recent meta-analyses showed that overall subjective and objective sleep quality was improved by BRA treatment.[2,17] In addition, sleep apnea activity and overnight oxygen saturation did not

significantly deteriorate with BRA treatment when compared with placebo. In general, subjects included in those studies did not experience severe SDB or significant comorbid respiratory disease. In contrast, in a subgroup analysis of 28 subjects, overnight transcutaneous carbon dioxide values were significantly increased by BRA, indicating respiratory impairment when compared with placebo treatment.[18] In obese patients, BRA use was associated with an increased risk for overnight oxygen desaturations.[19]

In contrast to the data from RCTs, data from pharmacovigilance databases strongly suggest that benzodiazepines may double the risk for sleep-disordered breathing as a severe adverse drug reaction.[3] It should be taken into consideration that known SDB constitutes a contraindication as stated in the summary of product characteristics of almost all BRAs. Therefore, any use of BRA hypnotics in patients with known but untreated sleep apnea is off-label.

ANABOLIC STEROIDS

Low testosterone levels are known in patients with sleep apnea and those low levels may increase with weight loss but not with CPAP treatment.[20,21] Initial studies reported an increase in sleep apnea activity after testosterone treatment when applied in quite high intramuscular dosages.[22–24] Therefore, current guidelines state untreated sleep apnea as a contraindication for testosterone treatment.

Use of anabolic steroids is known to reduce sleep duration and sleep quality.[21,22] The increase in arousal from sleep following anabolic steroid use may increase the risk for obstructive, mixed, and central sleep apneas.

GROWTH HORMONE

Acromegaly is characterized by an increased production of growth hormone (GH).[21] Macroglossia and impaired neuromuscular function have been suggested as the potential mechanisms behind the elevated prevalence of OSA. Initial data reported an increased prevalence of central apneas but could not be verified in a review of subsequent studies.[25] Surgical treatment of the GH-producing tumor reduces sleep apnea, although remaining elevated sleep apnea activity is documented in 40% of acromegaly patients after surgical cure of the disease.[21]

The effect of GH treatment in patients with GH deficiency (GHD) on sleep apnea activity is controversial. Whereas early small studies showed an aggravation of sleep apnea, a more recent study in a larger group of GHD subjects did not show any improvement or aggravation of sleep apnea.[26] Conversely, therapeutic application of GH in subjects with abdominal obesity without GHD was associated with an approximately 35% increase in the AHI after 1 year of treatment.[27] Obstructive apneas and hypopneas increased in number and this increase was accompanied by an increase in neck circumference in the GH treated group.

BACLOFEN

Baclofen is a γ-aminobutyric acid (GABA) B-receptor agonist used for its spasmolytic effects in neurologic disorders. In addition, baclofen has been used in an oral preparation for the treatment of alcohol dependency. In patients with known OSA, the apnea-hypopnea event frequency was increased after intrathecal baclofen administration in high doses.[28] Central apneas and severe central sleep apnea occurred when baclofen was applied by intrathecal or oral administration.[29,30] Pharmacovigilance data indicate increased prevalence of sleep apnea syndromes with baclofen when used in the treatment of alcohol addiction.[31] In essence, use of high oral and intrathecal dosages can aggravate or induce clinically significant sleep apnea.

PHOSPHODIESTERASE INHIBITORS

Phosphodiesterase inhibitors (PDIs), including sildenafil, vardenafil, and tadalafil, are widely used to treat erectile dysfunction. Several randomized studies using the PDI sildenafil demonstrated a significant increase in OSA events when compared with placebo.[22,32,33] Treatment of erectile dysfunction was generally more effective with the drug when compared with CPAP.[34] However, a recent study using vardenafil showed no change in the AHI.[35] Currently, it remains unclear whether the aggravation of sleep apnea is a substance-specific or a drug class effect of PDIs. Therefore, PDI treatment should be used with caution in untreated sleep apnea patients.

SODIUM OXYBATE

Sodium oxybate has the indication for treatment of cataplexy and excessive daytime sleepiness in patients with narcolepsy. The mode of action is incompletely understood but the effects are mediated through GABA-B and γ-hydroxybutyric acid receptors. It has a relative contraindication for patients with known SDB, for patients with COPD, and for individuals otherwise vulnerable to respiratory depression.[36,37] Uncontrolled data and pharmacovigilance reports indicate a marked increased risk for SDB as an adverse drug reaction.[3] The OR was very high (64). The risk may be specifically high in patients otherwise treated with hypnotic agents or central nervous system–depressant drugs (see previous discussion). The use of alcohol and sodium oxybate may have stronger depressive effects on respiratory drive. Notably, this negative effect of sodium oxybate on respiration during sleep was not verified in 2 RCTs.[2]

Management of Drug-Induced Respiratory Impairment During Sleep

To manage drug-induced respiratory impairment during sleep, a dose reduction or a complete termination of the drug treatment must first be considered. A follow-up of the effects of dose reduction on respiratory impairment is mandatory. If the treatment with the specific medication needs to be continued, specific treatment of sleep-disordered breathing must be initiated.[25] Treatments include CPAP or oral devices for OSA. Adaptive servo-ventilator treatment has shown superior efficacy for the treatment of central sleep apnea or combined obstructive and central sleep apnea. In case of sleep-related hypoventilation, treatment with noninvasive ventilation (eg, bilevel) is recommended.

The OSA phenotype with comorbid insomnia is rather frequent in typical clinical OSA cohorts and insomnia treatment is required for a subgroup of subjects.[38] The effect of BRA on respiratory function may be not clinically significant in otherwise heathy individuals with mild sleep-disordered breathing. Even subgroups of apnea patients may benefit from BRA intake with regard to a reduction of disturbed breathing during sleep. However, ventilation during sleep may be severely compromised in patients with severe OSA and comorbidities, which increases the risk for severe nocturnal hypoxia and hypoventilation. Therefore, BZA hypnotic use should be followed up by an objective sleep assessment in untreated OSA patients. On the other hand, BRA hypnotics can be used in patients in whom the SDB is treated.

SUMMARY

This short presentation of important drug classes with a potential harmful effect on breathing sleep shows that the variability of ventilatory impairment is highly variable. In many cases, no significant deterioration of respiration occurs and the patients report an improved sleep due to hypnotic or analgesic effects. However, the response pattern to those different drug entities is highly variable. Comorbidities, anthropometrics (age and body mass index), and preexisting SDB are the important factors that may cause severe harm to individual patients. Patient safety may be reassured by means of repetitive medical interview, clinical status, a specific sleep history, or an objective sleep test. The threshold for an overnight recording of breathing should be low. Because the detection of severe sleep apnea is the main target of such investigation, recordings from a limited channel device may be sufficient for the diagnosis.

REFERENCES

1. American Academy of Sleep Medicine. International classification of sleep disorders. 3rd edition. Darien (IL): American Academy of Sleep Medicine; 2014.
2. Mason M, Cates CJ, Smith I. Effects of opioid, hypnotic and sedating medications on sleep-disordered breathing in adults with obstructive sleep apnoea. Cochrane Database Syst Rev 2015;(7):CD011090.
3. Linselle M, Sommet A, Bondon-Guitton E, et al. Can drugs induce or aggravate sleep apneas? A case-noncase study in VigiBase®, the WHO pharmacovigilance database. Fundam Clin Pharmacol 2017; 31(3):359–66.
4. Lydic R, Keifer JC, Baghdoyan HA, et al. Opiate action on sleep and breathing. In: Kryger M, Roth T, editors. Principles and practice of sleep medicine. 6th edition. Philadelphia: Elsevier; 2017. p. 252–9 [Chapter 24].
5. Montandon G, Qin W, Liu H, et al. PreBotzinger complex neurokinin-1 receptor-expressing neurons mediate opioid-induced respiratory depression. J Neurosci 2011;31(4):1292–301.
6. Walker JM, Farney RJ, Rhondeau SM, et al. Chronic opioid use is a risk factor for the development of central sleep apnea and ataxic breathing. J Clin Sleep Med 2007;3:455–62.
7. Walker JM, Farney RJ. Are opioids associated with sleep apnea? A review of the evidence. Curr Pain Headache Rep 2009;13:120–6.
8. Farney RJ, McDonald AM, Boyle KM, et al. Sleep disordered breathing in patients receiving therapy with buprenorphine/naloxone. Eur Respir J 2013; 42:394–403.
9. Wang D, Teichtahl H. Opioids, sleep architecture, and sleep-disordered breathing. Sleep Med Rev 2007;11:35–46.
10. Webster LR, Choi Y, Desai H, et al. Sleep-disordered breathing and chronic opioid therapy. Pain Med 2008;9:425–32.
11. Feldman JL, Del Negro CA, Gray PA. Understanding the rhythm of breathing: so near, yet so far. Annu Rev Physiol 2013;75:423–52.
12. Doufas AG, Tian L, Davies MF, et al. Nocturnal intermittent hypoxia is independently associated with pain in subjects suffering from sleep-disordered breathing. Anesthesiology 2013;119:1149–62.
13. Khalid I, Roehrs TA, Hudgel DW, et al. Continuous positive airway pressure in severe obstructive sleep apnea reduces pain sensitivity. Sleep 2011;34(12): 1687–91.
14. Horner R. Respiratory physiology. In: Kryger M, Roth T, editors. Principles and practice of sleep medicine. 6th edition. Philadelphia: Elsevier; 2017. p. 155–66 [Chapter 15].
15. Eckert DJ, White DP, Jordan AS, et al. Defining phenotypic causes of obstructive sleep apnea. Identification of novel therapeutic targets. Am J Respir Crit Care Med 2013;188(8):996–1004.
16. Bonnet MH, Dexter JR, Arand DL. The effect of triazolam on arousal and respiration in central sleep apnea patients. Sleep 1990;13(1):31–41.
17. Lu XM, Zhu JP, Zhou XM. The effect of benzodiazepines on insomnia in patients with chronic obstructive pulmonary disease: a meta-analysis of treatment efficacy and safety. Int J Chron Obstruct Pulmon Dis 2016;11:675–85.
18. Midgren B, Hansson L, Skeidsvoll H, et al. The effects of nitrazepam and flunitrazepam on oxygen desaturation during sleep in patients with stable hypoxemic nonhypercapnic COPD. Chest 1989; 95(4):765–8.
19. Deflandre E, Kempeneers D, Degey S, et al. Risk factors for nocturnal hypoxemia in severe obstructive sleep apnea patients. Minerva Anestesiol 2017;83(5):449–56.
20. Grunstein RR, Handelsman DJ, Lawrence SJ, et al. Neuroendocrine dysfunction in sleep apnea: reversal by continuous positive airways pressure therapy. J Clin Endocrinol Metab 1989;68(2):352–8.
21. Ioachimescu AG, Ioachimescu OC. Endocrine disorders. In: Kryger M, Roth T, editors. Principles and practice of sleep medince. 6th edition. Philadelphia: Elsevier; 2017. p. 1300–12 [Chapter 132].
22. Liu PY, Yee B, Wishart SM, et al. The short-term effects of high-dose testosterone on sleep, breathing, and function in older men. J Clin Endocrinol Metab 2003;88(8):3605–13.
23. Cistulli PA, Grunstein RR, Sullivan CE. Effect of testosterone administration on upper airway collapsibility during sleep. Am J Respir Crit Care Med 1994; 149(2 Pt 1):530–2.
24. Matsumoto AM, Sandblom RE, Schoene RB, et al. Testosterone replacement in hypogonadal men: effects on obstructive sleep apnoea, respiratory drives, and sleep. Clin Endocrinol (Oxf) 1985; 22(6):713–21.

25. Randerath W, Verbraecken J, Andreas S, et al. Definition, discrimination, diagnosis and treatment of central breathing disturbances during sleep. Eur Respir J 2017;49(1) [pii:1600959].

26. Peker Y, Svensson J, Hedner J, et al. Sleep apnoea and quality of life in growth hormone (GH)-deficient adults before and after 6 months of GH replacement therapy. Clin Endocrinol (Oxf) 2006;65(1): 98–105.

27. Karimi M, Koranyi J, Franco C, et al. Increased neck soft tissue mass and worsening of obstructive sleep apnea after growth hormone treatment in men with abdominal obesity. J Clin Sleep Med 2010;6(3): 256–63.

28. Bensmail D, Marquer A, Roche N, et al. Pilot study assessing the impact of intrathecal baclofen administration mode on sleep-related respiratory parameters. Arch Phys Med Rehabil 2012;93(1):96–9.

29. Perogamvros L, Pépin JL, Thorens G, et al. Baclofen-associated onset of central sleep apnea in alcohol use disorder: a case report. Respiration 2015;90(6):507–11.

30. Olivier PY, Joyeux-Faure M, Gentina T, et al. Severe central sleep apnea associated with chronic baclofen therapy: a case series. Chest 2016;149(5): e127–31.

31. Revol B, Jullian-Desayes I, Bailly S, et al. Baclofen and sleep apnoea syndrome: analysis of VigiBase, the WHO pharmacovigilance database. Eur Respir J 2018;51(1) [pii:1701855].

32. Roizenblatt S, Guilleminault C, Poyares D, et al. A double-blind, placebo-controlled, crossover study of Sildenafil in obstructive sleep apnea. Arch Intern Med 2006;166:1763–7.

33. Neves C, Tufik S, Monteiro MA, et al. The effect of sildenafil on sleep respiratory parameters and heart rate variability in obstructive sleep apnea. Sleep Med 2010;11(6):545–51.

34. Steinke E, Palm Johansen P, Fridlund B, et al. Determinants of sexual dysfunction and interventions for patients with obstructive sleep apnoea: a systematic review. Int J Clin Pract 2016;70(1):5–19.

35. Melehan KL, Hoyos CM, Hamilton GS, et al. Randomised trial of CPAP and vardenafil on erectile and arterial function in men with obstructive sleep apnea and erectile dysfunction. J Clin Endocrinol Metab 2018. [Epub ahead of print].

36. Bazalakova M, Benca R. Wake-promoting medications: efficacy and adverse effects. In: Kryger M, Roth T, editors. Principles and practice of sleep medince. 6th edition. Philadelphia: Elsevier; 2017. p. 462–79 [Chapter 44].

37. George CF, Feldman N, Inhaber N, et al. A safety trial of sodium oxybate in patients with obstructive sleep apnea: acute effects on sleep-disordered breathing. Sleep Med 2010;11:38–42.

38. Saaresranta T, Hedner J, Bonsignore MR, et al, ESADA Study Group. Clinical phenotypes and comorbidity in European sleep apnoea patients. PLoS One 2016;11(10):e0163439.

Prescription Drugs Used in Insomnia

Sylvie Dujardin, MD[a], Angelique Pijpers, MD, PhD[a], Dirk Pevernagie, MD, PhD[a,b],*

KEYWORDS

- Chronic insomnia • Prescription drugs • Pharmacotherapy • Sleep-effect

KEY POINTS

- Several prescription drugs are available that at least temporarily improve sleep duration and continuity, objectively and subjectively, with acceptable side effects.
- Prescription drugs used for insomnia promote sleep by a limited number of different mechanisms: enhancing GABAergic neurotransmission, antagonizing receptors for the wake-promoting monoamines, or binding the melatonin receptors. Orexin receptor antagonists comprise a new class of hypnotic drugs.
- The ideal sleeping pill still does not exist.
- When available, cognitive behavioral therapy for insomnia remains the first-line therapy for chronic insomnia.

INTRODUCTION

Various studies have shown the efficacy of cognitive behavioral therapy for insomnia (CBT-I) and were recently confirmed by meta-analysis.[1] The American Academy of Sleep Medicine (AASM) clinical practice guideline and the European guideline for the treatment of insomnia state that this nonpharmacologic therapeutic approach is the treatment of choice for chronic insomnia in adults, regardless of age.[2,3] By acting on different sleep mechanisms, CBT-I helps to tilt the delicate neurobiologic balance from wakefulness to sleep.

Prescription of pharmacologic treatment is to be considered when CBT-I is not available or not effective. In the acute phase of CBT-I, adding pharmacotherapy may have a slightly better effect compared with CBT-I alone, provided the medication is discontinued in the maintenance phase of CBT-I.[4] However, pharmacotherapy is not indicated for chronic use and efforts at discontinuation should be made when this is the case.[3]

Moreover, discontinuation may improve rather than worsen the effects of CBT-I.[5]

Many studies have been conducted to evaluate the pharmacologic treatment of chronic insomnia. Unfortunately, large randomized controlled trials (RCTs) with representative patient populations are lacking. Studies are often weak from a methodologic point of view and, in addition, difficult to compare because of differences in patient samples, diagnostic and inclusion criteria, and outcome criteria. Finally, many studies are sponsored by the industry, which could lead to publication bias.

It is important to keep in mind that in the treatment of insomnia, whether pharmacologic or behavioral, a substantial placebo effect may confound clinical results. In a meta-analysis, the placebo effect was contended to account for almost two-thirds of the drug effect.[6] A recent meta-analysis comparing placebo with no treatment groups confirms the placebo effect in the subjective but not objective sleep measures.[7]

The authors have no disclosures to report.
[a] Sleep Medicine Center Kempenhaeghe, PO Box 61, Heeze 5590 AB, The Netherlands; [b] Department of Internal Medicine and Paediatrics, Faculty of Medicine and Health Sciences, Ghent University, Corneel Heymanslaan 10, 9000 Ghent, Belgium
* Corresponding author. Sleep Medicine Center Kempenhaeghe, PO Box 61, Heeze 5590 AB, The Netherlands.
E-mail address: pevernagied@kempenhaeghe.nl

Sleep Med Clin 13 (2018) 169–182
https://doi.org/10.1016/j.jsmc.2018.03.001
1556-407X/18/© 2018 Elsevier Inc. All rights reserved.

This article provides an overview of pharmacologic and biologic features of different hypnotic drugs, with a reference to medical practice in adults with chronic insomnia without comorbidities. The focus is on prescription drugs and discussed are benzodiazepines (BZDs), non-BZD BZD receptor agonists (NBBzRAs), melatonin receptor agonists, orexin receptor antagonists, antidepressants, and antipsychotics. Over-the-counter preparations, including antihistamines, are outside the scope of this article. The main characteristics of the reviewed drugs are summarized in **Table 1**.

The reviewed compounds all have an impact on the neurobiologic processes of sleep and may even change its normal macrostructure and microstructure. Because hypnotic drugs act via different pathways within the central nervous system, they have dissimilar neuropharmacologic profiles. Remarkably, these differential properties have not been translated into evidence that would facilitate clinical decision making based on the pharmacologic signature of the drug.[8]

Practical advice for optimization of drug treatment is outside the scope of this article. For further study, we refer the reader to other references.[9]

BENZODIAZEPINES
Neuropharmacology

BZD receptor agonists constitute the most important class of drugs prescribed for insomnia and encompass BZDs and NBBzRAs. Both groups intensify γ-aminobutyric acid (GABA)$_A$-mediated neurotransmission and are therefore GABA$_A$ agonists.

GABA is the most important and abundant inhibitory neurotransmitter in the nervous system. Stimulating GABAergic action promotes sleep, but the exact locations in the brain are not yet fully disclosed.[10] At very high dose, GABA$_A$ agonists suppress c-Fos expression in the entire central nervous system, including the sleep-wake control centers.[11] At lower dose, GABA$_A$ agonists increase c-Fos expression in ventrolateral preoptic area (VLPO) neurons, albeit less than in natural sleep. The VLPO (and the median preoptic nucleus) contain sleep-active GABAergic neurons that send anatomic projections to the arousal systems, in which GABA release has been shown to increase during sleep.[12] Besides, systemic injection of GABA$_A$ receptor agonists consistently suppressed the expression of c-Fos in the tuberomammillary nucleus (TMN).[11] The VLPO and the TMN mutually inhibit each other.[12] Thus GABA$_A$ agonists might stimulate sleep through reinforcing the relief of the inhibition of the VLPO by the TMN.[11] Microinjections of triazolam into the perifornical hypothalamus

containing hypocretin neurons significantly increased sleep.[13] BZDs might thus also act via inhibition of the hypocretin wake-promoting system.

Pharmacologic Properties

BZDs act as positive allosteric modulators of GABA$_A$ receptors: they increase the effect of GABA binding. GABA$_A$ receptors are located post-synaptically and consist of a pentameric complex forming a chloride channel. When the GABA is released in the synaptic cleft, the chloride channel opens. With BZD, the GABA$_A$ receptor increases the frequency of opening of its chloride-channel. By this mechanism, the cellular membrane of the post-synaptic neuron becomes hyperpolarized, thus inhibiting the activation of the neuron.[14]

The GABA$_A$ receptor carrying the α_1 subunit is believed to be the mediator of the sedative and amnesic effects of BZDs. The anxiolytic, myorelaxant, motor-impairing, and ethanol-potentiating effects are attributed to GABA$_A$ receptor, carrying other α subunits (α subunits 2, 3, 5).[15] Currently available BZDs are nonselective for GABA$_A$ receptors with different α subunits.[14]

Clinical Effects

BZDs have a positive effect on objective and subjective sleep parameters of people with insomnia. Recently, a meta-analysis was performed on two BZDs: triazolam and temazepam.[2] Two studies including a total of 72 patients addressed subjective sleep latencies (SL) and total sleep time (TST).[16,17] In the second study of 34 patients, objective SL and TST also were assessed.[17] Temazepam, 15 mg, decreased subjective SL by 20 minutes and objective SL by 37 minutes versus placebo. It increased subjective TST by 64 minutes and objective TST by 99 minutes versus placebo. The evidence for efficiency of triazolam is scarce. In a study of only subjective data with triazolam, 0.25 mg, improvements of subjective SL and TST (respectively −9 minutes and −25 minutes versus placebo) were not clinically relevant.[18]

Tolerance to hypnotic effect is a frequent manifestation in chronic use of BZDs. It has been shown that after 24 weeks of chronic BZD intake, the subjective sleep quality drops to a level below baseline. This was observed in BZDs with short and long half-life (lorazepam and nitrazepam, respectively).[19] Rebound insomnia is the most frequent symptom following acute withdrawal of BZDs, occurring in up to 71% of subjects.[20] Next to tolerance, dependence is of concern. The prevalence of misuse and dependency of BZDs and related Z-drugs has been estimated to be 5% in a German population. Approximately 20% of BZD users have a

Table 1
Prescription drugs used for insomnia: main characteristics

Drug (Class)	Predominant Mode of Action for Sedative Effect	T_{max} (h)	$T_{1/2}$ (h)	Recommended Use	Dose[a] (mg)	FDA Approved/ CSA IV
BZD						
Triazolam	Nonselective $GABA_A$ agonism	1–2	2–6	Sleep onset insomnia	0.125–0.25	+/+
Temazepam	Nonselective $GABA_A$ agonism	1–2	8–15	Sleep onset and sleep maintenance insomnia	7.5–30	+/+
Quazepam	Nonselective $GABA_A$ agonism	2–3	48–120	Not recommended		+/+
Estazolam	Nonselective $GABA_A$ agonism	1.5–2	8–24	Not recommended		+/+
Flurazepam	Nonselective $GABA_A$ agonism	1.5–4.5	48–120	Not recommended		+/+
NBBzRA						
Zopiclone	$GABA_A$ - $\alpha_{1,2,3}$ agonism	1.5–2	5	Sleep onset and sleep maintenance insomnia	3.75–7.5	+/+
Eszopiclone	$GABA_A$ - $\alpha_{1,2,3}$ agonism[b]	1–1.5	6	Sleep onset and sleep maintenance insomnia	1–3	+/+
Zolpidem	$GABA_A$ - α_1 agonism	1–2	2.6	Sleep onset and sleep maintenance insomnia	1.75–10 6.25–12.5 ER	+/+
Zaleplon	$GABA_A$ - α_1 agonism	~ 1	0.7–1.4	Sleep onset insomnia	5–20	+/+
Orexin receptor antagonists						
Suvorexant	OxR1 and OxR2 antagonism	2–3.5	12	Sleep onset and sleep maintenance insomnia	5–20	+/+
Melatonin and melatonin receptor agonists						
Ramelteon	Melatonin receptor agonism	0.75–1	1–2.5	Sleep onset insomnia	8	+/–
Melatonin	Melatonin receptor agonism	~0.75	~0.75	Not recommended		NA
Circadin®	Melatonin receptor agonism	0.75–3	3.5–4	Sleep onset and sleep maintenance insomnia, age >55 y	2	–/–[c]

(continued on next page)

Table 1
(continued)

Drug (Class)	Predominant Mode of Action for Sedative Effect	T$_{max}$ (h)	T$_{1/2}$ (h)	Recommended Use	Dose[a] (mg)	FDA Approved/ CSA IV
Antidepressants						
Doxepin	H1 antagonism	2–8	20	Sleep maintenance insomnia	3–6	+/–
Amitriptyline	H1, alpha1, M1 antagonism	2–8	30	Not recommended		–/–
Trazodone	5HT2A, alpha1 antagonism	1–2	9	Not recommended		–/–
Mirtazapine	H1, 5HT2A/2C antagonism	1–3	25	Not recommended		–/–
Antipsychotics						
Quetiapine	H1 but also alpha1, M1, 5HT, D2 antagonism	1–2	6	Not recommended		–/–
Olanzapine	H1 but also 5HT, M1, D2, alpha1 antagonism	4–6	20–54	Not recommended		–/–

Abbreviations: Alpha1, alpha-1 adrenergic receptor; CSA IV, Controlled Substance Act schedule IV controlled substances; D2, dopamine receptor D2; ER, extended release; FDA approved, U.S. Food and Drug Administration approved for the treatment of insomnia; GABA, γ-aminobutyric acid; GABA$_A$ - $\alpha_{1,2,3}$, GABA$_A$ receptor alpha subunits 1,2,3; H1, histamine receptor type 1; 5HT, 5-hydroxytryptamine (serotonin); M1, Muscarinic acetylcholine receptor 1; NA, not applicable; OxR1-2, orexin receptors type 1 and 2.

[a] The lowest effective dose should be used to minimize side effects.

[b] Precise mechanism unknown.

[c] European Medicines Agency approval.

Data from Refs.[26,31,74,77,97–99]

problematic intake. Overall, 50% of BZD users list insomnia as the reason for taking the drug.[20]

Important to highlight is that older adults are especially vulnerable, because BZDs increase the risk of cognitive impairment, delirium, falls, fractures, and motor vehicle accidents. Therefore, BZDs of any type should be avoided for the treatment of insomnia, according to the American Geriatrics Society Beers Criteria for Potentially Inappropriate Medication Use in Older Adults.[21] Sleep apnea is a contraindication for BZDs, although the available evidence indicates the effects on respiration are moderate.[22]

BZDs have an effect on the sleep macroarchitecture. Studies on healthy volunteers and those with insomnia have consistently shown that BZDs reduce the percentage of slow wave sleep.[23] Percentage of stage 2 sleep increases, and spectral power of the spindle frequency range (11–14 Hz) is enhanced.[24,25] The effect on rapid eye movement (REM) sleep is variable and less pronounced. In some individuals, a reduction of the amount of REM sleep has been reported.[26]

It seems paradoxic that BZDs improve subjective sleep quality while they decrease slow wave sleep. This paradox can possibly be explained by observations on the microstructure of sleep. In a recent study, the sleep of six chronic BZD abusers versus healthy control subjects was compared. The abusers had significantly more awakenings but fewer fast frequency arousals and lower indexes of non-REM (NREM) instability as measured by Cyclic Alternating Pattern rate. It has been hypothesized that chronic BZD use may affect the function of the thalamic filter. In normal subjects, incoming stimuli are able to produce arousals without awakenings. Potentially, the thalamic filter of chronic BZD users is less adaptive: the response to stimuli is either no reaction (no arousal) or a full awakening.[27]

Medical Prescription

Five BZDs are approved by the Food and Drug Administration (FDA) as prescription insomnia drugs: (1) quazepam, (2) estazolam, (3) flurazepam, (4) triazolam, and (5) temazepam. In Europe, approval varies across countries.

American guidelines support the prescription of triazolam, 0.25 mg, for sleep onset, and temazepam, 15 mg, for sleep onset and sleep maintenance insomnia versus no treatment in adults.[2] Because of lack of data appropriate for statistical analysis, the AASM could not give clinical practice recommendations for the other three FDA-approved drugs (quazepam, estazolam, flurazepam). Their long elimination half-life (>15 hours) is not favorable for use in insomnia.

In European guidelines, the use of BZDs is recommended for short-term treatment (less than 4 weeks), if CBT-I is not effective or not available. Shorter half-life drugs are favored and intermittent dosing is strongly recommended. Long-term treatment of insomnia with BZDs is not recommended because of lack of evidence, side effects, and risks of tolerance and dependence.[3] Prescription should be limited to cases where the impairment is clinically significant and the benefits are expected to outweigh the potential harms. When starting a prescription treatment, the clinician is encouraged to discuss the temporary nature of the prescription with the patient.[28]

NONBENZODIAZEPINE RECEPTOR AGONISTS
Neuropharmacology

NBBzRAs are thought to have a somewhat higher affinity for the $GABA_A$ α1 and α2 receptor subtypes or bind to the complex in a different way than BZDs. Therefore, NBBzRAs are considered to have a more favorable benefit-risk profile (fewer side effects, lower abuse potential) compared with BZDs.[29] The $GABA_A$ α_1 receptor subunit is associated with the most hypnotic effects. These receptors are primarily found on the lamina IV of the sensorimotor cortical regions, substantia nigra pars reticulata, olfactory bulb, ventral thalamic complex, the molecular layer of the cerebellum, pons, inferior colliculus, and globus pallidus.[30] This class of NBBzRAs, also referred to as "Z-drugs," comprise three compounds: (1) zopiclone and eszopiclone, (2) zolpidem, and (3) zaleplon.

Pharmacologic Properties

NBBzRAs are positive allosteric modulators at $GABA_A$ receptors, but they have a chemical structure that is unrelated to other hypnotics, including BZDs. They are all rapidly absorbed after oral administration. NBBzRAs, like BZDs, are primarily metabolized in the liver by the cytochrome P-450 (CYP) 3A4 enzyme.

Zopiclone and its active stereoisomer eszopiclone belong to the group of cyclopyrrolones. They bind to the $GABA_A$ $\alpha_{1, 2, 3}$ subunits. Eszopiclone has a time to maximal concentration (Tmax) of approximately 1 to 1.5 hours, with a half-life time of approximately 6 hours. Zopiclone has a Tmax of 1.5 to 2 hours and a half-life time of approximately 5 hours.

Zolpidem is an imidazopyridine and in therapeutic dosage binds selectively to the $GABA_A$ α_1 subunit. Tmax is 1 to 2 hours, with an additional 30 minutes for the extended-release formula. It has a short half-life time of approximately 2.6 hours.[31,32]

Zaleplon is a pyrazolopyrimidine. In therapeutic dosage, it binds selectively to the $GABA_A$ α_1 subunit. T max is 0.7 to 1.4 hours. It has an ultrashort half-life time of 1 hour and has therapeutic effects usually within 5 to 15 minutes after ingestion.[31,32]

Clinical Effects

Clinical effects of NBBzRAs in treatment of chronic insomnia, including discontinuation effects, are comparable with BZDs.[33,34] Side effects are partial comparable with BZDs.[35] Most commonly reported side effects are amnesia, dizziness, sedation, and headache.[36] An unpleasant, altered, or metallic taste is a typical side effect of (es)zopiclone.[37,38] Somnambulism has been reported with the use of zolpidem and zaleplon.[39,40] Like BZDs, Z-drugs have a potentially higher risk of falls, fractures, and injuries in elderly.[41] Data on whether or not Z-drugs are associated with an increased risk of motor vehicle accidents are controversial.[42,43]

Studies evaluating objective and subjective improvements of sleep parameters of insomniacs using NBBzRAs usually report favorable outcomes. However, many of those studies have methodologic flaws, making it difficult to draw definite conclusions.[2,36]

Of the cyclopyrrolones, the clinical effects of eszopiclone are more extensively studied than those of zopiclone. However, only six studies fit the criteria for systematic review in the AASM clinical practice guideline. In summary, a mean reduction in SL of 14 minutes was seen, TST improved up to 57 minutes, sleep quality was better, and there was less WASO. Studies with 2 mg eszopiclone yielded better statistical significant results than the 3 mg dose.[2]

Zolpidem, 10 mg, showed a mean reduction of SL of 5 to 12 minutes and improvement of TST by 29 minutes. In addition, improvements were seen in WASO, but not in sleep efficiency or number of awakenings.[2]

For zaleplon, only two studies met the inclusion criteria for review, of which one only reported subjective outcomes. Objective polysomnography data showed a significant reduction of SL of approximately 10 minutes. There were no significant differences in TST or sleep quality compared with placebo.[2]

Medical Prescription

The therapeutic dose of zopiclone ranges from 3.75 to 7.5 mg and of eszopiclone from 1 to 3 mg. The therapeutic dose of zolpidem mainly depends on the route of administration (oral tablets, spray, sublingual) varying from 1.75 to 10 mg or 6.25 to 12.5 mg extended-release tablets.[29]

Zaleplon is dosed at 5 to 20 mg. It is advised not to be taken within 4 hours of rise-time, because of the risk of residual sedation and memory impairment.[36] Because of its short half-life time, zaleplon is only suited for sleep-onset insomnia. The others are used for sleep onset and sleep maintenance insomnia. Eszopiclone is the only hypnotic sedative drug that is approved by the FDA for long-term use for the relief of insomnia.[37]

Availability and indication preferences for NBBzRAs vary worldwide. In the United States, NBBzRAs are considered as class IV drugs. As with BZDs and suvorexant, prescription of NBBzRAs should be considered only if nonpharmacologic treatments for insomnia are not available or ineffective. Similarly, prescription should be restricted to a short period of time and intermittent use is recommended when prescription is extended over a longer period of time. Like BDZ, caution should be taken when prescribing NBBzRAs to elderly and careful consideration in case of other drugs metabolized by CYP34A or simultaneous use of central nervous depressants.

OREXIN RECEPTOR ANTAGONISTS
Neuropharmacology

Orexin-producing neurons are located in specific parts of the hypothalamus. These neurons project to most parts of the brain and are active during wake. Orexins stabilize wake through a strong excitatory action on wake-promoting neurons. Orexin knockout mice have many more transitions among wake, NREM, and REM states than do wild-type mice, supporting this model. Similar patterns of sleep-wake disruption are present in human narcolepsy. In addition to promoting wakefulness, orexin plays a role in goal-directed, motivated behaviors.[44,45]

Pharmacologic Properties

There are two types of orexin receptors (OxR1 and OxR2), which are post-synaptic G-protein-coupled receptors. They are expressed in various parts of the brain: OxR1s are highly expressed in the locus coeruleus and OxR2s in the histaminergic TMN.[46,47] There are also two types of orexin neurotransmitters: type A and B (also known as hypocretin 1 and 2). Orexin neurotransmitter type A can bind to OxR1 and OxR2, whereas orexin neurotransmitter type B selectively binds to OxR2. The exact pathways by which dual orexin (hypocretin) receptor antagonists (DORAs) promote sleep, without causing narcoleptic features, are unknown. Presumably antagonism of OxR2s decreases histaminergic activity in the hypothalamus, and in addition antagonism of OxR1 decreases arousal from motivational states, therefore promoting sleep.

Suvorexant has a Tmax of approximately 2 to 3.5 hours, depending on the ingestion of food. It binds to plasma proteins and has a half-life time of approximately 12 hours. Its kinetics are not age-dependent, but gender and weight do play a role. Suvorexant is predominantly metabolized by CYP3A4 enzyme and some involvement of CYP2C19. Approximately 66% is eliminated in feces and 23% in urine.[48]

Clinical Effects

Orexin receptor antagonists are a novel drug class used to treat insomnia. So far, only suvorexant, a DORA, is registered in the United States, Japan, and Australia for the treatment of insomnia. Clinical data available for suvorexant are derived from a limited number of pivotal trials that could be subject to publication bias.[49–51]

In summary, clinical significant improvement was most noticeable in improvement of wake after sleep onset by 16 to 28 minutes, compared with placebo. This might favor suvorexant for sleep maintenance insomnia. However, the total number of awakenings was not statistically altered. TST increased by 10 minutes, compared with placebo, but this was not clinically significant. At higher doses (20 mg), it might improve sleep onset latency, with an average reduction of 22.3 minutes. Sleep efficiency at 20 mg increased on average with 10.4%. Available data were objectively controlled by polysomnography. Subjectively, TST improved but did not reach clinical significance.[49,51]

Reported side effects include somnolence, fatigue, abnormal dreams, and dry mouth, but these were not significantly different from placebo.[49–52] Polysomnographic data of patients with insomnia show a reduced REM latency and an increased REM sleep duration compared with placebo. There is a limited increase of the delta power band and a limited decrease in the γ and β power bands. The largest differences were seen in the first night and diminished over months 1 and 3. The clinical significance of these observations remains unclear.[53]

It should be noted that most of the presented data had an imprecision bias, mainly because of large confidence intervals. Furthermore, studies were sponsored by industry.

Medical Prescription

Suvorexant is FDA-approved for the treatment of insomnia characterized by sleep onset and/or sleep maintenance difficulties. The AASM clinical practice guideline recommends suvorexant only for the treatment of sleep maintenance insomnia.[2]

The recommended starting dose is 10 mg, taken approximately 30 minutes before bed time, with sleep opportunity of at least 7 hours. The drug is available in 5, 10, 15, and 20 mg tablets, with 20 mg being the maximum advised daily dose. Dose reduction should be considered in obesity. When patients use moderate CYP3A4 inhibitors, the recommended starting dose is 5 mg, and the highest dose should not exceed 10 mg.[52]

The use of suvorexant is not advised in patients using strong CYP3A4 inhibitors, those with severe hepatic impairment, or with a diagnosis of narcolepsy. There are no available data on use during pregnancy or lactation, which should therefore be avoided. It is not recommended to use suvorexant simultaneously with other central nervous system depressants, including alcohol. Available data suggest that suvorexant has no major respiratory depressant effects.[54–56] However, it is unclear if this is still the case in high-risk patients (severe sleep apnea, severe chronic obstructive pulmonary disease, concomitant use of muscle relaxants). To date, there are only a few postmarketing case reports on side effects.[57,58]

MELATONIN AND MELATONIN RECEPTOR AGONISTS
Neuropharmacology

Endogenous melatonin is secreted by the pineal gland. Melatonin secretion typically starts in late afternoon, reaches a peak in the first half of the night, and disappears on awakening. As such, melatonin secretion is a hormonal signal of the central nervous system that provides different end-organs with information on the nyctohemeral phase of the circadian cycle. The physiologic function of melatonin in humans has not been fully disclosed. It is hypothesized that melatonin entrains peripheral oscillators, but in vivo confirmation of this hypothesis is difficult, given the redundancy within the circadian system.[59]

Neurons of the suprachiasmaticus nucleus carry melatonin receptors, indicating that melatonin can act on the central master clock itself. In in vitro studies, exogenous melatonin had two distinct effects on neurons of the suprachiasmaticus nucleus: an acute inhibitory effect on neuronal firing and a phase-shifting effect.[59] The acute inhibitory effect may mediate the sleep-promoting properties of melatonin, whereas the phase-shifting properties may induce a delay or advance of the sleep phase, depending on the time of administration with respect to the actual circadian phase.[60,61]

Pharmacologic Properties

Natural melatonin and ramelteon are ligands with great affinity for MT1 and MT2 receptors.[61] They are present in various parts of the brain, but also in other tissues, including cardiac and peripheral vessels, retina, kidneys, and other organs.[62]

The pharmacokinetics of melatonin are characterized by a low and variable bioavailability (on average, 15%). Immediate-release melatonin has Tmax and elimination half-life close to 45 minutes.[63,64] The Tmax of prolonged-release melatonin is affected by food intake, and ranges from 45 minutes to 3 hours in the fed state. Its elimination half-life is 3.5 to 4 hours.

The pharmacokinetics of ramelteon are characterized by rapid absorption, with Tmax and elimination half-life, respectively, approximately 1 and 1.5 hours.[65]

Clinical Effects

Experience from patients in whom pinealectomy was performed for medical reasons has shown that melatonin is not an essential factor for inducing and maintaining sleep. Many of these patients do not experience changes in subjective sleep quality or polysomnographic sleep variables following resection of the pineal gland.[66]

The natural melatonin synthesis may be reduced by drugs (eg, BZDs, nonsteroidal anti-inflammatory drugs, calcium channel blockers, and β-blockers).[67] Oral administration of melatonin or ramelteon may reduce subjective SL and increase perceived sleep quality, although effects on sleep maintenance and duration are equivocal.[68]

In a dosage up to 10 mg given at 11:30 PM, short-acting melatonin induced no significant effect on sleep architecture in healthy subjects.[69] Neither were major changes in sleep architecture observed following exogenous administration of 2 mg melatonin with prolonged-release formulation.[70] In a clinical trial, ramelteon increased the percentage of time spent in N2 by approximately 2% points, at the expense of the percentage of time spent in slow wave sleep, but this is unlikely to be clinically significant.[71]

Melatonin and its agonists are considered safe drugs. Overall, side effects are not different from placebo.[2] One potential serious adverse effect with ramelteon, 8 mg, was a single case of reversible leukopenia out of 227 subjects with insomnia treated with the drug. Six-month nightly administration of prolonged-release 2 mg dose in a population of 65 to 80 year olds, and of ramelteon, 8 mg, in adults, did not produce tolerance, rebound insomnia, or withdrawal effects.[71,72] Biologic effects of melatonin outside sleep have been reviewed elsewhere.[61,73]

Medical Prescription

Ramelteon is FDA-approved for the treatment of insomnia characterized by difficulty with sleep onset.[74] Prolonged-release melatonin (Circadin®) is European Medicines Agency–approved for the short-term treatment of primary insomnia characterized by poor quality of sleep, in patients aged 55 or older. In addition, short-acting melatonin is available over-the-counter in many countries. Although evidence is limited, melatonin or ramelteon may be indicated to treat sleep-onset insomnia, because it slightly shortens the SL of patients with insomnia more than placebo.[2]

SEDATING ANTIDEPRESSANTS
Neuropharmacology

Sedating antidepressants promote sleep by antagonizing the effect of wake-promoting monoamines, including histamine, acetylcholine, noradrenaline, and serotonin. Evidence of the sleep-promoting effect of antagonizing histamine (H_1), muscarinic acetylcholine, noradrenaline receptors (α_1-adrenergic) and serotonin ($5HT_2$) receptors has been reviewed in a previous issue of *Sleep Medicine Clinics*.[75]

The neurons producing these monoamines are located in the ascending arousal system in the upper brainstem, its extension into the caudal hypothalamus, and in the basal forebrain. In wake (but not in REM sleep), histamine is released by neurons of the TMN and adjacent posterior hypothalamus, noradrenaline by neurons of the locus coeruleus, and serotonin by neurons of the dorsal and median raphe nuclei. Dopamine neurons located in the ventral periaqueductal gray matter are also part of this arousal system.[12]

Cholinergic neurons in the laterodorsal tegmental and pedunculopontine tegmental nuclei and the basal forebrain are active in wakefulness and REM sleep. Neurons forming the laterodorsal tegmental and pedunculopontine tegmental nuclei constitute an important modulator of the thalamic relay. In general, arousal systems project on multiple regions of the cerebrum, including the hypothalamus, thalamus, limbic system, and neocortex.[12]

Pharmacologic Properties

Doxepin and amitriptyline are sedative tricyclic antidepressants (TCAs) that also affect sleep. At doses recommended for treatment of depression, they are potent boosters of serotonergic and noradrenergic neurotransmission by blocking serotonin (5HT) and noradrenaline reuptake. They have more effect on the 5HT than on the noradrenaline reuptake, in contrast with TCAs that have stimulating effects.[76] Furthermore, doxepin and amitriptyline block histamine H_1 receptors, which accounts for their sedative and weight gain effects. They inhibit α_1-adrenergic receptors, causing hypotension, and muscarinic M_1 receptors, causing anticholinergic side effects.[29]

At low doses, doxepin and amitriptyline exert their sedating effect through potent H_1-antagonism. At 3 to 6 mg, doxepin almost acts as an H_1 selective antagonist. Low-dose amitriptyline is less selective and exhibits stronger anti-M_1 cholinergic as part of the sedating effect.[29]

Trazodone is chemically unrelated to tricyclic or other known antidepressant agents. Its antidepressant effect is probably caused by inhibition of serotonin uptake and $5HT_{2A/2C}$ antagonism. At lower (hypnotic) doses, $5HT_2$, α_1, and weak H_1 antagonism promotes sleep.[29,48]

Mirtazapine has a tetracyclic chemical structure. α_2-Antagonism results in disinhibition of 5HT and noradrenaline release. Therefore, mirtazapine is classified as a noradrenergic and specific serotonergic antidepressant. $5HT_{2A/2C}$ antagonism and potent H_1 antihistaminic action promote sleep.[48] The combined $5HT_{2C}$ and H_1 antagonism also promotes weight gain.[29] Contrarily to the TCAs, mirtazapine and trazodone have minimal to no effect on M_1 receptors.[48]

The pharmacokinetics of these drugs are diverse. Tmax is longer for doxepin and amitriptyline (2–8 hours) than for trazodone and mirtazapine (1–2 and 1–3 hours, respectively). Doxepin, amitriptyline, and mirtazapine all have elimination half-lives close to 24 hours. Trazodone has a significantly shorter elimination half-life of approximatively 8 to 9 hours.[77] Although the pharmacokinetic profile of trazodone is more apt for use in insomnia than the other antidepressant agents, residual sedation after awakening in the morning is a frequent complaint. Because of variability in clearance, trazodone may accumulate in some individuals over time.[48]

Clinical Effects

Doxepin has been shown to increase objective TST by 26 and 32 minutes (with the 3 and 6 mg dosage, respectively) mainly because of reductions in WASO.[2] Subjective increases in TST are comparable and maintained for up to 4 weeks.[78] Reductions in objective SL are less than clinical threshold with doxepin 3 mg and 6 mg. At these dosages, adverse effects are minimal.[2] Trials in the elderly population have shown no more adverse effects than placebo during up to 4 weeks of treatment with up to 6 mg and 12 weeks with 3 mg.[78-80]

Although a positive effect of amitriptyline has been shown on the sleep of depressed patients, there are no RCTs in the treatment of insomnia without comorbidities.[81]

Placebo-controlled studies of trazodone are also scarce in insomnia. In a study of patient-reported outcomes, trazodone, 50 mg, reduced subjective SL, TST, and WASO, but below threshold for clinical significance.[82] A polysomnography study of trazodone, 150 mg, administered to middle-aged self-reported poor sleepers failed to show a significant improvement in objective TST versus placebo, but confirms the subjective improvement in sleep quality.[83] Consistent with this observation, trazodone, 50 mg, administered to those with primary insomnia significantly improved the subjective ability to sleep. The change in polysomnographic variables was only significant for the number of night-time awakenings (20 awakenings after 7 days of placebo vs 13 after trazodone, 50 mg) and the amount of N1 sleep. Objective sleep efficiency was unchanged.[84]

There are no studies of mirtazapine in insomnia without comorbidities. In a study of depressed patients, TST improved and WASO decreased accordingly when compared with sleep parameters before mirtazapine administration, but there was no placebo control.[85] Acute administration of 30 mg mirtazapine to healthy volunteers did not improve TST versus placebo but improved other measures of sleep continuity.[86] Whether these findings are relevant for the sleep of those with insomnia is unproven.

Many antidepressants delay REM sleep and decrease its duration. This effect seems modest for low-dose doxepin, because it has been shown in some, but not all studies.[79,87] A study on amitriptyline, 75 mg, showed that the REM sleep period dropped to 19 minutes, versus 83 minutes with the use of placebo.[88] No significant REM sleep duration changes were shown for mirtazapine in healthy subjects or trazodone, 50 mg, in subjects with insomnia.[84,86]

In a minority of patients, antidepressants increase restless legs syndrome symptoms and/or periodic limb movements of sleep. This effect might be higher with mirtazapine and amitriptyline than with doxepin (at dose up to 50 mg) or trazodone, 100 mg.[89]

Medical Prescription

Doxepin, amitriptyline, trazodone, and mirtazapine are approved in the United States and many other countries as antidepressants. At much lower dose than needed for their antidepressant effect, they are prescribed for the treatment of insomnia. Only low-dose doxepin (3 to 6 mg) is FDA approved for that indication; any other use is off label.

In the American guidelines, the use of doxepin, 3 to 6 mg, is supported for sleep maintenance, but not for initiation of sleep. The use of amitriptyline, trazodone, or mirtazapine is not recommended.[2] The European guidelines report on sedating antidepressants as a group. These drugs are judged effective in the short-term treatment of insomnia, provided contraindications are carefully taken into account. Long-term treatment is not recommended.[3]

In older subjects, amitriptyline and doxepin greater than 6 mg are to be avoided, and mirtazapine is to be used with caution. Trazodone and doxepin up to 6 mg are not listed in the American Geriatrics Society Beers Criteria for Potentially Inappropriate Medication Use in Older Adults, and thus seem safer.[21] However, trazodone, 50 mg, slightly but significantly reduced next day memory, equilibrium, and muscle endurance versus placebo in subjects with primary insomnia younger than 65 years.[84]

ANTIPSYCHOTICS
Neuropharmacology

Antipsychotic drugs exert their sedative effects by antagonizing the activity of wake-stimulating neurotransmitters, similarly to the antidepressants.[75]

Pharmacologic Properties

All antipsychotic medications interact with dopamine D_2 receptors (most of them are D_2 blockers), and possess numerous other pharmacologic properties, among which various degrees of H_1 histamine, M_1 cholinergic, and α_1-adrenergic receptor antagonism. This triple action can be highly sedating.[29] The second-generation antipsychotics differ from the first generation, because they also possess $5HT_2$ antagonism. Therefore, they are expected to be better sleep promotors.[75]

Quetiapine is the most commonly used antipsychotic for insomnia.[90] Quetiapine is effective as an antipsychotic at doses of 300 to 800 mg. In much lower doses (25 to 50 mg), its hypnotic effect is preserved, because of its high affinity for H_1 receptors.[29]

Clinical Effects

The effects of antipsychotic medications on sleep have mostly been investigated in psychiatric patients. These studies are not relevant to insomnia without psychiatric comorbidity, and the doses given are often much higher than the ones needed for the sedating effect. Although quetiapine is used off label in insomnia, evidence is definitely lacking.[90] A small RCT including healthy people showed improvements in subjective and polysomnographic sleep with quetiapine, 25 mg and 100 mg.[91] In insomnia without psychiatric comorbidity, only one RCT has been published so far. In this study, seven patients took quetiapine, 25 mg daily, during 2 weeks versus six placebo control subjects. Compared with placebo, improvement of subjective TST and SL with quetiapine was not statistically significant.[92] Because of the small size of the study, no firm conclusion could be drawn. Although in these studies quetiapine, 25 to 75 mg, was well tolerated, a concern remains about serious adverse effects on the longer term, encompassing abuse, suicidal ideation, and metabolic adverse effects, even at low doses.[93,94] A significant increase in periodic leg movements during sleep was observed with quetiapine, 100 mg.[91]

No RCT exists on other antipsychotics prescribed for insomnia without psychiatric comorbidity.[94] Monti and colleagues[95] recently reviewed the effects of the second-generation antipsychotics in healthy subjects. The results were either nonsignificant or showed an improvement in measures of SL, WASO, and TST. Most consistent evidence of a positive effect on the sleep parameters of healthy subjects exists for olanzapine, 5 to 10 mg. Of note, the elimination half-life of olanzapine is more than 24 hours, whereas that of quetiapine is less than 8 hours.

Medical Prescription

Because of lack of evidence and potential harm even at low doses, antipsychotics are not approved or recommended for the treatment of insomnia without comorbidities.[3]

SUMMARY

Several prescription drugs are available that, at least temporarily, improve sleep duration and continuity objectively and subjectively, with acceptable side effects. Although new medication classes (eg, DORAs) are becoming available, the ideal sleeping pill still does not exist.

Will such a drug ever overthrow CBT-I as the first-line therapy for chronic insomnia? CBT-I targets many sleep mechanisms. Sleep restriction affects homeostatic sleep pressure, keeping strict bed and rise times, targets circadian timing and relaxation training reduces cognitive arousal. It is unlikely that a single drug will be able to modulate all these mechanisms simultaneously.

However, pharmacologic treatment will remain important for patients in whom CBT-I is not effective or not available. But even then, the use of medication should always be part of a broader treatment plan in which dysfunctional sleep habits are challenged, substance use is optimized, and comorbid conditions are addressed.

In insomnia, the subjective aspects of the sleep complaint are paramount in the diagnostic criteria. Epidemiologic studies increasingly point to a link between insomnia and somatic morbidity and mortality, but until now, only in the subgroup of objectively poor sleepers.[96–99] Although pharmacologic treatment might offer some benefits to this subgroup of insomnia patients, to date, there is no evidence that hypnotics can ameliorate their health risks. It is hoped that further unraveling of the neurobiology and genetics of sleep regulation and the pathophysiology of insomnia will help the development of drugs that not only improve subjective sleep complaints, but also objective health outcomes.

REFERENCES

1. van Straten A, van der Zweerde T, Kleiboer A, et al. Cognitive and behavioral therapies in the treatment of insomnia: a meta-analysis. Sleep Med Rev 2018; 38:3–16.
2. Sateia MJ, Buysse DJ, Krystal AD, et al. Clinical practice guideline for the pharmacologic treatment of chronic insomnia in adults: an American Academy of Sleep Medicine clinical practice guideline. J Clin Sleep Med 2017;13(2):307–49.
3. Riemann D, Baglioni C, Bassetti C, et al. European guideline for the diagnosis and treatment of insomnia. J Sleep Res 2017;26(6):675–700.
4. Morin CM, Vallieres A, Guay B, et al. Cognitive behavioral therapy, singly and combined with medication, for persistent insomnia: a randomized controlled trial. JAMA 2009;301(19):2005–15.
5. Zavesicka L, Brunovsky M, Matousek M, et al. Discontinuation of hypnotics during cognitive behavioural therapy for insomnia. BMC Psychiatry 2008;8:80.
6. Winkler A, Rief W. Effect of placebo conditions on polysomnographic parameters in primary insomnia: a meta-analysis. Sleep 2015;38(6):925–31.
7. Yeung V, Sharpe L, Glozier N, et al. A systematic review and meta-analysis of placebo versus no treatment for insomnia symptoms. Sleep Med Rev 2018; 38:17–27.
8. Krystal AD. A compendium of placebo-controlled trials of the risks/benefits of pharmacological treatments for insomnia: the empirical basis for U.S. clinical practice. Sleep Med Rev 2009;13(4):265–74.
9. Minkel J, Krystal AD. Optimizing the pharmacologic treatment of insomnia: current status and future horizons. Sleep Med Clin 2013;8(3):333–50.
10. Wafford KA, Ebert B. Emerging anti-insomnia drugs: tackling sleeplessness and the quality of wake time. Nat Rev Drug Discov 2008;7(6):530–40.
11. Lu J, Greco MA. Sleep circuitry and the hypnotic mechanism of GABAA drugs. J Clin Sleep Med 2006;2(2):S19–26.
12. Saper CB, Scammell TE, Lu J. Hypothalamic regulation of sleep and circadian rhythms. Nature 2005; 437(7063):1257–63.
13. Mendelson W, Laposky A. Effects of triazolam microinjections into the peri-fornicular region on sleep in rats. Sleep Hypnosis 2003;5(3):154–62.
14. Nestler EJ, Hyman S, Holtzmann DM, et al. Molecular neuropharmacology: a foundation for clinical neuroscience. 3rd edition. New York: McGraw-Hill Medical; 2015.
15. Rudolph U, Crestani F, Benke D, et al. Benzodiazepine actions mediated by specific gamma-aminobutyric acid(A) receptor subtypes. Nature 1999;401(6755):796–800.
16. Glass JR, Sproule BA, Herrmann N, et al. Effects of 2-week treatment with temazepam and diphenhydramine in elderly insomniacs: a randomized, placebo-controlled trial. J Clin Psychopharmacol 2008;28(2):182–8.
17. Wu R, Bao J, Zhang C, et al. Comparison of sleep condition and sleep-related psychological activity after cognitive-behavior and pharmacological therapy for chronic insomnia. Psychother Psychosom 2006;75(4):220–8.
18. Roehrs T, Bonahoom A, Pedrosi B, et al. Treatment regimen and hypnotic self-administration. Psychopharmacology (Berl) 2001;155(1):11–7.
19. Oswald I, French C, Adam K, et al. Benzodiazepine hypnotics remain effective for 24 weeks. Br Med J (Clin Res Ed) 1982;284(6319):860–3.
20. Janhsen K, Roser P, Hoffmann K. The problems of long-term treatment with benzodiazepines and related substances. Dtsch Arztebl Int 2015;112(1–2):1–7.
21. Campanelli C. American Geriatrics Society updated beers criteria for potentially inappropriate medication use in older adults: the American Geriatrics Society 2012 beers criteria update expert panel. J Am Geriatr Soc 2012;60(4):616–31.
22. Luyster FS, Buysse DJ, Strollo PJ Jr. Comorbid insomnia and obstructive sleep apnea: challenges for clinical practice and research. J Clin Sleep Med 2010;6(2):196–204.
23. Roehrs T, Roth T. Drug-related sleep stage changes: functional significance and clinical relevance. Sleep Med Clin 2010;5(4):559–70.
24. Bastien CH, LeBlanc M, Carrier J, et al. Sleep EEG power spectra, insomnia, and chronic use of benzodiazepines. Sleep 2003;26(3):313–7.
25. Borbely AA, Mattmann P, Loepfe M, et al. Effect of benzodiazepine hypnotics on all-night sleep EEG spectra. Hum Neurobiol 1985;4(3):189–94.
26. Kilduff T, Mendelson WB. Hypnotic medications: mechanisms of action and pharmacologic effects.

In: Kryger M, Roth T, editors. Principles and practice of sleep medicine. 6th edition. Philadelphia: Elsevier; 2017. p. 425–31.

27. Mazza M, Losurdo A, Testani E, et al. Polysomnographic findings in a cohort of chronic insomnia patients with benzodiazepine abuse. J Clin Sleep Med 2014;10(1):35–42.

28. Royant-Parola S, Brion A, Poirot I. Prise en charge de l'insomnie: guide pratique. Issy-les-Moulineaux (France): Elsevier Masson SAS; 2017.

29. Stahl SM. Stahl's essential psychopharmacology: neuroscientific basis and practical applications. Cambridge (England): Cambridge University Press; 2013.

30. Holm KJ, Goa KL. Zolpidem: an update of its pharmacology, therapeutic efficacy and tolerability in the treatment of insomnia. Drugs 2000;59(4): 865–89.

31. Wishart DS, Feunang YD, Guo AC, et al. DrugBank 5.0: a major update to the DrugBank database for 2018. Nucleic Acids Res 2018;46(D1):D1074–82.

32. Drover DR. Comparative pharmacokinetics and pharmacodynamics of short-acting hypnosedatives: zaleplon, zolpidem and zopiclone. Clin Pharmacokinet 2004;43(4):227–38.

33. Erman MK, Zammit G, Rubens R, et al. A polysomnographic placebo-controlled evaluation of the efficacy and safety of eszopiclone relative to placebo and zolpidem in the treatment of primary insomnia. J Clin Sleep Med 2008;4(3):229–34.

34. Walsh JK, Vogel GW, Scharf M, et al. A five week, polysomnographic assessment of zaleplon 10 mg for the treatment of primary insomnia. Sleep Med 2000;1(1):41–9.

35. Gunja N. In the Zzz zone: the effects of Z-drugs on human performance and driving. J Med Toxicol 2013;9(2):163–71.

36. Becker PM, Somiah M. Non-benzodiazepine receptor agonists for insomnia. Sleep Med Clin 2015; 10(1):57–76.

37. Krystal AD, Walsh JK, Laska E, et al. Sustained efficacy of eszopiclone over 6 months of nightly treatment: results of a randomized, double-blind, placebo-controlled study in adults with chronic insomnia. Sleep 2003;26(7):793–9.

38. Wadworth AN, McTavish D. Zopiclone. A review of its pharmacological properties and therapeutic efficacy as an hypnotic. Drugs Aging 1993;3(5): 441–59.

39. Toner LC, Tsambiras BM, Catalano G, et al. Central nervous system side effects associated with zolpidem treatment. Clin Neuropharmacol 2000;23(1): 54–8.

40. Chen YW, Tseng PT, Wu CK, et al. Zaleplon-induced anemsic somnambulism with eating behaviors under once dose. Acta Neurol Taiwan 2014;23(4): 143–5.

41. Treves N, Perlman A, Kolenberg Geron L, et al. Z-drugs and risk for falls and fractures in older adults: a systematic review and meta-analysis. Age Ageing 2018;47(2):201–8.

42. Orriols L, Philip P, Moore N, et al. Benzodiazepine-like hypnotics and the associated risk of road traffic accidents. Clin Pharmacol Ther 2011;89(4): 595–601.

43. Chang CM, Wu EC, Chen CY, et al. Psychotropic drugs and risk of motor vehicle accidents: a population-based case-control study. Br J Clin Pharmacol 2013;75(4):1125–33.

44. Mahler SV, Moorman DE, Smith RJ, et al. Motivational activation: a unifying hypothesis of orexin/hypocretin function. Nat Neurosci 2014;17(10): 1298–303.

45. Bonnavion P, de Lecea L. Hypocretins in the control of sleep and wakefulness. Curr Neurol Neurosci Rep 2010;10(3):174–9.

46. Sakurai T, Amemiya A, Ishii M, et al. Orexins and orexin receptors: a family of hypothalamic neuropeptides and G protein-coupled receptors that regulate feeding behavior. Cell 1998;92(4):573–85.

47. de Lecea L, Kilduff TS, Peyron C, et al. The hypocretins: hypothalamus-specific peptides with neuroexcitatory activity. Proc Natl Acad Sci U S A 1998; 95(1):322–7.

48. Law V, Knox C, Djoumbou Y, et al. DrugBank 4.0: shedding new light on drug metabolism. Nucleic Acids Res 2014;42(Database issue):D1091–7.

49. Herring WJ, Connor KM, Ivgy-May N, et al. Suvorexant in patients with insomnia: results from two 3-month randomized controlled clinical trials. Biol Psychiatry 2016;79(2):136–48.

50. Herring WJ, Snyder E, Budd K, et al. Orexin receptor antagonism for treatment of insomnia: a randomized clinical trial of suvorexant. Neurology 2012;79(23): 2265–74.

51. Michelson D, Snyder E, Paradis E, et al. Safety and efficacy of suvorexant during 1-year treatment of insomnia with subsequent abrupt treatment discontinuation: a phase 3 randomised, double-blind, placebo-controlled trial. Lancet Neurol 2014;13(5): 461–71.

52. Herring WJ, Connor KM, Snyder E, et al. Suvorexant in patients with insomnia: pooled analyses of three-month data from phase-3 randomized controlled clinical trials. J Clin Sleep Med 2016; 12(9):1215–25.

53. Snyder E, Ma J, Svetnik V, et al. Effects of suvorexant on sleep architecture and power spectral profile in patients with insomnia: analysis of pooled phase 3 data. Sleep Med 2016;19:93–100.

54. Sun H, Palcza J, Card D, et al. Effects of suvorexant, an orexin receptor antagonist, on respiration during sleep in patients with obstructive sleep apnea. J Clin Sleep Med 2016;12(1):9–17.

55. Sun H, Palcza J, Rosenberg R, et al. Effects of suvorexant, an orexin receptor antagonist, on breathing during sleep in patients with chronic obstructive pulmonary disease. Respir Med 2015; 109(3):416–26.

56. Uemura N, McCrea J, Sun H, et al. Effects of the orexin receptor antagonist suvorexant on respiration during sleep in healthy subjects. J Clin Pharmacol 2015;55(10):1093–100.

57. Tabata H, Kuriyama A, Yamao F, et al. Suvorexant-induced dream enactment behavior in parkinson disease: a case report. J Clin Sleep Med 2017; 13(5):759–60.

58. Petrous J, Furmaga K. Adverse reaction with suvorexant for insomnia: acute worsening of depression with emergence of suicidal thoughts. BMJ Case Rep 2017.

59. Pevet P. Melatonin receptors as therapeutic targets in the suprachiasmatic nucleus. Expert Opin Ther Targets 2016;20(10):1209–18.

60. Liu C, Weaver DR, Jin X, et al. Molecular dissection of two distinct actions of melatonin on the suprachiasmatic circadian clock. Neuron 1997;19(1): 91–102.

61. Liu J, Clough SJ, Hutchinson AJ, et al. MT1 and MT2 melatonin receptors: a therapeutic perspective. Annu Rev Pharmacol Toxicol 2016;56:361–83.

62. Pandi-Perumal SR, Trakht I, Srinivasan V, et al. Physiological effects of melatonin: role of melatonin receptors and signal transduction pathways. Prog Neurobiol 2008;85(3):335–53.

63. Andersen LP, Werner MU, Rosenkilde MM, et al. Pharmacokinetics of oral and intravenous melatonin in healthy volunteers. BMC Pharmacol Toxicol 2016; 17:8.

64. Harpsoe NG, Andersen LP, Gogenur I, et al. Clinical pharmacokinetics of melatonin: a systematic review. Eur J Clin Pharmacol 2015;71(8):901–9.

65. Sateia MJ, Kirby-Long P, Taylor JL. Efficacy and clinical safety of ramelteon: an evidence-based review. Sleep Med Rev 2008;12(4):319–22.

66. Slawik H, Stoffel M, Riedl L, et al. Prospective study on salivary evening melatonin and sleep before and after pinealectomy in humans. J Biol Rhythms 2016; 31(1):82–93.

67. Auld F, Maschauer EL, Morrison I, et al. Evidence for the efficacy of melatonin in the treatment of primary adult sleep disorders. Sleep Med Rev 2017;34:10–22.

68. Ferracioli-Oda E, Qawasmi A, Bloch MH. Meta-analysis: melatonin for the treatment of primary sleep disorders. PLoS One 2013;8(5):e63773.

69. Stone BM, Turner C, Mills SL, et al. Hypnotic activity of melatonin. Sleep 2000;23(5):663–9.

70. Arbon EL, Knurowska M, Dijk DJ. Randomised clinical trial of the effects of prolonged-release melatonin, temazepam and zolpidem on slow-wave activity during sleep in healthy people. J Psychopharmacol 2015;29(7):764–76.

71. Mayer G, Wang-Weigand S, Roth-Schechter B, et al. Efficacy and safety of 6-month nightly ramelteon administration in adults with chronic primary insomnia. Sleep 2009;32(3):351–60.

72. Wade AG, Ford I, Crawford G, et al. Nightly treatment of primary insomnia with prolonged release melatonin for 6 months: a randomized placebo controlled trial on age and endogenous melatonin as predictors of efficacy and safety. BMC Med 2010;8:51.

73. Tordjman S, Chokron S, Delorme R, et al. Melatonin: pharmacology, functions and therapeutic benefits. Curr Neuropharmacol 2017;15(3):434–43.

74. Available at: https://www.fda.gov/Drugs/DrugSafety. Accessed January 22, 2018.

75. Krystal AD. Antidepressant and antipsychotic drugs. Sleep Med Clin 2010;5(4):571–89.

76. DeMartinis NA, Winokur A. Effects of psychiatric medications on sleep and sleep disorders. CNS Neurol Disord Drug Targets 2007;6(1):17–29.

77. Buysse DJ, Tyagi S. Clinical pharmacology of other drugs used as hypnotics. In: Kryger M, Roth T, editors. Principles and practice of sleep medicine. 6th edition. Philadelphia: Elsevier; 2017. p. 432–45.

78. Lankford A, Rogowski R, Essink B, et al. Efficacy and safety of doxepin 6 mg in a four-week outpatient trial of elderly adults with chronic primary insomnia. Sleep Med 2012;13(2):133–8.

79. Scharf M, Rogowski R, Hull S, et al. Efficacy and safety of doxepin 1 mg, 3 mg, and 6 mg in elderly patients with primary insomnia: a randomized, double-blind, placebo-controlled crossover study. J Clin Psychiatry 2008;69(10):1557–64.

80. Krystal AD, Durrence HH, Scharf M, et al. Efficacy and safety of doxepin 1 mg and 3 mg in a 12-week sleep laboratory and outpatient trial of elderly subjects with chronic primary insomnia. Sleep 2010;33(11):1553–61.

81. Liu Y, Xu X, Dong M, et al. Treatment of insomnia with tricyclic antidepressants: a meta-analysis of polysomnographic randomized controlled trials. Sleep Med 2017;34:126–33.

82. Walsh JK, Erman M, Erwin CW, et al. Subjective hypnotic efficacy of trazodone and zolpidem in DSMIII-R primary insomnia. Hum Psychopharmacol 1998; 13(3):191–8.

83. Montgomery I, Oswald I, Morgan K, et al. Trazodone enhances sleep in subjective quality but not in objective duration. Br J Clin Pharmacol 1983;16(2): 139–44.

84. Roth AJ, McCall WV, Liguori A. Cognitive, psychomotor and polysomnographic effects of trazodone in primary insomniacs. J Sleep Res 2011;20(4): 552–8.

85. Schmid DA, Wichniak A, Uhr M, et al. Changes of sleep architecture, spectral composition of sleep

EEG, the nocturnal secretion of cortisol, ACTH, GH, prolactin, melatonin, ghrelin, and leptin, and the DEX-CRH test in depressed patients during treatment with mirtazapine. Neuropsychopharmacology 2006;31(4):832–44.

86. Aslan S, Isik E, Cosar B. The effects of mirtazapine on sleep: a placebo controlled, double-blind study in young healthy volunteers. Sleep 2002; 25(6):677–9.

87. Krystal AD, Lankford A, Durrence HH, et al. Efficacy and safety of doxepin 3 and 6 mg in a 35-day sleep laboratory trial in adults with chronic primary insomnia. Sleep 2011;34(10):1433–42.

88. Goerke M, Cohrs S, Rodenbeck A, et al. Differential effect of an anticholinergic antidepressant on sleep-dependent memory consolidation. Sleep 2014; 37(5):977–85.

89. Kolla BP, Mansukhani MP, Bostwick JM. The influence of antidepressants on restless legs syndrome and periodic limb movements: a systematic review. Sleep Med Rev 2018;38:131–40.

90. Walsh JK. Drugs used to treat insomnia in 2002: regulatory-based rather than evidence-based medicine. Sleep 2004;27(8):1441–2.

91. Cohrs S, Rodenbeck A, Guan Z, et al. Sleep-promoting properties of quetiapine in healthy subjects. Psychopharmacology (Berl) 2004;174(3): 421–9.

92. Tassniyom K, Paholpak S, Tassniyom S, et al. Quetiapine for primary insomnia: a double blind, randomized controlled trial. J Med Assoc Thai 2010; 93(6):729–34.

93. Coe HV, Hong IS. Safety of low doses of quetiapine when used for insomnia. Ann Pharmacother 2012; 46(5):718–22.

94. Thompson W, Quay TAW, Rojas-Fernandez C, et al. Atypical antipsychotics for insomnia: a systematic review. Sleep Med 2016;22:13–7.

95. Monti JM, Torterolo P, Pandi Perumal SR. The effects of second generation antipsychotic drugs on sleep variables in healthy subjects and patients with schizophrenia. Sleep Med Rev 2017; 33:51–7.

96. Vgontzas AN, Fernandez-Mendoza J, Liao D, et al. Insomnia with objective short sleep duration: the most biologically severe phenotype of the disorder. Sleep Med Rev 2013;17(4):241–54.

97. Stahl SM. Temazepam. In: Stahl SM, editor. Stahl's Essential Pharmacology: The prescriber's guide. 6th ed. Cambridge (UK): Cambridge University Press; 2017. p. 703–6.

98. Yasui-Furukori N, Takahata T, Kondo T, et al. Time effects of food intake on the pharmacokinetics and pharmacodynamics of quazepam. Br J Clin Pharmacol 2003;55(4):382–8.

99. Available at: https://www.drugs.com. Accessed February 19, 2018.

Drugs Used in Narcolepsy and Other Hypersomnias

Gert Jan Lammers, MD, PhD[a,b,*]

KEYWORDS

- Narcolepsy • Idiopathic hypersomnia • Nonpharmacological treatment • Pharmacologic treatment
- Stimulants • Sodium oxybate • Pitolisant

KEY POINTS

- State-of-the-art treatment of narcolepsy and hypersomnias of central origin consists of a combination of facilitating acceptance of the disorder, lifestyle advice, and pharmacologic treatment.
- The treatment goal of pharmacologic treatment must be improved performance and avoidance of side effects.
- Even when optimally treated, excessive daytime sleepiness will never completely disappear. In contrast, cataplexy, hypnagogic hallucinations, and sleep paralysis may completely disappear.

INTRODUCTION

Hypersomnolence may have various expressions and lead to a variety of complaints, including a subjective feeling of sleepiness, difficulty in sustaining attention, impaired performance, memory complaints, automatic behavior, unintended naps, irritability, and/or an increased amount of sleep. Regarding sleep, usually 1 of 2 distinctive phenotypes is predominantly present: an inability to stay awake during the day or an increased need for sleep. This distinction may not only guide the underlying diagnosis but may also predict efficacy of certain (pharmacologic) treatment interventions. By definition, the complaint is present each and every day.

Narcolepsy with cataplexy is a typical example of a disorder characterized by an inability to stay awake during the day, usually accompanied by an inability to stay asleep at night but without a significant increase in the hours spent asleep during the 24 hours of the day. The classic form of idiopathic hypersomnia (IH) is the typical example of an increased need for sleep: there is an irresistible need for an increased number of hours spent asleep during the night and, despite this increase, there are complaints of sleepiness during the day. This latter phenotype is more difficult to treat.

It must be kept in mind that by far the most prevalent cause of excessive daytime sleepiness (EDS) is sleep deprivation. Complaints caused by sleep deprivation are neither quantitatively nor qualitatively different from complaints caused by sleep disorders, which may cause diagnostic challenges. In case of doubt, patients must always be first advised to extend sleep to assess whether sleep deprivation is the likely cause of their complaints. It is also important to realize that if a sleep disorder is the cause for EDS, sleep apnea is a much more prevalent cause than narcolepsy or IH because of its much higher prevalence.

THE COMPLAINTS TO BE TREATED

The key problem of most patients who suffer from narcolepsy or IH is their inability to remain fully alert and/or even awake during longer periods of the day, relentlessly present each and every day of their life.[1,2] In narcolepsy with cataplexy in addition, the strict physiologic boundaries of specific

Disclosure: Consultant or member of the international advisory boards on narcolepsy of UCB International, Jazz Pharmaceuticals, and Bioprojet.
[a] Department of Neurology, Leiden University Medical Center, Albinusdreef 2, Leiden 2333 AA, The Netherlands;
[b] Sleep-Wake Centers of SEIN, Achterweg 5, 2103 SW Heemstede, The Netherlands
* Department of Neurology, Leiden University Medical Center, Albinusdreef 2, Leiden 2333 AA, The Netherlands.
E-mail address: G.J.Lammers@LUMC.nl

components of wake and sleep stages are fluid. This leads to partial expressions, particularly identifiable in rapid eye movement (REM) sleep, explaining such symptoms as cataplexy, hypnagogic hallucinations (HHs), and sleep paralysis (SP).[2] The loss of state boundaries leads to more symptoms that are not always mentioned in textbooks, such as automatic behavior, memory complaints, and dream delusions.

COMORBIDITY

Patients who suffer from narcolepsy with cataplexy clearly bear a risk to become obese, and those who suffer from narcolepsy and IH have an increased chance to develop complaints of fatigue and psychiatric comorbidities, such as anxiety and depression.[2,3]

It may be important to treat these comorbidities as well; however, that is beyond the scope of this article.

BURDEN

It is not difficult to imagine that narcolepsy and IH have a severe negative impact on daily functioning and the experienced quality of life. It is even more detrimental when it starts during childhood because of the additional negative impact on social development and achievements at school.[2,4]

EPIDEMIOLOGY

Narcolepsy with cataplexy has an estimated prevalence of 25 to 50 per 100,000 population. The incidence is estimated to be 0.74 to 1.37 per 100,000 person-years.[5–7] There are no reliable prevalence or incidence estimations of narcolepsy without cataplexy and IH but the prevalence is probably lower than for narcolepsy with cataplexy.

The age of onset is usually between 15 and 35 years but it may start at any age. There is a trend for a diagnosis at younger age and, probably, also for an earlier symptom onset during the last decade.

CURRENTLY AVAILABLE TREATMENTS

Before starting treatment, it is of paramount importance that patients and their relatives are informed about the consequences of their chronic disease and learn to accept the diagnosis. This greatly facilitates the implementation of the behavioral modifications and decreases the burden of the disease. Accepting the diagnosis implies implementing behavioral or lifestyle modifications. Initiating pharmacologic treatment only after the implementation of lifestyle changes will prevent medication being used to compensate for a lack of lifestyle adjustment and will optimize treatment response. Only when medication is added to lifestyle adjustments can optimal and long-term improvement be established.

In addition, a supportive social environment (eg, family members, friends, employer, colleagues, patient group organizations, and support groups) is highly valuable.

TREATMENT GOALS

Unfortunately, there is currently only symptomatic treatment of narcolepsy and IH. Although symptomatic, it may lead to profound improvement. There are 2 known effective treatment modalities: behavioral modification and pharmacologic therapy. As a rule, both are needed to achieve sufficient improvement.[2]

Therapy for EDS as expression of narcolepsy or IH should focus on the key problem: improving sustained attention and, therefore, performance, and reducing the chance for involuntary sleep attacks or naps. Because treatment is symptomatic, EDS complaints will never completely disappear. It should be explained to patients that the treatment goal is to improve the quality and duration of wakefulness during the day. They must be warned that there will usually remain a high chance of falling asleep in sedentary situations.

When initiating treatment of cataplexy, HHs, and SP, the intention should be to let them disappear. To reach this, pharmacologic treatment is almost always needed. HHs may sometimes be less prevalent when falling asleep in the supine position is avoided.

Behavioral Modification

Patients should be advised to live a regular life, go to bed at the same hour each night, and get up at the same time each morning as much as possible. Scheduled daytime naps, usually less than 20 minutes, may temporarily alleviate and prevent daytime sleepiness, and a short nap just before certain activities demanding a high degree of attention may facilitate the proper completion. The optimal frequency, duration, and timing of these naps must be established on an individual basis. In most narcoleptic patients, longer naps have no better or longer lasting refreshing properties. Moreover, it is more difficult and inconvenient to wake up after a longer nap because, in most instances, deep sleep will occur. However, some patients only do well with longer naps. Unfortunately, there are few published studies regarding this important topic.[8]

Many particularly narcoleptic patients experience an influence from diet. They feel better when avoiding (large amounts of) carbohydrates during the day. Unfortunately, there also are few scientific data regarding this observation.[9] Alcohol consumption should preferably be avoided.

Pharmacological Therapy

Despite these behavioral measures, most patients will need adjuvant pharmacologic treatment. A variety of substances can be used. This observation already indicates that no drug is efficacious in all. Because most drugs predominantly act on either EDS or cataplexy, combinations are often needed to control both symptoms in those who suffer from narcolepsy with cataplexy. The only available drug that may improve all major symptoms of narcolepsy is sodium oxybate (SXB). Combinations of SXB with, for example, stimulants may have a synergetic effect for the amelioration of EDS and, therefore, may be preferred over monotherapy.

What should be kept in mind when making a choice for a certain drug or combinations of drugs in an individual patient, and how to evaluate its efficacy?

- EDS will never be completely alleviated, whereas cataplexy, HHs, and SP may completely disappear in some patients.
- Improvement of daytime performance is a much more important treatment goal than a reduction of the total amount of daytime sleep.
- Long-term improvement of nocturnal sleep can only be reached with SXB.
- History taking from both the patients and partners or relatives is the best way to guide and adjust therapy.
- Individual differences in efficacy, side-effects, and tolerability of drugs seem to be extensive. Knowledge about the efficacy of a drug as assessed in groups is, therefore, of relative importance for making a choice in an individual.
- Pharmacokinetic aspects, that is, short-acting and fast-acting versus slow-acting and long-acting drugs, may be more important than the expected efficacy.

Treatment of excessive daytime sleepiness

Stimulants still are the mainstay of the treatment of EDS.[10,11] They enhance release and inhibit the reuptake of catecholamines and, to a lesser extent, serotonin in the central nervous system and the periphery. They are also weak inhibitors of monoamine oxidase. These include dextroamphetamine (5–60 mg/d; usually in 1–3 doses per day), methylphenidate (10–60 mg/d; usually in 2–4 doses per day), and mazindol (1–6 mg/d; usually in 1–2 doses per day). Side-effects and tolerance are drawbacks in the use of stimulants. The most important side effects include irritability, agitation, headache, and peripheral sympathetic stimulation. These are usually dose-related. Although addiction does not seem to be a problem in narcolepsy or presumably in IH, some patients tend to increase their dosage because they prefer high alertness.[12] Tolerance develops in about one-third of patients.[12,13] Mazindol has been withdrawn from the market in most countries owing to observed uncommon but severe side-effects in related drugs that suppress appetite, in particular fenfluramines. The side effects were pulmonary hypertension and valvular regurgitation.[14] Because some patients respond better to mazindol than to any other drug, it may be considered, provided treatment is closely monitored.

Modafinil (100–400 mg/d; usually in 1 or 2 doses) is usually grouped with stimulants but is chemically unrelated to amphetamine.[11] It blocks the dopamine reuptake but the mode of action is not yet fully explained. The efficacy is probably equal to that of the stimulants, although direct comparisons are lacking. The clinical impression of most experts in the field is that during treatment with modafinil all the described side-effects, as well as tolerance, of stimulants may occur but are less frequent and less severe in general. More specific side effects of modafinil are headache and nausea. However, they usually disappear after 2 to 3 weeks of treatment. Although the experts are probably right, this opinion is not very relevant for deciding for a certain stimulant or modafinil in an individual patient: the interindividual differences in experienced response and side effects are too widespread to guide treatment only on opinions regarding efficacy on a group level. When prescribed to women of childbearing age, it must be kept in mind that there is interaction with oral contraceptives. Dose adjustment is required.

The European Medicines Agency (EMA) completed a remarkable review of the safety and effectiveness of modafinil in 2010.[15] The Agency's Committee for Medicinal Products for Human Use concluded that the benefits of modafinil-containing medicines continue to outweigh their risks but that their use should be restricted to the treatment of adults suffering from narcolepsy. It is not exactly clear on which data this advice was based, or why apparently narcolepsy was generally considered to be a more relevant or more invalidating disorder than IH. Moreover, it contained no risk evaluation when replacing modafinil with another stimulant.[15] Because of these unanswered questions, most national and international guidelines, including in Europe, still recommend the use of modafinil in IH.[16–18]

Armodafinil is the R-enantiomer of modafinil and has very similar effects. It is not available in most European countries. Caffeine may alleviate sleepiness but has a weak effect: the alerting effect of

6 cups of strong coffee is comparable with that of 5 mg of dexamphetamine.

Long-acting agents (modafinil, armodafinil, dexamphetamine, methylphenidate, controlled release) are generally better tolerated than the short-acting ones. The quick and short-acting agents can be used to good effect when targeted at social events or difficult periods during the day. For this reason, combinations of stimulants may be tailored to the circumstances. Unfortunately, there are no studies assessing the advantages or disadvantages of combinations of stimulants.

Pitolisant, a selective histamine-3 receptor antagonist, has recently been approved by the EMA. Pitolisant was the first histamine-3 receptor antagonist to reach the market. It is an advantage to have an additional option for the treatment of EDS with a different and selective mode of action when compared with stimulants. The dose range is 9 to 36 mg. Published studies show efficacy, particularly regarding improvement of EDS, but also regarding improvement of cataplexy.[19,20] On a group level, the efficacy for EDS is comparable to modafinil; the same holds true for side effects.[19] Because of the different mode of action, it can be combined with other stimulants and with SXB. However, scientific data regarding combination with other stimulants are currently lacking. Pitolisant is not registered for the treatment of IH, although there are encouraging results in a published study with subjects suffering from IH.[21]

Pitolisant shares with modafinil the disadvantage of interaction with oral contraceptives, requiring dose adjustment of the oral contraceptives. However, recently, new studies have been initiated to assess whether the interaction is indeed clinically relevant.

SXB, the sodium salt of gamma-hydroxybutyrate (GHB), is a hypnotic and, therefore, prescribed for use during the night, with a shown beneficial effect on nocturnal sleep, EDS, and cataplexy.[22–24] It is a naturally occurring substance in the human brain and GHB receptors have been identified in the brain. However, the therapeutic effect of SXB seems to be mediated by the gamma-aminobutyric acid (GABA)-B receptor. Because of its very short half-life, 2 separate doses are required during the night. The usual starting dose is 2.25 g twice a night. The dose must be gradually increased, keeping in mind that the optimal daytime effects after a dose increase will reveal after weeks. Therefore, it usually takes several months to reach an optimal situation. Moreover, a relevant improvement of EDS is, in most patients, achieved only with higher doses (6–9 g/night).[24] Efficacy for

nocturnal sleep and/or cataplexy usually already occurs on lower dosages. The effect on EDS of higher doses seems to be similar to that of modafinil and side effects are, if present, usually mild.[24] The combination of both of these substances is even more effective.[24] The most frequent side effect is nausea, and the most disabling are enuresis, sleep walking, and uncommon but possible mood disturbance, including depression. Lowering the dose usually ends the enuresis and sleep walking. Mood disturbance may be a reason to discontinue the medication. Weight loss may also occur.[25]

In follow-up studies, there is no indication that tolerance develops and abrupt cessation does not induce rebound cataplexy. However, long-term clinical experience shows that a substantial proportion of patients may develop (some) tolerance for the sleep-promoting effects, although efficacy for the other symptoms remains.

SXB should not be used in conjunction with other sedatives or alcohol. If patients have consumed alcohol in the evening, they should omit 1 or both doses afterward. In patients with comorbid obstructive sleep apnea syndrome (OSAS), treatment should be closely monitored because SXB may worsen OSAS. Cotreatment with continuous positive airway pressure may be indicated.[26]

Unfortunately, there may be concern for misuse. Although potential threats related to misuse may result in hesitation in patients to take, and in physicians to prescribe, the substance, it is important to realize that when the drug is properly used it is safe and bears no risk for dependence, at least when used in the treatment of narcolepsy. There are few data for the use in IH and it is not registered for the treatment of IH.[17,27]

Treatment of cataplexy

Most studies concerning the treatment of the REM dissociation phenomena focused on cataplexy. Amelioration of cataplexy is generally associated with improvement of HHs and SP.[11] SXB and tricyclic antidepressants are the most effective treatments. The different tricyclic antidepressants all inhibit the reuptake of norepinephrine and serotonin, and are potent REM sleep inhibitors. The most commonly used ones are clomipramine in a low dose (10–50 mg/d) and imipramine, also in a relatively low dose.[11] As with stimulants, side effects are a drawback. Side effects are largely due to the anticholinergic properties. The most frequently reported are dry mouth, increased sweating, sexual dysfunction (impotence, delayed orgasm, and erection and ejaculation dysfunction), weight gain, tachycardia, constipation, blurred vision, and urinary retention. However, very low doses, up to 20 mg, are often remarkably effective and are seldom accompanied by significant side effects. Therefore, many clinicians consider clomipramine to be the treatment of choice. The most relevant drawback, even with low doses, is the occurrence of tolerance. Moreover, tricyclic antidepressants should never be stopped abruptly because of the risk of severe aggravation of cataplexy, which may lead to a status cataplecticus.

Many alternative antidepressants have been studied, especially selective serotonin reuptake inhibitors, and more selective noradrenergic reuptake inhibitors, such as fluoxetine, zimelidine, viloxazine, femoxetine, fluvoxamine, and paroxetine. These should be prescribed in the same dosages as used in the treatment of depression and, therefore, their side-effect profile seems not favorable compared with the side effects with low dosages of clomipramine. All these substances seem to act mainly via less selective desmethyl metabolites. In recent years, venlafaxine and atomoxetine have become very popular in the treatment of cataplexy, although there are no randomized placebo-controlled studies available. Acute withdrawal of these substances will also lead to rebound cataplexy.

SXB is the best studied drug in the treatment of cataplexy and is probably the most potent inhibitor in most patients.[23] It has never been compared with any antidepressant, so it is difficult to know whether it is really most effective in most patients. However, the relatively mild side-effect profile, as well as the broader action on the other symptoms of narcolepsy, such as disturbed nocturnal sleep and EDS, makes it a favorable option.

Several drugs may theoretically be expected to aggravate cataplexy but only prazosin, an alpha 1 antagonist, is reliably documented to treat arterial hypertension.

In recent studies, the recently registered histamine-3 antagonist pitolisant also showed to be effective in the treatment of cataplexy. However, its exact place in the treatment of cataplexy needs to be established.

Treatment of disturbed nocturnal sleep
Disturbed nocturnal sleep can be a major complaint of patients. Unfortunately, treatment options are limited because SXB is the only drug with a proven long-term effect on nocturnal sleep.[22] Short-term beneficial effects of benzodiazepines have been described. Although nocturnal sleep may (temporarily) be improved with benzodiazepines, improvement of EDS is not the rule. The efficacy of

baclofen, another GABA-B receptor agonist, has not been convincingly proved.[28] However, there are anecdotal reports of its efficacy. Occasionally, patients report on improvement when using cannabis or cannabidiol oil but there are no scientific studies performed with these substances or for this indication.

Treatment in children
Treatment of children suffering from narcolepsy does not differ significantly from treatment in adulthood, although hardly any treatment studies have focused on children. Behavioral problems as expressions of narcolepsy only occur at young age. There are indications that treatment of EDS may have a positive impact on behavior but studies focusing on this important symptom are urgently needed.

RECOMMENDATIONS FOR THE INITIATION OF PHARMACOLOGIC TREATMENT

Patients should continue the scheduled daytime naps and always start with 1 medication at a time. It is usually best to treat the most invalidating symptoms first. If this clearly is EDS, start with a stimulant, if it clearly is cataplexy and/or HHs, start with a low dose of clomipramine. If both disturbed nocturnal sleep and/or cataplexy are severe, SXB may be considered as first choice. Always start with a low dose and increase the dose based on history taking, keeping in mind the trade-off between efficacy and side effects. The exact place of pitolisant has to be determined. It may very well become a first-line drug in a subgroup of patients.

FUTURE PHARMACOLOGIC TREATMENTS
Idiopathic Hypersomnia

There are studies reporting on subjective improvement of EDS with clarithromycin, a negative allosteric modulator of the GABA-A receptor. However, its use is still controversial.[17] These studies need replication and, preferably, evidence for objective improvement and long-term safety.[17]

Flumazenil, an antagonist of benzodiazepine-binding domain in GABA-A receptors, improved subjective sleepiness and reaction time in a single-blind trial.[29] Also, its use is controversial. A phase II, dose-finding study of pentylenetetrazole (BTD-001–NCT02512588), another GABA-A antagonist for EDS in IH, is currently running.[17]

One observational study has shown SXB to be a potential effective treatment of IH.[27]

Narcolepsy

Because narcolepsy with cataplexy is presumed to be an autoimmune disorder, various immune modulating treatments have been proposed. Some have been applied in individual cases in which the diagnosis was made shortly after symptom onset, up to now without real convincing or promising results. Although these therapies may potentially prevent progression of the disorder and/or rescue cells that are attacked but not yet destroyed, the timing of such treatment is very difficult. Application after the appearance of cataplexy may already be too late because cataplexy probably occurs when more than 80% of the hypocretin (also named orexin) cells are lost. Initiation in an earlier phase is very difficult because there currently are no clinical signs or laboratory findings that reliably predict the evolution of narcolepsy without cataplexy to narcolepsy with cataplexy. Another problem is that immune modulating therapies may have serious side effects. With the currently available nonimmunologic treatments known to be safe and effective in most patients, and a normal life expectancy for those who suffer from narcolepsy, it is difficult from an ethical perspective to initiate studies with risk-bearing immune modulating therapies. Last, but not least, clinicians can currently only speculate about the autoimmune mechanisms involved in the development of narcolepsy. Therefore, it is impossible to make a rational choice for a specific immune-modulating therapy.

The most effective symptomatic treatment of narcolepsy would be expected to be treatment with hypocretin. Unfortunately, this is not as easy as may be expected. In a normal situation, hypocretin is locally produced in the brain and, as far as is known, only acts in the brain. When applied as a drug, it can hardly pass the blood brain barrier. Nasal application has been suggested as an alternative but this route may only be effective if active transport of hypocretin can be facilitated. Without such facilitation, the mucosa surface of the human nose will probably be too small to allow the uptake of enough hypocretin to induce a clinically significant effect. Currently, it is more probable that hypocretin agonists will be developed for therapeutic use than that nasal application will turn out to be feasible and effective.

Alternative symptomatic treatments currently under study include

- A new psychostimulant JZP-110 (solriamfetol), a dopaminergic and noradrenergic phenylalanine derivative: First results in narcolepsy are encouraging.[30] Several phase 3 studies will be completed soon.
- Long-acting SXB: A phase 3 study is currently being performed.
- Low-sodium formulation of SXB: A phase 3 study is currently running.

- In an animal study, it has been shown that modafinil, when coadministered with a connexin inhibitor, flecainide, is more effective than when administered alone.[31] Follow-up studies are expected.

SUMMARY

Lifestyle adjustment, in combination with symptomatic pharmacologic treatment, allows most patients, particularly those with an inability to stay awake, to live a relatively normal life. New pharmacologic substances show encouraging results in phase 2 and 3 studies to improve the current situation. More dedicated studies in IH, particularly in those who suffer from an increased need for sleep, are needed.

REFERENCES

1. American Academy of Sleep Medicine. The international classification of sleep disorders. 3rd edition. Darien (IL): American Academy of Sleep Medicine; 2014.
2. Overeem S, Mignot E, van Dijk JG, et al. Narcolepsy: clinical features, new pathophysiologic insights, and future perspectives. J Clin Neurophysiol 2001;18: 78–105.
3. Ruoff CM, Reaven NL, Funk SE, et al. High rates of psychiatric comorbidity in narcolepsy: findings from the burden of narcolepsy disease (BOND) study of 9,312 patients in the United States. J Clin Psychiatry 2017;78(2):171–6.
4. Postiglione E, Antelmi E, Pizza F, et al. The clinical spectrum of childhood narcolepsy. Sleep Med Rev 2018;38:70–85.
5. Silber MH, Krahn LE, Olson E, et al. The epidemiology of narcolepsy in Olmsted County, Minnesota: a population-based study. Sleep 2002;25:197–202.
6. Longstreth WT, Koepsell TD, Ton TG, et al. The epidemiology of narcolepsy. Sleep 2007;30:13–26.
7. Wijnans L, Lecomte C, de Vries C, et al. The incidence of narcolepsy in Europe: before, during, and after the influenza A(H1N1) pandemic and vaccination campaigns. Vaccine 2013;31(8): 1246–54.
8. Mullington J, Broughton R. Scheduled naps in the management of daytime sleepiness in narcolepsy-cataplexy. Sleep 1993;16:444–56.
9. Bruck D, Armstrong S, Coleman G. Sleepiness after glucose in narcolepsy. J Sleep Res 1994;3:171–9.
10. Wise MS, Arand DL, Auger RR, et al. Treatment of narcolepsy and other hypersomnias of central origin. Sleep 2007;30:1712–27.
11. Billiard M, Bassetti C, Dauvilliers Y, et al. EFNS guidelines on management of narcolepsy. Eur J Neurol 2006;13:1035–48.

12. Parkes JD, Dahlitz M. Amphetamine prescription. Sleep 1993;16:201–3.
13. Mitler MM, Aldrich MS, Koob GF, et al. Narcolepsy and its treatment with stimulants. ASDA standards of practice. Sleep 1994;17:352–71.
14. Ryan DH, Bray GA, Helmcke F, et al. Serial echocardiographic and clinical evaluation of valvular regurgitation before, during, and after treatment with fenfluramine or dexfenfluramine and mazindol or phentermine. Obes Res 1999;7:313–22.
15. Available at: http://www.ema.europa.eu/docs/en_GB/document_library/Referrals_document/Modafinil_31/WC500105597.pdf. Accessed March 26, 2018.
16. Lopez R, Arnulf I, Drouot X, et al. French consensus. Management of patients with hypersomnia: which strategy? Rev Neurol (Paris) 2017;173(1–2):8–18.
17. Evangelista E, Lopez R, Dauvilliers Y. Update on treatment for idiopathic hypersomnia. Expert Opin Investig Drugs 2018;27(2):187–92.
18. Mayer G, Benes H, Young P, et al. Modafinil in the treatment of idiopathic hypersomnia without long sleep time—a randomized, double-blind, placebo-controlled study. J Sleep Res 2015;24:74–81.
19. Dauvilliers Y, Bassetti C, Lammers GJ, et al, HARMONY I study group. Pitolisant versus placebo or modafinil in patients with narcolepsy: a double-blind, randomised trial. Lancet Neurol 2013;12(11):1068–75.
20. Szakacs Z, Dauvilliers Y, Mikhaylov V, et al, HARMONY-CTP study group. Safety and efficacy of pitolisant on cataplexy in patients with narcolepsy: a randomised, double-blind, placebo-controlled trial. Lancet Neurol 2017;16(3):200–7.
21. Leu-Semenescu S, Nittur N, Golmard J-L, et al. Effects of pitolisant, a histamine H3 inverse agonist, in drug-resistant idiopathic and symptomatic hypersomnia: a chart review. Sleep Med 2014;15:681–7.
22. Black J, Pardi D, Hornfeldt CS, et al. The nightly use of sodium oxybate is associated with a reduction in nocturnal sleep disruption: a double-blind, placebo-controlled study in patients with narcolepsy. J Clin Sleep Med 2010;6(6):596–602.
23. U.S. Xyrem Multicenter Study Group. Sodium oxybate demonstrates long-term efficacy for the treatment of cataplexy in patients with narcolepsy. Sleep Med 2004;5:119–23.
24. Black J, Houghton WC. Sodium oxybate improves excessive daytime sleepiness in narcolepsy. Sleep 2006;29:939–46.
25. Schinkelshoek MS, Smolders IM, Donjacour CE, et al. Decreased body mass index during treatment with sodium oxybate in narcolepsy type 1. J Sleep Res 2018. [Epub ahead of print].
26. Feldman NT. Clinical perspective: monitoring sodium oxybate-treated narcolepsy patients for the development of sleep-disordered breathing. Sleep Breath 2010;14(1):77–9.
27. Leu-Semenescu S, Louis P, Arnulf I. Benefits and risk of sodium oxybate in idiopathic hypersomnia versus narcolepsy type 1: a chart review. Sleep Med 2016;17:38–44.
28. Brown MA, Guilleminault C. A review of sodium oxybate and baclofen in the treatment of sleep disorders. Curr Pharm Des 2011;17(15):1430–5.
29. Trotti LM, Saini P, Koola C, et al. Flumazenil for the treatment of refractory hypersomnolence: clinical experience with 153 patients. J Clin Sleep Med 2016;12:1389–94.
30. Ruoff C, Swick TJ, Doekel R, et al. Effect of oral JZP-110 (ADX-N05) on wakefulness and sleepiness in adults with narcolepsy: a phase 2b study. Sleep 2016;39(7):1379–87.
31. Duchêne A, Perier M, Zhao Y, et al. Impact of astroglial connexins on modafinil pharmacological properties. Sleep 2016;39(6):1283–92.

Drugs Used in Parasomnia

Paola Proserpio, MD[a], Michele Terzaghi, MD[b], Raffaele Manni, MD[b],
Lino Nobili, MD, PhD[a,c],*

KEYWORDS

- Disorders of arousal • REM behavior disorder • Sleep-related eating disorder • Sleep enuresis
- Benzodiazepines • Clonazepam • Melatonin • Antidepressant drugs

KEY POINTS

- Nonrapid eye movement (NREM) parasomnias, especially during childhood, are often benign conditions, and pharmacologic therapy is usually unnecessary.
- There are no properly powered randomized controlled studies evaluating the efficacy of pharmacologic therapy for NREM parasomnias.
- The most commonly used drugs for NREM parasomnias are intermediate- and long-acting benzodiazepines and antidepressants. Anecdotal cases reported the efficacy of melatonergic agents and hydroxytryptophan.
- The pharmacologic treatment of rapid eye movement sleep behavior disorder is symptomatic, and the most commonly used drugs are clonazepam and melatonin.

INTRODUCTION

Parasomnias are defined as "undesirable physical events or experiences that occur during entry into sleep, within sleep, or during arousal from sleep."[1] Depending on the sleep stage of occurrence, they are classified as nonrapid eye movement (NREM)-related parasomnias (confusional arousals, sleepwalking, sleep terrors, and sleep-related eating disorder), rapid eye movement (REM)-related parasomnias (REM sleep behavior disorder [RBD], recurrent isolated sleep paralysis, and nightmare disorder), and other parasomnias (exploding head syndrome [EHS], sleep-related hallucinations, and sleep enuresis [SE]).[1]

Parasomnias are not generally associated with a primary complaint of insomnia or excessive sleepiness, although this last one may be present in some of them. On the other hand, parasomnias can be associated with possible resulting injuries, adverse health, and negative psychosocial effects. Moreover, the clinical consequences of parasomnias can affect the patient, parents, or both.

Parasomnias, especially disorders of arousal (DOA) during childhood, are often relatively benign and transitory and do not usually require a pharmacologic therapy. A relevant aspect in both NREM and REM parasomnia treatment is to prevent sleep-related injuries by maintaining a safe environment. Physicians should always evaluate the possible presence of favoring and precipitating factors (sleep disorders and drugs). A pharmacologic treatment may be indicated in case of frequent, troublesome, or particularly dangerous events. The aim of this article is to review current available evidence on pharmacologic treatment of different forms of parasomnia.

NON RAPID EYE MOVEMENT PARASOMNIAS
Disorder of Arousal from Non Rapid Eye Movement Sleep

DOA are the subgroup of parasomnias arising from NREM sleep, encompassing confusional arousals, sleep terrors, and sleep walking.[1] They are most prevalent during childhood and normally cease

[a] Department of Neuroscience, Centre of Sleep Medicine, Centre for Epilepsy Surgery, Niguarda Hospital, Piazza Ospedale Maggiore, Milan 3-20162, Italy; [b] Sleep Medicine and Epilepsy, IRCCS Mondino Foundation, Via Mondino, Pavia 2-27100, Italy; [c] Department of Neuroscience (DINOGMI), University of Genoa, Child neuropsychiatry, Gaslini Institute, Via Gerolamo Gaslini, Genoa 5-16147, Italy
* Corresponding author. Department of Neuroscience, Centre of Sleep Medicine, Niguarda Hospital, Piazza Ospedale Maggiore, Milan 3-20162, Italy
E-mail address: lino.nobili@ospedaleniguarda.it

Sleep Med Clin 13 (2018) 191–202
https://doi.org/10.1016/j.jsmc.2018.02.003

by adolescence, but onset or persistence during adulthood is well recognized.[2] More than one type may coexist within the same patient.[3] Many clinical features are common to these manifestations.[4,5] First, they generally occur during deep NREM sleep (N3) and, thus, most often take place in the first third of the night. During the episode, patients are usually unresponsive to the environment and completely or partially amnestic after the event. A positive family history is frequently found in DOA. Finally, any factor that deepens (sleep deprivation, stress, febrile illness, medications, alcohol) or fragments sleep (external or internal stimuli, sleep disorders, mental activity) may increase the occurrence of DOA.

DOA are generally considered benign phenomena. However, especially in adults, they can be characterized by complex behavior with potentially violent or injurious features[6] or be associated with significant functional impairment, such as daytime sleepiness, fatigue, and distress.[7] Therefore, evaluation and treatment are recommended in these cases, especially when violent manifestations are frequent or very disturbing for the patient or other family members.

The management of DOA is not well codified. No drug has yet been approved, and there are no properly powered randomized controlled studies evaluating the efficacy of behavioral or pharmacologic interventions for DOA.[8] Current treatment recommendations are based on scarce evidence derived from expert opinions, case reports, and only few case series. To date, the largest retrospective case series, analyzing treatment options and efficacy in DOA, refers to a population of 103 adults.[9]

Only recently, a self-administered scale has been developed with the aim of providing a valid and reliable tool able to assess the diagnosis and severity of NREM parasomnia as well as to monitor the efficacy of treatment.[10] Considering that evidence is lacking for off-label use of pharmacologic agents, clinicians may wish to ensure that patients are fully informed about all therapeutic options.[8]

Nonpharmacologic treatment
As previously discussed, if the episodes are rare, or not associated with harm potential, treatment is often unnecessary. Management includes reassuring patients about the usual benign nature of the episodes. Parents or bed partners should be instructed to keep calm and not to insist in trying to awaken the patient because this may aggravate or lengthen the episodes.[11] Precautions should be taken to ensure a safe sleep environment. Simple safety measures can include the removal of

obstructions in the bedroom, securing windows, sleeping on the ground floor, and installing locks or alarms on windows, doors, and stairways.[4,11]

Every priming or triggering factor should be investigated and avoided. For instance, every effort should be made to ensure regular and adequate sleep routines, to prevent sleep loss or disruption of the sleep-wake cycle. Sleep disorders (sleep apnea or periodic leg movements) must be recognized and treated.[12] Moreover, patients should avoid the intake of drugs or substances that could favor the occurrence of episodes (alcohol, hypnotics, antipsychotics, antidepressants, antihistamines).

Some investigators proposed "scheduled awakenings" in the case of DOA occurring nightly and consistently at or around the same time each night.[13] In adults, a psychological approach may be considered (hypnosis, relaxation therapy, or cognitive behavioral therapy), although studies evaluating its efficacy have provided contrasting results.[14,15]

Pharmacologic treatment
The main indications for a pharmacologic treatment in patients with DOA encompass the following: (1) persistence of frequent episodes despite resolution and removal of all potential predisposing and precipitating factors; (2) high risk of injury for the patient or the family; (3) significant functional impairment (such as insomnia, daytime sleepiness, weight gain from nocturnal eating); (4) potential legal consequences related to sexual or violent behavior.

As illustrated above, if drug therapy is planned, patients or their parents should be advised that drugs for DOA are considered "off label" and, if the decision is to prescribe, a patient's written consent is recommended.

Benzodiazepines Intermediate and long-acting agents in the benzodiazepine class of sedative hypnotics (BZD) are the most frequently used treatment of DOA.[4,11,16] although they have never been approved for this indication. They act by increasing the chloride conductance through GABA A receptors,[17] thus inducing a hypnotic-sedative effect. It is worth reminding that BDZ may have muscle-relaxing properties and should be used with caution if comorbid sleep-disordered breathing is suspected. The use of BZD in the treatment of DOA is apparently paradoxic, considering that other sedative-hypnotics such as non-BZD receptor agonists can induce amnestic nocturnal behavior.[18] The exact mechanism by which BZD suppress DOA is unknown. Probably, their effectiveness may be related to sedative effects or to decreases in slow-wave sleep.[19] Alternatively, they may work through the suppression of cortical arousals.[16]

Among the BZD class, clonazepam at 0.5 to 2 mg is the most common medication used in the treatment of DOA. However, studies (mainly conducted in adults) in the last 2 decades showed conflicting results. To date, only small case series, analyzing the efficacy of BDZ in children,[20] have been published. In 1989, Schenck and colleagues[21] studied 100 consecutive adults referred to their sleep disorders center for repeated nocturnal injury. All patients underwent full polysomnographic recordings. Fifty-four of these patients were diagnosed with either sleep terrors or sleepwalking. Clonazepam was prescribed for 28 of these patients and a rapid and sustained response was observed in 83.6% of them. A few years later, the same group published the results of a study designed to look for safety and abuse of BZDs taken for sleep disorders.[22] They analyzed 170 adults with sleep-related injuries of whom 69 had either sleepwalking or sleep terrors and were treated with BDZ, essentially clonazepam (n = 58) but also alprazolam. Most patients (86%) reported good control after an average follow-up of 3.5 years. The mean dose for clonazepam at the end of the study was 1.10 ± 0.96 mg. Interestingly, the risk of dosage escalation was low. In a more recent case series, Attarian and Zhu[9] analyzed the response to various therapeutic modalities in 103 adults with DOA. They found that clonazepam (0.5–2 mg) was used in 55% of the patients with a high response to treatment (73.7%).

Conversely, in another report, 5 patients with sleepwalking treated with clonazepam reported persistence of nocturnal episodes after 1 year of follow-up.[15]

Clonazepam has also been used successfully in somnambulism induced by neuroleptics,[23] and in DOA with behaviors such as driving and sleep violence.[22,24]

Anecdotal data have shown that patients with DOA respond to diazepam (2 to 5 mg).[25] However, in a small double-blind placebo-controlled crossover study of diazepam in sleepwalking, results failed to show significant difference between placebo and diazepam,[26] although investigators stated that in some participants, there was an alleviation of self-reported symptoms. Other BZDs that have been shown to be effective include triazolam (0.25 mg) at bedtime[27] and flurazepam.[28]

Antidepressant drugs Antidepressant drugs are occasionally effective in the treatment of DOA.[4,29] In the already mentioned recent largest

case series study,[9] 4 patients responded to sertraline and 2 responded to clomipramine.

Anecdotal data reported efficacy of tricyclic antidepressant (imipramine or clomipramine) and trazodone. For instance, 2 patients with a history of sleep terrors and sleepwalking, in both of whom diazepam therapy failed, responded well to imipramine.[30] Conversely, trazodone provided a remarkable relief of symptoms in a 7-year-old girl who suffered from a severe sleep terror disorder, previously treated unsuccessfully with imipramine.[31]

Serotoninergic antidepressants, especially paroxetine, have been reported to be particularly effective in the treatment of sleep terrors. Indeed, a small case series showed a significant reduction of sleep terror events in 6 patients.[32] The investigators suggested that selective serotonin reuptake inhibitors (SSRI) may improve sleep terrors by virtue of serotonergic effects on the mesencephalic periaqueductal gray matter. Considering sleepwalking, a single case report showed the efficacy of paroxetine,[33,34] whereas other evidence reported a paroxetine inducing somnambulism.[35]

The mechanism by which antidepressant medications would influence DOA remains unclear, especially in light of these contradictory results. Indeed, the different efficacy of serotonin in sleepwalking and sleep terrors could suggest possible distinct pathophysiologic mechanisms at the basis of these manifestations.[4]

Other drugs Single case reports have shown the efficacy of other pharmacologic treatments, such as melatonin, hydroxytryptophan, and ramelteon.

Melatonin (N-acetyl-5-methoxytryptamine) is an endogenous hormone produced by the pineal gland and released exclusively at night. Exogenous melatonin supplementation is well tolerated and has no significant adverse effects and a low potential for dependence. Melatonin has been shown to synchronize the circadian rhythms and improve the onset, duration, and quality of sleep. Thus, melatonin seems to represent an alternative treatment of sleep disorders with significantly less side effects.[36] Moreover, melatonin has been shown to be particularly useful for treatment of sleep disorders in children with neurodevelopmental disabilities.[37] To date, only 2 case reports showed its efficacy in the treatment of DOA. In particular, Jan and colleagues[38] described a 12-year-old patient affected by Asperger syndrome and a chronic sleep-phase onset delay in whom melatonin was effective in the treatment of sleepwalking and sleep terror episodes. However, its efficacy could be related mainly to the correction of the circadian disorder and the consequent improvement of the underlying sleep deprivation. More recently, Özcan and Dönmez[39] reported the efficacy of treatment with melatonin for 2 weeks in a 36-month-old patient with sleep terror.

An open pharmacologic trial conducted in 45 children with sleep terror demonstrated the efficacy of L-5-hydroxytryptophan, a precursor of serotonin, in 83.9% of patients after 6 months of therapy.[40] The investigators hypothesized that this drug could induce a long-term improvement of sleep terrors through a stabilization of the sleep microstructure and a modulation of the arousal level in children.

Finally, Sasayama and colleagues[41] recently reported a boy with attention-deficit/hyperactivity disorder whose night terrors and sleepwalking were effectively treated with ramelteon, a melatonin receptor agonist, probably improving sleep deprivation.

SLEEP-RELATED EATING DISORDER

Sleep-related eating disorder (SRED) is an NREM sleep parasomnia characterized by frequent episodes of dysfunctional and involuntary eating and drinking that occur after an arousal during NREM sleep associated with diminished levels of consciousness and subsequent recall, with problematic health consequences.[1] This sleep disorder generally starts in young adults, with a female predominance.[42] SRED is sometimes associated with the use of psychotropic drugs (triazolam, zolpidem, amitriptyline, olanzapine, and risperidone) and other sleep disorders, including parasomnias, narcolepsy, restless legs syndrome, and periodic leg movements.[43] Thus, the first goal of treatment is to eliminate any precipitating factors and to recognize and treat any comorbid sleep disorders. Indeed, removal of any offending drug together with treatment of sleep disturbances has been shown to resolve many cases of SRED.[43,44] Moreover, the nonpharmacologic treatment plan should also include education regarding proper sleep hygiene, the maintenance of a safe sleep environment, and the limitation of other precipitating factors, such as cigarette smoking or alcohol intake.[45–47]

The preferred drugs used for treatment of SRED are represented by dopamine agonists, BZDs, topiramate, and SSRI.[47,48(p2)]

A randomized, double-blind, placebo-controlled crossover study of pramipexole (0.18–0.36 mg/d) on 11 SRED subjects demonstrated improvement in sleep quality and actigraphic measures.[49] Nevertheless, number and duration of waking episodes related to eating behaviors were unchanged, and no weight loss was observed. A more recent work confirmed the efficacy of dopamine agonist in 3 patients with SRED.[50] Interestingly, other dopaminergic agents, such as carbidopa/L-dopa and bromocriptine as monotherapy, were effective in 25% of the patients with SRED associated with sleepwalking, and in combination with BZDs (mainly clonazepam), opiates, or both in approximately 87% of subjects.[51]

SSRI (fluoxetine, paroxetine, and fluvoxamine) were reportedly effective in 2 different studies.[51,52]

Substantial reduction of sleep-related eating episodes and significant weight loss have been achieved in subjects treated with topiramate, an antiepileptic drug that induces weight loss.[50,53–55] In particular, Winkelman[55] reported that 68% of patients responded to topiramate, with a mean dose of 135 mg/d, but the discontinuation rate was high, because of side effects, including dullness, paresthesia, and daytime sleepiness. In a more recent study, 20 patients with SRED were treated with topiramate, 17 of whom showed cessation or a clear reduction in night eating episodes, whereas 6 (30%) had to discontinue medication because of adverse effects (eg, dizziness, visual problems, and worsening of preexisting depressive symptoms).[50] Physicians should follow up patients regularly with SRED treated with topiramate in order to promptly recognize and treat side effects.[47] It is unclear how topiramate works to decrease SRED manifestations. It was hypothesized that the drug may work by suppressing arousals produced by underlying sleep disorders or by acting as an anorexigenic agent, either through glutamatergic antagonism or serotonergic agonism.[54] Moreover, topiramate has been reported to stimulate insulin release and increase insulin sensitivity, both of which may contribute to appetite regulation and weight loss.[56]

Zapp and colleagues[57] recently described a case of a patient with SRED associated with the use of various antidepressants and sleep apnea that completely vanished after treatment with agomelatine or melatonin extended release.

RAPID EYE MOVEMENT PARASOMNIAS
Rapid Eye Movement Sleep Behavior Disorder

RBD treatment is currently based on a symptomatic approach, because interventions to prevent or slow the conversion toward neurodegenerative diseases in susceptible subjects are not available at the moment.

Sleep-related injuries are frequent and reported in up to 65% of RBD cases,[58–60] so that RBD subjects should be offered a treatment immediately following the diagnosis. Symptomatic treatment is aimed at preventing injuries to the patient and/or to the bed partner by reducing the frequency and severity of dream-enacted behaviors. Effects on dream content and sleep quality should also be considered when optimizing RBD pharmacologic interventions.

In the management of RBD subjects, clinicians should also be aware of the possibility that ongoing pharmacologic treatment with antidepressants, particularly SSRIs, can have an impact on RBD, worsening its manifestations.[61]

Despite the importance of establishing treatment, research found a limited number of drugs effective in RBD, and current knowledge about efficacy and tolerability profile of drugs used in RBD subjects is still based on low-level evidence data based on case reports and case series.[62] Thus, adequately powered controlled trials addressing drug effects in this category are needed.

Clonazepam

The effectiveness of clonazepam on RBD was reported in the seminal paper from Schenck and colleagues,[63] and since then, it has been widely used for RBD treatment as first-choice therapy. Its efficacy is reflected in a complete remission of symptoms in 55% to 90% of RBD subjects.[60] In a recent open-label study of the effect of clonazepam up to 3 mg, the figure of RBD subjects defined as responders (ie, absence of injuries and potential injurious behaviors to self and/or to bed partner) was reported to be 66.7%.[64] Clonazepam doses are between 0.25 and 4.0 mg at bedtime, with 0.5 mg appearing to be a suitable dosage for most of the subjects.[65]

Although RBD symptoms occur after discontinuation of clonazepam,[62] they usually are easily controlled by the resumption of therapy. Tolerance and withdrawal symptoms only rarely occur, even if complaints of insomnia and unsatisfactory sleep quality can be reported.[62] Main side effects, such as early morning sedation, incoordination, falls, confusion, memory impairment, sexual dysfunctions, and worsening of sleep-disordered breathing, can occur.[62] Clonazepam does not influence the occurrence of dreams with emotional or sorrowful content, but results in a reduction of the frequency of nightmares and dreams with violent and frightening content, paralleled by the reduction in potential injurious behaviors.[64] In consideration of the side-effect profile of the drug, caution is needed in elderly subjects for the possibility to impair both postural instability and cognitive performances, up to the occurrence of confusional states in subjects with cognitive decline.[66]

Furthermore, clonazepam should be prescribed at the lowest effective dose in patients with sleep apnea, and respiratory pattern should be assessed during treatment.

Melatonin

Exogenous melatonin has been shown as being approximately equally effective at reducing RBD severity in respect to clonazepam.[62,65,67] In a comparative study to clonazepam, melatonin resulted in better tolerability, with subjects taking clonazepam reporting more frequently drowsiness, instability, and neuropsychological impairment.[65] Differently from clonazepam, melatonin has univocal evidence of restoring REM sleep muscle atonia.[68] Melatonin dosages are 2 mg to 12 mg at bedtime. Melatonin at a median dosage of 6 mg proved to be as effective in reducing RBD behavior as clonazepam (0.5 mg).[65] These doses are usually well tolerated, despite dose-dependent side effects, such as morning headache, sleepiness, delusions, and hallucinations.[69]

Because of its profile of effectiveness and tolerability, melatonin is a valid option in RBD subjects and can be preferred to clonazepam in the case of background disease features, consisting of sleep-disordered breathing, disorders of gait and unsteadiness, or cognitive impairment.

Melatonergic agents

On the basis of the effectiveness and tolerability profile of exogenous melatonin, melatoninergic agents are expected to benefit RBD subjects. Effects of ramelteon at doses of 8 mg/d (in improving RBD control in subjects affected by extrapyramidal disorders[70]) were not confirmed on objective polysomnographic assessment of RBD behavior and REM sleep without atonia (RSWA), despite a subjective reduction in dream enactment frequency and severity.[71,72] In the same way, agomelatine (25 mg) proved to improve RBD symptoms in idiopathic RBD, but did not change RBD motor events frequency and RSWA on polysomnographic assessment.[73]

Dopamine agonists

Controversial results were carried out by efforts in treating RBD with pramipexole. Pramipexole was reported to reduce RBD symptoms[74–76] and seems to be effective mainly in the form of RBD with limited loss of atonia.[75] However, no changes were found in RBD subjects with extrapyramidal disorders on clinical or polysomnographic grounds.[77] All in all, pramipexole should be considered when other treatments have failed to control RBD. Since its efficacy in restless legs syndrome, pramipexole can be considered initial treatment of subjects with comorbid restless legs syndrome, but deserves a short-interval follow-up visit to assess RBD evolution.

Acetylcholinesterase inhibitors

Use of acetylcholinesterase inhibitors for RBD treatment is based on the notion that cholinergic mechanisms are central for the initiation and co-ordination of REM sleep.[78] Furthermore, in dementia with Lewy bodies, in which cholinergic transmission is impaired, administration of acetylcholinesterase inhibitor was reported to potentially restore correct sleep patterns and resolve nocturnal confusional events.[79,80]

However, conflicting data are reported in the literature about acetylcholinesterase inhibitor's efficacy in RBD.

Acetylcholinesterase inhibitors donepezil and rivastigmine were reported to reduce RBD behavior.[62,81–84] On the other hand, no changes in RBD in subjects with comorbid neurodegenerative diseases could be found,[69] and even the occurrence of de novo RBD was reported in a patient with Alzheimer disease.[85] Altogether, considering the limited and conflicting data about the efficacy of acetylcholinesterase inhibitors in RBD, these drugs should be used as a third-line treatment analogously to pramipexole, in cases of clonazepam or melatonin failure. Because the possibility that RBD occurs in the context of cognitive impairment, acetylcholinesterase inhibitors can be used in symptomatic RBD patients requiring concurrent treatment of cognitive impairment or hallucinations (ie, dementia with Lewy bodies and Parkinson disease dementia).

Cannabidiol

There has been evidence that suggests that cannabis may have therapeutic potential in several neurologic disorders, and sleep in particular.[86] Data on the effect of cannabinoids on RBD are limited, but the efficacy of cannabidiol, the nonintoxicating constituent of cannabis, in ameliorating RBD in subjects with Parkinson disease was reported, together with a good tolerability profile.[87]

Miscellaneous

For BZDs other than clonazepam, temazepam as monotherapy or in association to zopiclone,[88,89] triazolam,[60] and alprazolam[22] were used in RBD, suggesting that they may have a class-specific effect. Zopiclone appears to be effective and well tolerated in reducing RBD symptoms.[88] Herbal derivates, as Yi-Gan San[90] or Yokukansan, which contain exactly measured mixtures of dried herbs, can be effective in improving RBD symptoms. Sodium oxybate can be an effective add-on option for the treatment of idiopathic RBD, refractory to conventional therapies, despite a lack of improvement in polysomnographic parameters.[91,92]

Nightmare Disorder

The therapeutic approach to nightmares encompasses nonpharmacologic as well as pharmacologic options. Although psychotherapy and cognitive behavior interventions have traditionally been the treatment of choice, drugs alone or in combination therapy can be used as an alternative to psychological interventions.

In the evaluation of nightmares, it should be kept in mind that numerous drugs can trigger nightmares and vivid dreams, among which are catecholaminergic agents, β-blockers, barbiturates, dopaminergic agents, and alcohol and even some antidepressants. Several drugs classes, including SSRIs, tricyclic antidepressants, antipsychotics, and adrenergic agonists, were studied in nightmare disorder.[93–95] Some lines of evidence show that risperidone, trazodone, clonidine, quetiapine, fluvoxamine, mirtazapine, and terazosin can be helpful.[95] However, data are limited, and the quality of evidence is poor.[62]

Prazosin

Prazosin is a centrally acting selective α1-adrenergic antagonist and has been considered efficacious as pharmacologic treatment of nightmares, especially in cases of posttraumatic nightmares, with a good profile of tolerability.[96–98] The relapse of nightmares following discontinuation of prazosin was reported, showing the need for long-term use.[99] However, recent data put into discussion the results from previous studies,[100] and data showing no effect of prazosin on nightmare frequency were reported.[95]

Cannabinoids

The use of tetrahydrocannabinol in the treatment of nightmares associated with posttraumatic stress disorder was reported to result in the reduction of nightmare recurrence and intensity.[101–104] A good profile of tolerability accompanied the drug,[104] with dry mouth, headache, and dizziness being the more frequently reported symptoms.

RECURRENT ISOLATED SLEEP PARALYSIS

It should be carefully considered whether to pharmacologically treat sleep paralysis episodes or not. Most of the patients with sleep paralysis do not experience clinically significant distress, and basic treatment is avoidance of sleep deprivation and other precipitants. In the case of recurrent sleep paralysis and significant clinical distress, the cost/benefit balance of drug therapy should be considered. A substantial lack of systematic data in this field leads personal experience to have a central role in the choice of the drug.

Pharmacologic intervention is based on the possibility of suppressing REM sleep, and tricyclic antidepressants (clomipramine, imipramine, desmethylimipramine)[105–107] and SSRIs (fluoxetine, femoxetine, and viloxazine)[107–109] can be considered. Sodium oxybate is a possible therapy for sleep paralysis in narcolepsy.[110]

OTHER PARASOMNIAS
Exploding Head Syndrome

EHS is characterized by a "sudden, loud imagined noise or sense of a violent explosion in the head occurring as the patient is falling asleep or waking during the night."[1]

To date, no open or controlled clinical trials for EHS treatment are available, but several case studies of effective treatment have been conducted.[111,112] In many cases, reassurance about the benign nature of EHS could lead to a remission of EHS episodes. Tricyclic antidepressants (clomipramine, amitriptyline) are reported to decrease the frequency and intensity of attacks in some patients.[111,113] Moreover, calcium channel blockers (flunarizine and slow-release nifedipine) may also be useful.[114,115] Finally, anticonvulsants have been prescribed in some cases. Topiramate reduced the intensity of auditory sounds from loud bangs to much softer buzzing sounds, but without a complete remission.[116] Carbamazepine was described to be effective in 3 cases.[112]

Sleep-Related Hallucinations

Sleep-related hallucinations are "hallucinatory experiences that occur at sleep onset (hypnagogic) or on awakening from sleep (hypnopompic)."[1] They can be associated with narcolepsy, but a high prevalence in the normal population is also described. Complex nocturnal visual hallucinations are often associated with different disorders, especially in elderly, such as visual loss (Charles Bonnet syndrome), Lewy body disorders, and pathologic abnormality of the mesencephalon and diencephalon (peduncular hallucinosis).

Little objective information is available regarding the management of sleep-related hallucinations. Reassurance is frequently sufficient. Tricyclic antidepressants have been suggested for hypnagogic and hypnopompic hallucinations.

Sleep Enuresis

SE is characterized by "recurrent involuntary voiding that occurs during sleep. In primary SE,

recurrent involuntary voiding occurs at least twice a week during sleep after 5 years of age in a subject who has never been consistently dry during sleep for 6 consecutive months. SE is considered secondary in a child or adult who had previously been dry for 6 consecutive months and then began wetting at least twice a week. Both primary and secondary enuresis must be present for a period of at least 3 months."[1] Moreover, SE is defined as *monosymptomatic* when the subject has no associated daytime symptoms of bladder dysfunction (such as wetting, increased voiding frequency, urgency, jiggling, squatting, and holding maneuvers). However, usually, when a meticulous history is obtained, most children have at least some mild daytime void symptoms, and their SE is classifiable as *non-monosymptomatic*.[117]

The management of SE starts from some simple strategies, such as lifting or wakening, rewarding dry nights, bladder training (including retention control training), and fluid restriction.[117–119] On the other hand, it has been suggested that children should be encouraged to maintain an adequate fluid intake, because fluid restriction can worsen bladder function.[120] Alarm systems that alert and awaken the child if any moisture is detected are considered a first-line treatment, and its effect seems to be more gradual but sustained with respect to drugs.[121]

The established drug treatment for polyuric bedwetting is desmopressin, a synthetic analogue of the pituitary hormone arginine vasopressin, which reduces urine production by increasing water absorption.[119,120] It is available in tablet or fastmelting oral lyophilisate form. Desmopressin should be taken 1 hour before going to sleep. Treatment begins with a 0.2-mg desmopressin tablet or 120 µg of the melt tablet. If the starting dose does not lead to a clinical response, after 14 days the dose can be increased up to 0.4 mg or 240 µg. If treatment is successful, it can continue to be prescribed in 3-month blocks.[119] The sudden discontinuation of desmopressin results in a high recurrence of enuresis.[122] Desmopressin is considered a safe drug. The rare and most severe side effect of oral desmopressin therapy is the risk of "water intoxication" (if medication intake coincides with drinking large volumes) with symptoms of vomiting, headache, decreased consciousness, possible seizures, and hyponatremia. Therefore, fluid intake in the evening should be restricted to 250 mL, and night-time drinking is not recommended. This complication seems to be more frequent during therapy with intranasal formulation of desmopressin.[123] Desmopressin is mostly indicated in children with nocturnal polyuria and normal bladder reservoir function and in those in whom alarm therapy has failed or who are thought to be unlikely to comply with alarm therapy.[124] It is frequently used as a stopgap (sleepovers and school camps) rather than cure for long term. About 30% of children with enuresis are full responders, and 40% have a partial response to desmopressin.[124] However, the long-lasting curative effect is low.[125]

The tricyclic antidepressant imipramine has anticholinergic, antispasmodic, and local anesthetic effects, and possibly a central nervous system effect on voiding, and has been approved for use in treating nocturnal enuresis in children aged 6 years and older.[126] It is effective in about 40% of patients with enuresis, but only 25% of them experience complete dryness once the medication is withdrawn.[127] Side effects encompass cardiac arrhythmias, hypotension, hepatotoxicity, central nervous system depression, interaction with other drugs, and the danger of intoxication by accidental overdose. Therefore, screening for a long QT syndrome with electrocardiogram before starting treatment is recommended.

Anticholinergic drugs are used for SE, mainly for non-monosymptomatic cases.[117–120] They are thought to act by increasing the functional bladder capacity and enabling patients affected to achieve better control over micturition. The anticholinergic drug most frequently used is represented by oxybutynin (0.1–0.3 mg/kg/d), although it has considerable risk of side effects (flushing, blurred vision, constipation, tremor, decreased salivation, and decreased ability to sweat) because of its relatively nonspecific affinity for several cholinergic receptor isoforms. The fourth International Consultation on Incontinence[128] recommended the use of propiverine (0.8–1 mg/kg/d) as first-line medication for non-monosymptomatic SE (level of evidence 1, grade of recommendation B/C). Recent studies have shown the efficacy and safety of other anticholinergic drugs, such as trospium chloride, solifenacin,[129] and tolterodine[130] in children.

Although anticholinergic monotherapy could be ineffective, it can improve treatment response when combined with other established treatments, such as imipramine, desmopressin, or enuresis alarms, particularly in treatment-resistant cases.[131] Indeed, a recent meta-analysis demonstrated that the combination therapy, comprising desmopressin plus an anticholinergic agent, was more effective compared with desmopressin monotherapy for the treatment of SE in children.[132]

REFERENCES

1. American Academy of Sleep Medicine. International classification of sleep disorders-third edition (ICSD-3). Darien (Illinois); 2014.
2. Stallman HM, Kohler M. Prevalence of sleepwalking: a systematic review and meta-analysis. PLoS One 2016;11(11):e0164769.
3. Derry CP, Harvey AS, Walker MC, et al. NREM arousal parasomnias and their distinction from nocturnal frontal lobe epilepsy: a video EEG analysis. Sleep 2009;32(12):1637–44.
4. Howell MJ. Parasomnias: an updated review. Neurotherapeutics 2012;9(4):753–75.
5. Zadra A, Desautels A, Petit D, et al. Somnambulism: clinical aspects and pathophysiological hypotheses. Lancet Neurol 2013;12(3):285–94.
6. Siclari F, Khatami R, Urbaniok F, et al. Violence in sleep. Brain 2010;133(12):3494–509.
7. Lopez R, Jaussent I, Scholz S, et al. Functional impairment in adult sleepwalkers: a case-control study. Sleep 2013;36(3):345–51.
8. Harris M, Grunstein RR. Treatments for somnambulism in adults: assessing the evidence. Sleep Med Rev 2009;13(4):295–7.
9. Attarian H, Zhu L. Treatment options for disorders of arousal: a case series. Int J Neurosci 2013;123(9):623–5.
10. Arnulf I, Zhang B, Uguccioni G, et al. A scale for assessing the severity of arousal disorders. Sleep 2014;37(1):127–36.
11. Attarian H. Treatment options for parasomnias. Neurol Clin 2010;28(4):1089–106.
12. Tinuper P, Bisulli F, Provini F. The parasomnias: mechanisms and treatment: the parasomnias: mechanisms and treatment. Epilepsia 2012;53:12–9.
13. Kotagal S. Treatment of dyssomnias and parasomnias in childhood. Curr Treat Options Neurol 2012;14(6):630–49.
14. Galbiati A, Rinaldi F, Giora E, et al. Behavioural and cognitive-behavioural treatments of parasomnias. Behav Neurol 2015;2015:786928.
15. Guilleminault C, Kirisoglu C, Bao G, et al. Adult chronic sleepwalking and its treatment based on polysomnography. Brain 2005;128(Pt 5):1062–9.
16. Cochen De Cock V. Sleepwalking. Curr Treat Options Neurol 2016;18(2):6.
17. Rudolph U, Möhler H. GABA-based therapeutic approaches: GABAA receptor subtype functions. Curr Opin Pharmacol 2006;6(1):18–23.
18. Dolder CR, Nelson MH. Hypnosedative-induced complex behaviours: incidence, mechanisms and management. CNS Drugs 2008;22(12):1021–36.
19. Mason TBA, Pack AI. Sleep terrors in childhood. J Pediatr 2005;147(3):388–92.
20. Allen RM. Attenuation of drug-induced anxiety dreams and pavor nocturnus by benzodiazepines. J Clin Psychiatry 1983;44(3):106–8.
21. Schenck CH, Milner DM, Hurwitz TD, et al. A polysomnographic and clinical report on sleep-related injury in 100 adult patients. Am J Psychiatry 1989;146(9):1166–73.

22. Schenck CH, Mahowald MW. Long-term, nightly benzodiazepine treatment of injurious parasomnias and other disorders of disrupted nocturnal sleep in 170 adults. Am J Med 1996;100(3):333–7.
23. Goldbloom D, Chouinard G. Clonazepam in the treatment of neuroleptic-induced somnambulism. Am J Psychiatry 1984;141(11):1486.
24. Schenck CH, Mahowald MW. A polysomnographically documented case of adult somnambulism with long-distance automobile driving and frequent nocturnal violence: parasomnia with continuing danger as a noninsane automatism? Sleep 1995; 18(9):765–72.
25. Remulla A, Guilleminault C. Somnambulism (sleepwalking). Expert Opin Pharmacother 2004;5(10): 2069–74.
26. Reid WH, Haffke EA, Chu CC. Diazepam in intractable sleepwalking: a pilot study. Hillside J Clin Psychiatry 1984;6(1):49–55.
27. Berlin RM, Qayyum U. Sleepwalking: diagnosis and treatment through the life cycle. Psychosomatics 1986;27(11):755–60.
28. Kavey NB, Whyte J, Resor SR, et al. Somnambulism in adults. Neurology 1990;40(5):749–52.
29. Kierlin L, Littner MR. Parasomnias and antidepressant therapy: a review of the literature. Front Psychiatry 2011;2:71.
30. Cooper AJ. Treatment of coexistent night-terrors and somnambulism in adults with imipramine and diazepam. J Clin Psychiatry 1987;48(5):209–10.
31. Balon R. Sleep terror disorder and insomnia treated with trazodone: a case report. Ann Clin Psychiatry 1994;6(3):161–3.
32. Wilson SJ, Lillywhite AR, Potokar JP, et al. Adult night terrors and paroxetine. Lancet 1997; 350(9072):185.
33. Frölich Alfred Wiater Gerd Lehmkuhl J. Successful treatment of severe parasomnias with paroxetine in a 12-year-old boy. Int J Psychiatry Clin Pract 2001; 5(3):215–8.
34. Lillywhite AR, Wilson SJ, Nutt DJ. Successful treatment of night terrors and somnambulism with paroxetine. Br J Psychiatry 1994;164(4):551–4.
35. Kawashima T, Yamada S. Paroxetine-induced somnambulism. J Clin Psychiatry 2003;64(4):483.
36. Xie Z, Chen F, Li WA, et al. A review of sleep disorders and melatonin. Neurol Res 2017;39(6): 559–65.
37. Jan JE, Freeman RD. Melatonin therapy for circadian rhythm sleep disorders in children with multiple disabilities: what have we learned in the last decade? Dev Med Child Neurol 2004;46(11): 776–82.
38. Jan JE, Freeman RD, Wasdell MB, et al. A child with severe night terrors and sleep-walking responds to melatonin therapy. Dev Med Child Neurol 2004;46(11):789.
39. Özcan Ö, Dönmez YE. Melatonin treatment for childhood sleep terror. J Child Adolesc Psychopharmacol 2014;24(9):528–9.
40. Bruni O, Ferri R, Miano S, et al. l-5-Hydroxytryptophan treatment of sleep terrors in children. Eur J Pediatr 2004;163(7):402–7.
41. Sasayama D, Washizuka S, Honda H. Effective treatment of night terrors and sleepwalking with ramelteon. J Child Adolesc Psychopharmacol 2016; 26(10):948.
42. Winkelman JW, Johnson EA, Richards LM. Sleep-related eating disorder. Handb Clin Neurol 2011; 98:577–85.
43. Inoue Y. Sleep-related eating disorder and its associated conditions: clinical implication of SRED. Psychiatry Clin Neurosci 2015;69(6):309–20.
44. Howell MJ, Schenck CH. Restless nocturnal eating: a common feature of Willis-Ekbom Syndrome (RLS). J Clin Sleep Med 2012;8(4):413–9.
45. Auger RR. Sleep-related eating disorders. Psychiatry (Edgmont) 2006;3(11):64.
46. Brion A, Flamand M, Oudiette D, et al. Sleep-related eating disorder versus sleepwalking: a controlled study. Sleep Med 2012;13(8):1094–101.
47. Chiaro G, Caletti MT, Provini F. Treatment of sleep-related eating disorder. Curr Treat Options Neurol 2015;17(8):361.
48. Howell MJ, Schenck CH. Treatment of nocturnal eating disorders. Curr Treat Options Neurol 2009; 11(5):333–9.
49. Provini F, Albani F, Vetrugno R, et al. A pilot double-blind placebo-controlled trial of low-dose pramipexole in sleep-related eating disorder. Eur J Neurol 2005;12(6):432–6.
50. Santin J, Mery V, Elso MJ, et al. Sleep-related eating disorder: a descriptive study in Chilean patients. Sleep Med 2014;15(2):163–7.
51. Schenck CH, Hurwitz TD, O'Connor KA, et al. Additional categories of sleep-related eating disorders and the current status of treatment. Sleep 1993; 16(5):457–66.
52. Miyaoka T, Yasukawa R, Tsubouchi K, et al. Successful treatment of nocturnal eating/drinking syndrome with selective serotonin reuptake inhibitors. Int Clin Psychopharmacol 2003;18(3): 175–7.
53. Martinez-Salio A, Soler-Algarra S, Calvo-Garcia I, et al. Nocturnal sleep-related eating disorder that responds to topiramate. Rev Neurol 2007;45(5): 276–9 [in Spanish].
54. Winkelman JW. Treatment of nocturnal eating syndrome and sleep-related eating disorder with topiramate. Sleep Med 2003;4(3):243–6.
55. Winkelman JW. Efficacy and tolerability of open-label topiramate in the treatment of sleep-related eating disorder: a retrospective case series. J Clin Psychiatry 2006;67(11):1729–34.

56. Wilkes JJ, Nelson E, Osborne M, et al. Topiramate is an insulin-sensitizing compound in vivo with direct effects on adipocytes in female ZDF rats. Am J Physiol Endocrinol Metab 2005;288(3):E617–24.

57. Zapp AA, Fischer EC, Deuschle M. The effect of agomelatine and melatonin on sleep-related eating: a case report. J Med Case Rep 2017;11(1):275.

58. Comella CL, Nardine TM, Diederich NJ, et al. Sleep-related violence, injury, and REM sleep behavior disorder in Parkinson's disease. Neurology 1998;51(2):526–9.

59. McCarter SJ, St Louis EK, Boswell CL, et al. Factors associated with injury in REM sleep behavior disorder. Sleep Med 2014;15(11):1332–8.

60. Olson EJ, Boeve BF, Silber MH. Rapid eye movement sleep behaviour disorder: demographic, clinical and laboratory findings in 93 cases. Brain J Neurol 2000;123(Pt 2):331–9.

61. Postuma RB, Gagnon J-F, Tuineaig M, et al. Antidepressants and REM sleep behavior disorder: isolated side effect or neurodegenerative signal? Sleep 2013;36(11):1579–85.

62. Aurora RN, Zak RS, Maganti RK, et al. Best practice guide for the treatment of REM sleep behavior disorder (RBD). J Clin Sleep Med 2010;6(1):85–95.

63. Schenck CH, Bundlie SR, Ettinger MG, et al. Chronic behavioral disorders of human REM sleep: a new category of parasomnia. Sleep 1986;9(2):293–308.

64. Li SX, Lam SP, Zhang J, et al. A prospective, naturalistic follow-up study of treatment outcomes with clonazepam in rapid eye movement sleep behavior disorder. Sleep Med 2016;21:114–20.

65. McCarter SJ, Boswell CL, St Louis EK, et al. Treatment outcomes in REM sleep behavior disorder. Sleep Med 2013;14(3):237–42.

66. Terzaghi M, Sartori I, Rustioni V, et al. Sleep disorders and acute nocturnal delirium in the elderly: a comorbidity not to be overlooked. Eur J Intern Med 2014;25(4):350–5.

67. Kunz D, Mahlberg R. A two-part, double-blind, placebo-controlled trial of exogenous melatonin in REM sleep behaviour disorder. J Sleep Res 2010;19(4):591–6.

68. Kunz D, Bes F. Melatonin as a therapy in REM sleep behavior disorder patients: an open-labeled pilot study on the possible influence of melatonin on REM-sleep regulation. Mov Disord 1999;14(3):507–11.

69. Boeve BF, Silber MH, Ferman TJ. Melatonin for treatment of REM sleep behavior disorder in neurologic disorders: results in 14 patients. Sleep Med 2003;4(4):281–4.

70. Nomura T, Kawase S, Watanabe Y, et al. Use of ramelteon for the treatment of secondary REM sleep behavior disorder. Intern Med 2013;52(18):2123–6.

71. Esaki Y, Kitajima T, Koike S, et al. An open-labeled trial of ramelteon in idiopathic rapid eye movement sleep behavior disorder. J Clin Sleep Med 2016;12(5):689–93.

72. St. Louis EK, McCarter SJ, Boeve BF. Ramelteon for idiopathic REM sleep behavior disorder: implications for pathophysiology and future treatment trials. J Clin Sleep Med 2016;12(05):643–5.

73. Bonakis A, Economou N-T, Papageorgiou SG, et al. Agomelatine may improve REM sleep behavior disorder symptoms. J Clin Psychopharmacol 2012;32(5):732–4.

74. Fantini ML, Gagnon J-F, Filipini D, et al. The effects of pramipexole in REM sleep behavior disorder. Neurology 2003;61(10):1418–20.

75. Sasai T, Matsuura M, Inoue Y. Factors associated with the effect of pramipexole on symptoms of idiopathic REM sleep behavior disorder. Parkinsonism Relat Disord 2013;19(2):153–7.

76. Schmidt MH, Koshal VB, Schmidt HS. Use of pramipexole in REM sleep behavior disorder: results from a case series. Sleep Med 2006;7(5):418–23.

77. Kumru H, Iranzo A, Carrasco E, et al. Lack of effects of pramipexole on REM sleep behavior disorder in Parkinson disease. Sleep 2008;31(10):1418–21.

78. McCarley RW. Neurobiology of REM and NREM sleep. Sleep Med 2007;8(4):302–30.

79. Fernandez HH, Wu C-K, Ott BR. Pharmacotherapy of dementia with Lewy bodies. Expert Opin Pharmacother 2003;4(11):2027–37.

80. Terzaghi M, Rustioni V, Manni R, et al. Agrypnia with nocturnal confusional behaviors in dementia with Lewy bodies: immediate efficacy of rivastigmine. Mov Disord 2010;25(5):647–9.

81. Brunetti V, Losurdo A, Testani E, et al. Rivastigmine for refractory REM behavior disorder in mild cognitive impairment. Curr Alzheimer Res 2014;11(3):267–73.

82. Di Giacopo R, Fasano A, Quaranta D, et al. Rivastigmine as alternative treatment for refractory REM behavior disorder in Parkinson's disease. Mov Disord 2012;27(4):559–61.

83. Massironi G, Galluzzi S, Frisoni GB. Drug treatment of REM sleep behavior disorders in dementia with Lewy bodies. Int Psychogeriatr 2003;15(4):377–83.

84. Ringman JM, Simmons JH. Treatment of REM sleep behavior disorder with donepezil: a report of three cases. Neurology 2000;55(6):870–1.

85. Yeh S-B, Yeh P-Y, Schenck CH. Rivastigmine-induced REM sleep behavior disorder (RBD) in a 88-year-old man with Alzheimer's disease. J Clin Sleep Med 2010;6(2):192–5.

86. Babson KA, Sottile J, Morabito D. Cannabis, cannabinoids, and sleep: a review of the literature. Curr Psychiatry Rep 2017;19(4):23.

87. Chagas MHN, Eckeli AL, Zuardi AW, et al. Cannabidiol can improve complex sleep-related behaviours

associated with rapid eye movement sleep behaviour disorder in Parkinson's disease patients: a case series. J Clin Pharm Ther 2014;39(5):564–6.

88. Anderson KN, Shneerson JM. Drug treatment of REM sleep behavior disorder: the use of drug therapies other than clonazepam. J Clin Sleep Med 2009;5(3):235–9.

89. Bonakis A, Howard RS, Ebrahim IO, et al. REM sleep behaviour disorder (RBD) and its associations in young patients. Sleep Med 2009;10(6): 641–5.

90. Jung Y, St Louis EK. Treatment of REM sleep behavior disorder. Curr Treat Options Neurol 2016;18(11):50.

91. Moghadam KK, Pizza F, Primavera A, et al. Sodium oxybate for idiopathic REM sleep behavior disorder: a report on two patients. Sleep Med 2017;32: 16–21.

92. Shneerson JM. Successful treatment of REM sleep behavior disorder with sodium oxybate. Clin Neuropharmacol 2009;32(3):158–9.

93. Detweiler MB, Pagadala B, Candelario J, et al. Treatment of post-traumatic stress disorder nightmares at a Veterans Affairs medical center. J Clin Med 2016;5(12) [pii: E117].

94. Jeffreys M, Capehart B, Friedman MJ. Pharmacotherapy for posttraumatic stress disorder: review with clinical applications. J Rehabil Res Dev 2012;49(5):703–15.

95. Miller KE, Brownlow JA, Woodward S, et al. Sleep and dreaming in posttraumatic stress disorder. Curr Psychiatry Rep 2017;19(10):71.

96. George KC, Kebejian L, Ruth LJ, et al. Meta-analysis of the efficacy and safety of prazosin versus placebo for the treatment of nightmares and sleep disturbances in adults with posttraumatic stress disorder. J Trauma Dissociation 2016;17(4):494–510.

97. Kung S, Espinel Z, Lapid MI. Treatment of nightmares with prazosin: a systematic review. Mayo Clin Proc 2012;87(9):890–900.

98. Raskind MA, Peterson K, Williams T, et al. A trial of prazosin for combat trauma PTSD with nightmares in active-duty soldiers returned from Iraq and Afghanistan. Am J Psychiatry 2013;170(9): 1003–10.

99. Hudson SM, Whiteside TE, Lorenz RA, et al. Prazosin for the treatment of nightmares related to posttraumatic stress disorder: a review of the literature. Prim Care Companion CNS Disord 2012;14(2) [pii: PCC.11r01222].

100. Khachatryan D, Groll D, Booij L, et al. Prazosin for treating sleep disturbances in adults with posttraumatic stress disorder: a systematic review and meta-analysis of randomized controlled trials. Gen Hosp Psychiatry 2016;39:46–52.

101. Cameron C, Watson D, Robinson J. Use of a synthetic cannabinoid in a correctional population for posttraumatic stress disorder-related insomnia and nightmares, chronic pain, harm reduction, and other indications: a retrospective evaluation. J Clin Psychopharmacol 2014;34(5):559–64.

102. Fraser GA. The use of a synthetic cannabinoid in the management of treatment-resistant nightmares in posttraumatic stress disorder (PTSD). CNS Neurosci Ther 2009;15(1):84–8.

103. Jetly R, Heber A, Fraser G, et al. The efficacy of nabilone, a synthetic cannabinoid, in the treatment of PTSD-associated nightmares: a preliminary randomized, double-blind, placebo-controlled crossover design study. Psychoneuroendocrinology 2015;51:585–8.

104. Roitman P, Mechoulam R, Cooper-Kazaz R, et al. Preliminary, open-label, pilot study of add-on oral Δ9-tetrahydrocannabinol in chronic post-traumatic stress disorder. Clin Drug Investig 2014;34(8): 587–91.

105. Guilleminault C, Raynal D, Takahashi S, et al. Evaluation of short-term and long-term treatment of the narcolepsy syndrome with clomipramine hydrochloride. Acta Neurol Scand 1976;54(1):71–87.

106. Hishikawa Y, Ida H, Nakai K, et al. Treatment of narcolepsy with imipramine (tofranil) and desmethylimipramine (pertofran). J Neurol Sci 1966;3(5): 453–61.

107. Mitler MM, Hajdukovic R, Erman M, et al. Narcolepsy. J Clin Neurophysiol 1990;7(1):93–118.

108. Koran LM, Raghavan S. Fluoxetine for isolated sleep paralysis. Psychosomatics 1993;34(2): 184–7.

109. Schrader H, Kayed K, Bendixen Markset AC, et al. The treatment of accessory symptoms in narcolepsy: a double-blind cross-over study of a selective serotonin re-uptake inhibitor (femoxetine) versus placebo. Acta Neurol Scand 1986;74(4): 297–303.

110. Abad VC, Guilleminault C. New developments in the management of narcolepsy. Nat Sci Sleep 2017;9:39–57.

111. Frese A, Summ O, Evers S. Exploding head syndrome: six new cases and review of the literature. Cephalalgia 2014;34(10):823–7.

112. Sharpless BA. Exploding head syndrome. Sleep Med Rev 2014;18(6):489–93.

113. Sachs C, Svanborg E. The exploding head syndrome: polysomnographic recordings and therapeutic suggestions. Sleep 1991;14(3):263–6.

114. Chakravarty A. Exploding head syndrome: report of two new cases. Cephalalgia 2008;28(4):399–400.

115. Jacome DE. Exploding head syndrome and idiopathic stabbing headache relieved by nifedipine. Cephalalgia Int J Headache 2001;21(5):617–8.

116. Palikh GM, Vaughn BV. Topiramate responsive exploding head syndrome. J Clin Sleep Med 2010; 6(4):382–3.

117. Harari MD. Nocturnal enuresis: nocturnal enuresis. J Paediatr Child Health 2013;49(4):264–71.

118. Jain S, Bhatt GC. Advances in the management of primary monosymptomatic nocturnal enuresis in children. Paediatr Int Child Health 2016;36(1):7–14.

119. Kuwertz-Bröking E, von Gontard A. Clinical management of nocturnal enuresis. Pediatr Nephrol 2017. [Epub ahead of print].

120. Caldwell PHY, Deshpande AV, Gontard AV. Management of nocturnal enuresis. BMJ 2013; 347(oct29 11):f6259.

121. Glazener CMA, Evans JHC, Peto RE. Alarm interventions for nocturnal enuresis in children. Cochrane Database Syst Rev 2005;(2):CD002911.

122. Hjalmas K, Arnold T, Bower W, et al. Nocturnal enuresis: an international evidence based management strategy. J Urol 2004;171(6 Pt 2): 2545–61.

123. Robson WLM, Leung AKC, Norgaard JP. The comparative safety of oral versus intranasal desmopressin for the treatment of children with nocturnal enuresis. J Urol 2007;178(1):24–30.

124. Neveus T, Eggert P, Evans J, et al. Evaluation of and treatment for monosymptomatic enuresis: a standardization document from the International Children's Continence Society. J Urol 2010;183(2): 441–7.

125. Glazener CM, Evans JH. Desmopressin for nocturnal enuresis in children. Cochrane Database Syst Rev 2002;(3):CD002112.

126. Nevéus T. Nocturnal enuresis-theoretic background and practical guidelines. Pediatr Nephrol 2011;26(8):1207–14.

127. Caldwell PHY, Sureshkumar P, Wong WCF. Tricyclic and related drugs for nocturnal enuresis in children. Cochrane Database Syst Rev 2016;(1): CD002117.

128. International Consultation on Incontinence, Abrams P, Cardozo L, et al, editors. Incontinence. 4th edition. Paris: Health Publication; 2009.

129. Hoebeke P, De Pooter J, De Caestecker K, et al. Solifenacin for therapy resistant overactive bladder. J Urol 2009;182(4 Suppl):2040–4.

130. Raes A, Hoebeke P, Segaert I, et al. Retrospective analysis of efficacy and tolerability of tolterodine in children with overactive bladder. Eur Urol 2004; 45(2):240–4.

131. Deshpande AV, Caldwell PHY, Sureshkumar P. Drugs for nocturnal enuresis in children (other than desmopressin and tricyclics). Cochrane Database Syst Rev 2012;(12):CD002238.

132. Yu J, Yan Z, Zhou S, et al. Desmopressin plus anticholinergic agent in the treatment of nocturnal enuresis: a meta-analysis. Exp Ther Med 2017; 14(4):2875–84.

Drug Therapy in Obstructive Sleep Apnea

Jan Hedner, MD, PhD*, Ding Zou, MD, PhD

KEYWORDS

- Sleep • Obstructive sleep apnea • Drug • Medication • Therapy

KEY POINTS

- Current, mainly mechanical, therapies in obstructive sleep apnea (OSA) are frequently hampered by limited compliance (continuous positive airway pressure) or efficacy (mandibular advancement devices).
- Previous attempts to identify a drug therapy in OSA, in order to overcome these limitations, have been unsuccessful; there is currently no available pharmacologic alternative in this condition.
- Relevant experimental models of OSA are lacking, as sleep disordered breathing is a heterogeneous condition that involves multiple dominating pathophysiological traits.
- The current trend is to identify drug candidates that address selective mechanisms in OSA. This approach will provide a better understanding of the OSA condition and enable phenotyping OSA patients in future drug development programs.

GENERAL ASPECTS OF DRUGS IN OBSTRUCTIVE SLEEP APNEA

Overview

Obstructive sleep apnea (OSA) is a common condition that has turned out to provide a major challenge for physicians and the health care systems. This form of sleep disordered breathing is characterized by recurrent episodes of complete or partial obstruction of the upper airway, which causes periodic hypoxia and hypercapnia during sleep.[1] OSA leads to not only transient cortical arousals and sleep fragmentation but also to increased oxidative stress, autonomic dysregulation, and hemodynamic changes during sleep.[2] These consequences have been linked to daytime sleepiness as well as increased cardiovascular/metabolic morbidities in terms of arterial hypertension, coronary heart disease, stroke, type 2 diabetes and mortality in patients with OSA.[3]

Despite the high prevalence, treatment options for OSA are limited. So far there is no generally effective drug available for this condition. Nevertheless, several drug candidates have been proposed; there are currently steps taken toward more strategic development programs in OSA. Previous attempts to generate a drug therapy were more or less serendipity driven, and the literature in the area is characterized by small-scale studies. These studies have been reviewed in several publications in the area[4,5] as well as in a recent Cochrane review.[6] There are now better designed trials, which adequately address many of the potential pitfalls encountered in previous studies, under way. There is also considerable literature on interventional strategies that reside on the physiologic mechanisms, which appear during upper airway collapse in sleep.[7,8]

Disclosure Statement: Dr J. Hedner reports grants from the Swedish Heart-Lung Foundation and from the University of Gothenburg, grants from ResMed and from PhilipsRespironics related to European database work (ESADA), and personal fees from Itamar and AstraZeneca outside the submitted work. Dr J. Hedner has 2 patents related to OSA therapy, one pending and one issued. Dr D. Zou reports no conflicts of interest.
Department of Internal Medicine and Clinical Nutrition, Center for Sleep and Vigilance Disorders, Sahlgrenska Academy, University of Gothenburg, Medicinaregatan 8B, Box 421, Gothenburg SE-40530, Sweden
* Corresponding author.
E-mail address: Jan.hedner@lungall.gu.se

Sleep Med Clin 13 (2018) 203–217
https://doi.org/10.1016/j.jsmc.2018.03.004
1556-407X/18/© 2018 Elsevier Inc. All rights reserved.

This article addresses some major methodologic problems encountered when designing clinical drug trials in OSA. The authors describe some major outcomes addressed in previous and ongoing studies, which more specifically include drugs with a potential effect on the various pathophysiologic mechanisms that have been associated with the sleep and breathing disorder. The authors also briefly address drugs with an effect on associated conditions, including sleepiness, obesity, arterial hypertension, gastroesophageal reflux, and conditions of the oronasal airway. Finally, the authors review endocrine mechanisms, including menopausal hormone replacement therapy, hypothyroidism, and acromegaly, that may be relevant to OSA pathophysiology.

Current Treatment Options

OSA is known to, pathophysiologically, during sleep involve anatomic predisposition for airway collapse, reduced compensatory neuromuscular control of the upper airway, and labile central neurochemical ventilatory control.[1] Continuous positive airway pressure (CPAP), a highly efficacious treatment in OSA, splints the upper airway but does not seem to modulate these fundamental underlying mechanisms. Moreover, the clinical utility of CPAP has been extremely well established for many years, but CPAP therapy is clearly limited by the incomplete tolerability and poor compliance.[9] Not only do several patients reject this form of therapy completely but there are also many who use CPAP only during part of the night. Partial use of the device will frequently leave several hours of residual sleep apnea every night and thereby tentatively only provide partial therapy for the sleep and breathing disorder.[10] Most outcome studies in the area have introduced a cutoff threshold of 4 hours per night, and there is evidence that this amount of use represents a minimum for long-term efficacious therapy.[11] However, there is considerable interindividual variation in the subjective sleep need, which probably should be better accounted for. Although the 4 hours may be close to adequate in some patients, they may only represent a fraction of a relevant sleep period in others.

With these limitations in mind, there is certainly an incentive to identify potential pharmacologic remedies in OSA. In fact, in a comparative sense, it may be argued that a drug therapy with only partial efficacy, for example, 50% reduction of OSA but present during 8 hours of sleep (alleviation of 50% of OSA), may result in a better therapeutic response than a mechanical device that induces a 100% reduction of OSA but only during 2 hours (alleviation of 25% of OSA) in an 8-hour sleeper. Clearly, future trials of pharmacologic therapies in OSA should introduce the component habitual sleep length in order to adequately compute effectiveness and the influence of therapy on various outcomes.[12] Incomplete compliance is also relevant for other mechanical therapies, such as intraoral devices, whereby the possibility to monitor and quantify use is in fact even more restricted compared with in CPAP.

Obstructive Sleep Apnea as a Target in Clinical Trials

There are no established regulatory guidelines related to the design of clinical trial programs in sleep disordered breathing. There is also uncertainty about appropriate clinical endpoints in trials and whether these should be focused on frequency markers, such as the apnea hypopnea index (AHI), markers of hypoxia, such as the oxygen desaturation index (ODI) or mean nocturnal oxygen saturation, daytime symptoms such as excessive daytime sleepiness, or comorbid disorders such as hypertension or metabolic disease.

Multicenter trials need to observe the risk of interscorer variability in studies using polysomnography and potentially apply centralized scoring functions. The choice of the recording technique applied, for instance, use of thermistor or pressure cannula in protocols, may markedly influence the results. Other challenges in clinical trials in OSA include night-to-night variability of the breathing disorder, variability resulting from the influence of body position change, variability related to differences between nights in sleep stage distribution (particularly in those with sleep stage–dependent apnea) or changes in OSA severity induced by external factors, such as drug or alcohol intake (**Table 1**). Although there are guidelines addressing scoring rules of sleep and breathing events, there is a need to better define general standards to be applied in large-scale clinical trials. Finally, as discussed later in this article, there is emerging evidence for distinct subphenotypes of OSA. This finding suggests that a particular pharmacologic remedy may be specifically effective in some patients but not in others. Hence, insights gained in clinical trials may help us to subselect and better define such specific groups of patients. The stricter, with respect to subphenotype, our protocols are designed, the better the efficacy of the intervention will be in this context.

Another problematic dimension related to drug development in OSA is the choice of appropriate outcome variables in clinical drug trials. Most

Table 1
Challenges in clinical trials in obstructive sleep apnea

Specific to recordings or measurements	Interscorer variability in polysomnography Inconsistent use or choice of sensors Incomplete sleep classification in polygraphy studies
Specific to the OSA disorder	Night-to-night variability of the breathing disorder Position-dependent OSA Sleep stage–dependent OSA Variation due to drug or alcohol intake
Specific to subphenotypes	Anatomic predisposition for airway collapse Poor compensatory neuromuscular control of the upper airway Labile central neurochemical ventilatory control Low arousal threshold
Specific to end-points	Efficacy OSA variable (eg, AHI, ODI, or similar) Efficacy variable related to comorbidity (eg, arterial hypertension, obesity) Efficacy variable related to sleepiness, cognition

previous trials have used the AHI as a primary measure of efficacy. However, it should be noted that this measure is only weakly associated with, for instance, sleepiness, cognitive dysfunction, or cardiovascular morbidity, blood pressure elevation or coronary artery disease. Other metrics, such as hypoxemia or sleep fragmentation, may be more relevant and closely associated with the vascular or metabolic sequels of OSA.[13] Moreover, a drug used for treatment of sleep apnea could also be designed to address comorbid conditions, such as cardiovascular or metabolic disease, daytime cognitive function, or daytime sleepiness; this could represent a useful end point in clinical trials. This possibility has rarely been systematically explored in currently published studies. Hence, future interventional trials in this area should benefit from a global evaluation that includes breathing events during sleep, daytime symptoms, vascular sequels, and disease-specific outcome measurements of quality of life.

The Phenotype Approach

At least 4 physiologic traits that may result in OSA have been described.[14] Interestingly, these traits differ in several fundamental aspects and may pave the way for specific therapeutic approaches in OSA (**Fig. 1**).[8] A small or narrow upper airway provides an anatomic predisposition to airway collapse during sleep; factors, such as local fat deposition, hypertrophied tonsils, or adenoids, may contribute in this dominating trait in OSA. A

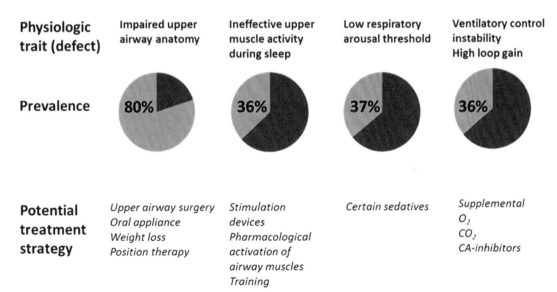

Fig. 1. Physiologic phenotyping in 69 random patients with OSA and 21 controls. Please note that a single patient may appear in more than one category. CA, carbonic anhydrase. (*Data from* Eckert DJ, White DP, Jordan AS, et al. Defining phenotypic causes of obstructive sleep apnea. Identification of novel therapeutic targets. Am J Respir Crit Care Med 2013;188(8):1002; with permission.)

stronger dominance of this trait would be less likely to be responsive to drug therapy in a dynamic sense. However, therapies like pharmacologically induced weight loss may certainly provide a therapeutic potential at least in a subgroup of these patients.

A second trait is that of ineffective upper airway muscle responsiveness during sleep. The state of sleep per se is known to induce a reduction of dilatory muscle activity, which increases the risk of airway collapse. This effect is counteracted by arousing phenomena and increased central respiratory drive induced by, for example, mild hypercapnia. The net effect of such activation, increased pharyngeal upper airway dilating muscle activity, seems to be compromised in at least one-third of patients with clinical OSA.[14] Several drugs that might increase this activity have been explored in OSA, and this should certainly provide a potential target in drug development.

The third mechanism relates to the threshold for arousal from sleep. This important mechanism tends to stabilize respiration by providing a constant input to upper airway dilator muscles.[15] A modified arousal threshold may cause a mismatch between increased respiratory drive (as a consequence of a respiratory event) and upper airway muscle recruitment which would likely induce a breathing instability. A particular clinical focus has been directed toward hypnotic agents found to increase the arousal threshold; but the potential beneficial effect on OSA, which might be expected in approximately one-third of patients with OSA with a low threshold, is modest.[16]

Finally, OSA was found to be associated with instability of the respiratory control system (high loop gain).[17] The oscillation of the ventilatory drive may diminish pharyngeal dilatory muscle activity and contribute to pathogenesis of OSA. Loop gain may be pharmacologically modified; therefore, this mechanism has been studied quite extensively in this condition.[8]

SPECIFIC PHARMACOLOGIC STRATEGIES APPLIED IN OBSTRUCTIVE SLEEP APNEA

A substantial body of literature on drug therapies in OSA is available.[6] As mentioned earlier, most of the trials in OSA are limited in size; but there are also larger studies that meet more stringent quality criteria. Most studies have addressed the direct interventional effects on sleep disordered breathing, whereas others focused the effects on OSA following treatment of associated conditions, such as obesity, arterial hypertension, or gastroesophageal reflux disease.

Noradrenaline and Dopamine Mechanisms

The central noradrenergic system is highly state dependent and influenced by sleep and arousal mechanisms. The major source of noradrenergic neurons and activity is in the locus coeruleus of the brain stem; there is widespread distribution of adrenergic receptors throughout the brain and spinal cord. Arousals from sleep are associated with periodic activation of autonomic activity, which spills over on cardiovascular and respiratory regulation, importantly in the form of a tonic excitatory influence on hypoglossal motoneurons. This mechanism would provide a rationale for the use of adrenergic agents in OSA. Tricyclic antidepressant drugs increase central adrenergic neuronal activity by inhibition of noradrenaline reuptake. Protriptyline was in fact one of the first drugs tested in OSA.[18,19] Pilot studies suggested improved oxygen saturation in parallel with changes in sleep architecture, but this was not confirmed in subsequent controlled studies.[20] The early studies of protriptyline also suggested that the drug reduces rapid eye movement (REM) sleep, a sleep stage associated with more severe apneic events. Subsequent studies also demonstrated a specific reduction of REM sleep and nocturnal hypoxemia after protriptyline in patients with chronic obstructive pulmonary disease.[21] However, these effects were not maintained at long-term follow-up.[22] Together with disrupting effects on the sleep pattern, these weak long-term effects clearly limit the usefulness of protriptyline in OSA.

Only a few studies have dealt with dopamine-related mechanisms in OSA. Dopamine is recognized as an inhibitory neurotransmitter in the mammalian carotid body and may, therefore, be involved in respiratory control mechanisms in OSA. Domperidone, a peripherally acting dopamine antagonist, increased the hypercapnic ventilatory response in patients with OSA.[23] An uncontrolled study looking at the combination of domperidone and pseudoephedrine reported beneficial effects on sleepiness and possibly fewer apneas as well as improved oxygenation.[24] However, the observed effects may have been caused by concomitant weight reduction. Further controlled randomized studies are needed.

Potassium Channel Blockers

Potassium channels are widely distributed ion channels that control a variety of cell functions. Potassium channel blockade has been shown to modulate hypoglossal motoneuron activity and is identified as a potential mechanism for muscle activation in all stages of sleep. Studies in a rat model, using local application, have demonstrated a considerable activation of genioglossal activity.[25] However, administration of a voltage-gated potassium channel blocker 4-aminopyridine showed only a small increase in tonic genioglossus muscle activity during REM sleep in healthy subjects.[26]

In a spontaneously breathing anesthetized pig model, Wirth and coworkers[27] investigated the potassium channel blocker AVE-0118 administered topically in the upper airway. AVE-0118 was found to, with a duration of more than 4 hours, dose-dependently inhibit upper airway collapsibility in a manner that was abolished by upper airway lidocaine anesthesia. The relevance of this model was supported by the finding that intravenous administration of either naloxone or acetazolamide was ineffective. Paroxetine and mirtazapine were weakly effective and fluoxetine moderately effective, in line with reported clinical efficacy. AVE-0118 has also been investigated for its potential as an antiarrhythmic drug.[28,29] These data on AVE-0118 are promising, in particular the potential to administer a drug with documented effects on upper airway muscle tone during sleep in those OSA patients who have that physiologic defect.

Serotonin Modulation

Brainstem raphe nuclei constitute the principal source of central serotonin (5-hydroxytryptamine [5-HT]). Axons from these neurons extend to almost every part of the central nervous system. There are at least 7 different serotonin receptor families that mediate either excitatory or inhibitory neurotransmission. The various receptor subtypes, either G protein-coupled receptors or a ligand-gated ion channel, are located in the central and peripheral nervous systems. Several of these receptors have been intimately associated with different aspects of sleep. There is also a link to other physiologic mechanisms, such as appetite, cognition, respiration, and cardiovascular function. Serotonin activity modulates several neurotransmitters, including glutamate, γ-aminobutyric acid (GABA), dopamine, adrenalin/noradrenalin, and acetylcholine.

Tonic 5-HT input to the hypoglossal motoneurons from the medullary raphe decreases from wakefulness to non-REM sleep to reach a minimum during REM sleep. Mono-amino oxidase A–deficient transgenic mice have increased rates of central apnea, which is sharply reduced after the administration of ondansetron or fluoxetine.[30]

Hypoglossal nerve firing and genioglossus muscle activity are facilitated by 5-HT, which is reduced during REM sleep.[31] This finding may be physiologically relevant in patients with REM sleep–dependent OSA but would leave less of a therapeutic window during REM sleep for 5-HT reuptake inhibitors. A Chinese association study found a lower AHI along with lower plasma concentrations of 5-HT and 5-hydroxyindolacetic acid (5-HT metabolite) in male patients carrying an S-12 haplotype constructed by polymorphisms of the serotonin transporter gene.[32]

Animal experiments have facilitated the characterization of serotonin receptors potentially involved in respiration. For instance, the 5-HT2A and 5-HT2C subtypes are the predominant postsynaptic receptors on dilator motor neurons. 5-HT1A (inhibitory) and 5-HT2 are found in central respiratory controller areas. Stimulation of these receptors, as well as the 5-HT3 receptor, induced respiratory inhibition; this effect may have involved the nodose ganglion.[33] These mechanisms also seem to be determined by species differences and animal preparations. For instance, ondansetron (a 5-HT3 receptor antagonist) reduced sleep disordered breathing during REM sleep by 54% in an English bulldog model[34] but had no effect in human OSA.[35] Also, serotonin-mediated effects are claimed to be overestimated in vagotomized animal preparation.[36]

Clinical data suggest that selective serotonin reuptake inhibitor drugs might reduce AHI, mainly during non-REM sleep. Fluoxetine reduced AHI by approximately 40% in a small uncontrolled study[37] and a double-blind controlled study of paroxetine demonstrated a 20% reduction of the AHI during non-REM sleep.[38] Human experimental studies also report an increased genioglossus muscle activity after paroxetine during wake.[39] Indeed, serotonergic medullary raphe activity is particularly low during REM sleep; this could explain a lower effect of this drug class during this sleep phase.[40]

A particular focus in this area has been placed on mirtazapine, a drug with 5-HT1 agonistic and 5-HT2/5-HT3 receptor antagonistic properties. Mirtazapine is known to promote slow-wave sleep in men,[41] and animal data suggest that this is accompanied by increased genioglossus activity[42] and, consequently, a reduction of sleep apnea.[43] Early human studies also reported a prominent reduction of OSA,[44] but this effect was not confirmed in subsequent randomized controlled trials.[45] Side effects, including sedation and weight gain, limit the usefulness of mirtazapine in OSA.

It may be summarized that animal data demonstrate a potential association between serotonergic mechanisms and control of breathing, but there is yet no evidence that modulation of these mechanisms has any impact on human sleep apnea.

Acetylcholine Mechanisms

Drugs that modulate acetylcholinergic activity might theoretically affect OSA by multiple mechanisms. Acetylcholine functions as a neurotransmitter in the peripheral and the central nervous systems. Cholinergic mechanisms regulate autonomic nervous function and constitute one of the main active neurotransmitter systems during REM sleep. Indeed, animal studies have demonstrated a reduction of genioglossal muscle tone after hypoglossal motor nucleus application of compounds that facilitate acetylcholinergic tone.[46] The procholinergic respiratory stimulant nicotine is known to activate upper airway muscle activity in animals, but the effects were inconsistent in patients with OSA. Nicotine gum taken at bedtime reduced the AHI in one study,[47] but this was not confirmed in 2 subsequent randomized trials exploring the effects of nicotine patches.[48,49] In addition, sleep quality deteriorated after nicotine.[48] Another study on healthy awake participants did not find a consistent increase of genioglossal muscle activity after a transmucosal nicotine patch.[50] Drugs with anticholinergic properties do not seem to influence OSA to any particular extent.

Other studies suggest that increased cholinergic activity may be beneficial and in fact reduce OSA. Acetylcholine is known to modulate secretory activity in the upper airway, and this may result in a reduction of airway compliance and reduced collapsibility during sleep. Other indirect evidence demonstrated that a reduced thalamic cholinergic nerve terminal density was associated with OSA severity in patients with multisystem atrophy, potentially as a result of reduced pontine cholinergic mechanisms.[51]

The cholinesterase inhibitory drug physostigmine increases both muscarinic and nicotinic activity by a reduced enzymatic degradation of acetylcholine. A double-blind, placebo-controlled, randomized, crossover trial of infused physostigmine in lean patients with OSA demonstrated a reduction of AHI particularly during REM sleep.[52] Improvement of OSA was also reported in a small randomized controlled study using the orally available cholinesterase inhibitor donepezil administered for 4 weeks.[53] However, more recent data have not confirmed these initial promising findings.[54] There are no ongoing studies in this area at the moment, but future investigations that account for potential intraindividual differences in OSA pathophysiology may result in the identification of a specific therapeutic target for drugs of this class.

Tetrahydrocannabinols

Animal data suggest that Δ9-tetrahydrocannabinol might improve spontaneous sleep disordered breathing presumably by stabilization of autonomic output and reduced serotonin-induced exacerbation of sleep apnea.[55] Dronabinol, an exogenous cannabinoid type 1 and type 2 receptor agonist, at dosages of 2.5 to 10.0 mg daily reduced sleep disordered breathing in a pilot study of 17 patients with moderate to severe OSA.[56] In a subsequent placebo-controlled trial of OSA patients receiving 2.5 or 10.0 mg for up to 6 weeks, the AHI was dose-dependently reduced with approximately 40%, along with a reduced Epworth sleepiness scale score.[57] The maintenance of wakefulness test sleep latency, gross sleep architecture, and overnight oxygenation remained unchanged after therapy.

The potential underlying mechanisms of this drug class remain unresolved, and there is no information on possible specific target groups based on physiologic mechanisms considered in OSA. Future studies are needed in order to fully explore a possible potential of this drug class in OSA.

Xanthines

The respiratory stimulant caffeine is a frequently used xanthine for the treatment of apnea in premature infants. Caffeine reduces, but does not eliminate, apnea. Other xanthines, like theophylline and aminophylline, are known to influence ventilation by multiple effects, including an antagonistic action on adenosine in the central nervous system. There is also a peripheral effect that involves a stimulation of diaphragm contractility.

OSA was reduced by 20% in an early placebo-controlled trial of theophylline, but this was accompanied by a deterioration of sleep quality.[58] Similar, but smaller, reductions of AHI were reported in other trials[59,60]; but the residual AHI and CPAP pressure were not significantly affected by sustained-release theophylline in patients with OSA under CPAP treatment.[61] Hence, the effect of xanthines generally seems to be weak in OSA. However, there are data investigating the role of theophylline in patients with complex breathing disorders and central sleep apnea. In a placebo-controlled trial of 15 patients with compensated heart failure and central sleep apnea, AHI decreased by approximately 50%; but there was no effect on the ventricular ejection fraction.[62] These findings were confirmed in an uncontrolled trial of oral theophylline in 13 patients with compensated heart failure and periodic breathing.[63] Yet, another controlled trial of theophylline in patients with congestive heart failure reported an increase in plasma renin concentration and improved ventilation (lowered transcutaneous carbon dioxide), whereas the sympathetic activity that was monitored remained unaffected.[64] These findings are interesting for the understanding of sleep disordered breathing in heart failure, but theophylline cannot be generally recommended in these patients because of a potential proarrhythmogenic effect.

Carbonic Anhydrase Inhibitors

High loop gain, as previously described, refers to an unstable respiratory control system that responds sharply to only small changes in local P_{CO_2} concentration. Pronounced oscillations may periodically lead to low ventilatory drive and a propensity to airway collapse, particularly in patients with a narrow upper airway. The carbonic anhydrase inhibitor acetazolamide was found to cause a marked reduction of loop gain in 12 out of 13 tested subjects, and this change was paralleled with a 50% reduction of the AHI.[65] The effect was seen during both REM and non-REM sleep. Other physiologic traits, such as the arousal threshold or upper airway muscle activity, were unaffected. These data aligned well with previous studies involving carbonic anhydrase inhibition. For instance, a placebo-controlled study of acetazolamide in high-altitude induced sleep disordered breathing demonstrated almost complete restoration of ventilation during sleep, along with an improvement of oxygenation.[66] Another high altitude study addressed subjects with severe sleep apnea off CPAP at 490 m and at altitudes of 1860 m and 2590 m. Exposure to altitude leads to a sharp increase in AHI and periodic hypoxia during sleep, whereas acetazolamide 2×250 mg daily reduced the AHI, improved the oxygen saturation, nocturnal transcutaneous P_{CO_2}, sleep efficiency, and subjective insomnia.[67] Acetazolamide also prevented excessive blood pressure elevations at altitude. There are also smaller short-term studies of acetazolamide that demonstrated an almost 50% reduction of central

apneas[68] and a 20% reduction of obstructive events.[69]

The exact mechanisms behind the effect of acetazolamide on sleep disordered breathing are unknown but may involve an altered acid-base mechanism that can be affected by the drug (eg, metabolic acidosis). There are data suggesting that carbonic anhydrase activity, either primarily or secondarily, is increased in patients with OSA in relation to the severity of the condition.[70] It is also possible that other linked comorbidities in OSA may be affected as a result of this altered activity. Parati and colleagues[71] demonstrated an increased diastolic and mean arterial blood pressure in 21 healthy volunteers receiving placebo exposed to a high altitude. This effect was inhibited in the group of 21 controls receiving acetazolamide 2×250 mg daily. These findings may have implications for blood pressure control in patients with OSA and periodic hypoxemia at sea level. Indeed, the most recent trial in this field recruited hypertensive patients with OSA and evaluated the effect on both blood pressure and respiration during sleep in a crossover fashion, comparing CPAP, acetazolamide, and CPAP plus acetazolamide treatment.[72] Following washout of antihypertensive medication acetazolamide, contrary to CPAP, induced a significant reduction of systolic blood pressure and vascular stiffness. Sleep disordered breathing was reduced with approximately 40%. The data lead to the speculation that increased carbonic anhydrase activity may have additive or synergistic effects on blood pressure elevation in OSA.

Other carbonic anhydrase inhibitors, like topiramate[73,74] and zonisamide,[75] have also been shown to reduce OSA, suggesting that this beneficial effect on OSA is a drug class–specific effect (**Fig. 2**). Finally, besides effects on the breathing disorder and potentially on blood pressure, there are reports on body weight reduction following these drugs, which may add to the overall treatment effect in OSA.[76] It remains that neurologic side effects may limit the usefulness of drugs with carbonic anhydrase inhibition properties. A study that further investigates the safety profile of this drug class in OSA is ongoing (EudraCT number: 2017-004767-13).

The γ-Aminobutyric Acid–Benzodiazepine Receptor Complex

GABA is the main inhibitory neurotransmitter in the central nervous system. This amino acid regulates neuronal excitability by binding to specific transmembrane receptors referred to as the

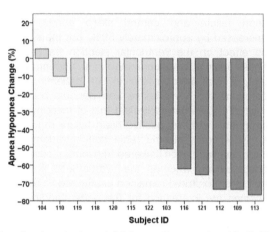

Fig. 2. Reduction of the AHI after 2 different drugs with carbonic anhydrase inhibitory effect, zonisamide (*left*) and acetazolamide (*right*), after 4 weeks' treatment. Shown is the relative effect in individual subjects with OSA. Green bars signify subjects reaching an AHI less than 10 or with a 50% AHI reduction. Note the superior effect after acetazolamide, as all subjects except one in fact reduced the AHI. The variability in the treatment response may reflect that these subjects have different pathophysiologic traits. ID, identification.

(GABA)-benzodiazepine receptor complex both presynaptically and postsynaptically.[77] This complex has been implicated for the modulation of arousal threshold in OSA. In addition, episodic hypoxia has been speculated to accelerate the progression of OSA by GABAergic mechanisms via impairment of neural control of upper airway patency and respiratory contractile function.[78] Hence, agonists at this receptor, including various short- and long-acting benzodiazepines and benzodiazepine-like drugs, have been regarded as potentially contraindicated in patients with OSA. However, there are data suggesting that a higher arousal threshold in fact may be beneficial in the therapy of OSA in certain patients.[79] Any medication that increases the arousal threshold may have the potential to buy time for the upper airway muscle recruitment and possibly stabilization of airway patency.[7] Several of the compounds in this class had only minor effects on sleep apnea, and the effects were quite variable.[80–82] Nevertheless, Eckert and coworkers[83] found a reduction of the AHI from 31 to 24 in a study administering eszopiclone in patients with moderate to severe OSA. The greatest reductions in the AHI occurred in those with a low arousal threshold. These findings suggest that improved phenotyping of patients with OSA may prove to be useful for detection of patients potentially at risk on sedative drugs. They also open the perspective of a mechanism that may be used, alone or in combination, to tailor pharmacologic therapies in OSA.

TREATMENTS ADDRESSING ASSOCIATED CONDITIONS IN OBSTRUCTIVE SLEEP APNEA
Reduction of Daytime Sleepiness in Sleep Disordered Breathing

Although most daytime somnolence in OSA is eliminated by conventional therapy, there is a subset of patients with residual daytime sleepiness. The exact size of this group remains unknown, but approximately 15% of patients may be affected. There have been several studies on the efficacy and usefulness of pharmacologic therapy addressing sleepiness in such patients.[84] The analeptic modafinil, which is widely used for this indication, has multiple pharmacologic effects, including facilitation of monoamine release and promotion of hypothalamic histamine levels, which may be relevant to promotion of wakefulness.

Modafinil reduces subjective and objective sleepiness, vigilance, and quality of life in CPAP-treated patients with OSA; but there are no effects on sleep disordered breathing.[85] Modafinil has also been documented in the context of driving and neurocognitive performance as well as sleepiness in patients with OSA under short-term CPAP withdrawal.[86] Armodafinil, the R-isomer of racemic modafinil, has been documented in a randomized placebo-controlled study of CPAP-adherent patients with OSA.[87] However, an European Medicines Agency pharmacovigilance program has alerted on the link between modafinil and serious skin reactions, especially in children, as well as psychiatric/cardiovascular adverse reactions. This finding has led to a restriction of the recommendation of modafinil outside the use in narcolepsy.

Pitolisant is a novel antagonist/inverse agonist of the histamine H3 receptor, which is indicated in adults for the treatment of narcolepsy with or without cataplexy.[88] The effect in various conditions, in particular narcolepsy, on excessive diurnal sleepiness is well documented. However, there are currently less efficacy data on sleepiness related to OSA. The prevailing indication for pitolisant in the European Union is treatment of narcolepsy with or without cataplexy.

Solriamfetol is a recently U.S. Food and Drug Administration approved drug for the treatment of excessive daytime sleepiness.[89] This norepinephrine-dopamine reuptake inhibitor has undergone phase III clinical trials for narcolepsy and sleep apnea and phase II clinical trials for hypersomnia. A 6-week randomized-withdrawal trial demonstrated an increase of objectively assessed sleepiness and a placebo corrected Epworth sleepiness scale score of approximately 4.5 units in patients with OSA and excessive sleepiness.[90] Side effects were moderately common, most prominently headache in about 10% of studied patients.

Hence, there are pharmacologic strategies that may be considered in the treatment of excessive sleepiness related to OSA, but drugs are relatively infrequently used in this context. It is possible that arguments like treating somnolence alone with an effective pharmacotherapy would result in a tendency among patients to give up conventional mechanical therapies like CPAP.

Body Weight Reduction and Sleep Disordered Breathing

Moderate to severe OSA is present in at least 50% of obese patients, and approximately 50% of patients with OSA are obese. A more or less linear relationship between body mass index and OSA severity was described earlier.[91] There is a wealth of weight-reduction study data suggesting that the AHI is reduced by approximately 3% for every 1% of body weight that is lost.[92] Protocols that address pharmacologic weight reductions suggest not only that OSA is modifiable by weight loss but also that added metabolic benefits may be achieved in patients with a combination of the two conditions. A 6-month, open, uncontrolled cohort study of sibutramine in 87 obese men with OSA reported a 35% reduction in sleep-disordered breathing (respiratory disturbance index from 46.0 to 16.3 events per hour) along with a body weight loss of approximately 8.5%.[93] Multiple metabolic indices, including insulin resistance, high-density lipoprotein cholesterol, visceral and subcutaneous abdominal fat, and liver fat, were improved in parallel, whereas heart rate and blood pressure were unchanged.[94] However, weight reduction was less pronounced in a subsequent smaller study comparing sibutramine treatment with conventional CPAP; the effects on sleep-disordered breathing were small and inferior to those induced by CPAP.[95]

The lipase inhibitor orlistat and the cannabinoid receptor antagonist rimonabant represent other drugs that are used for weight management but have not been explored in OSA. The long-acting glucagon-like peptide-1 receptor agonist liraglutide was investigated in a large-scale sleep apnea study during 32 weeks.[96] During dietary deficit, a dose of 3 mg caused a 5.7% weight loss (placebo 1.6%) and 12.2 events per hour reduction of AHI (placebo 6.1 events per hour, baseline 49.2 events per hour) along with an improvement of systolic blood pressure and hemoglobin A1c. Another approach includes the combination of phentermine and a carbonic anhydrase inhibitor topiramate in obese patients with OSA. In this 28-week placebo-controlled study, body weight dropped by 10.3% (placebo 4.2%), whereas the AHI decreased by 69% (placebo 38%).[74] Again, there were beneficial effects on blood pressure, sleep fragmentation, and sleep quality. To summarize, there is little doubt that drug-induced weight loss is feasible in obese patients with sleep apnea, and the added beneficial effects on comorbid conditions in these patients may compete with those induced by conventional mechanical therapies like CPAP.[97]

Antihypertensive Therapy and Obstructive Sleep Apnea

More than 50% of the adult to elderly population with sleep apnea, investigated in European sleep laboratories, receive treatment with antihypertensive drugs.[98] Conversely, at least 30% hypertensive patients and 80% of those with resistant hypertension exhibit moderate to severe OSA.[99] An experimental study showed that acute changes in systemic blood pressure adversely influenced genioglossus activity.[100] The question has been raised as to whether blood pressure reduction per se, or medications specifically used for the treatment of arterial hypertension, may influence sleep apnea. Few clinical trials have been conducted to address this issue, and the results are inconsistent. Both the angiotensin-converting enzyme inhibitor cilazapril and the β-blocker metoprolol were found to moderately reduce apnea frequency during sleep in an early double-blind trial.[101] However, no effect on AHI was found on celiprolol compared with the placebo in a more subsequent study.[102] Another double-blind randomized trial addressing cilazapril reported a marginal reduction of the respiratory disturbance index and the apnea index during non-REM but not during REM sleep.[103] This finding was not confirmed in a controlled trial comparing CPAP and the angiotensin II receptor antagonist valsartan.[104] A randomized study that compared the effect of atenolol, amlodipine, enalapril, hydrochlorothiazide, and losartan in 40 hypertensive patients with OSA found no effect on sleep disordered breathing by any of the studied compounds, although the degree of blood pressure reduction achieved by treatment varied between the therapies.[105] Finally, in a meta-analysis of 11 studies evaluating the effect of antihypertensive medications on the severity of OSA, a small but significant reduction of AHI was demonstrated.[106] The effect is more pronounced with the use of diuretics, suggesting volume control by promoting diuresis[107] or suppressing aldosterone[108] may be important for hypertensive patients with OSA.

Gastroesophageal Reflux and Sleep Disordered Breathing

Gastroesophageal reflux disease is common in patients with OSA. The exact mechanistic relationship between the two conditions is unclear but may, besides common predisposing factors, such as obesity and alcohol, involve the periodic reduction of intrathoracic pressure caused by OSA during sleep. Alternatively, acid reflux in gastroesophageal reflux disease may produce arousals and night choking as well as acid-induced long-term pharyngeal tissue swelling, which promotes upper airway obstruction during sleep. Indeed, a 50% reduction of AHI after short-term combined antireflux therapy for cisapride and omeprazole was described in patients with the two combined conditions.[109] A small parallel group study using nizatidine reported a decrease in the arousal index, but not in the AHI, after 1 month of treatment,[110] whereas omeprazole produced reductions in the apnea index and the AHI by 31% and 25%, respectively, in a preliminary study.[111] These findings are not supported by a more recent study, in which rabeprazole significantly improved objective and subjective measures of sleep quality in patients with OSA and gastroesophageal reflux disease, but the AHI remained unchanged.[112]

Other Specific Therapies that May Influence Obstructive Sleep Apnea

Several studies have attempted to reduce upper airway compliance by compounds that lower surface tension of liquids in the upper airway lining. These studies are generally small, and the effect size is moderate.[113–115] The effect of fluticasone on nasal airflow resistance–induced reduction of AHI was approximately 25% in patients with mild OSA and coexisting rhinitis.[116] However, the effectiveness could not be shown in a trial of nasal decongestant in moderate OSA.[117]

A different approach is that of various hormone replacement therapies in OSA. For instance, sex-related steroids have been speculated to mediate a protective effect against OSA which may be related to an oscillation of genioglossus electromyographic activity in menstrual cycle.[118] Other potential mechanisms include respiratory stimulation, improved chemosensitivity, or a modification of the arousal threshold. However, replacement with estrogen and progesterone to postmenopausal women has produced inconsistent data. Smaller studies showed a shortening of apnea duration,[119] whereas subsequent randomized controlled studies found a marginal reduction of the AHI.[120] In other studies, various combinations of estrogen and progesterone were ineffective[121] or reduced OSA.[122–124] Progesterone alone was also effective in postmenopausal women with documented upper airway obstruction.[125] Although these data suggest a potential for hormone replacement therapy after menopause with respect to sleep disordered breathing, there is a lack of a cost-benefit assessment that takes potential side effects into account.

The effect of substitution therapy on OSA in hypothyroidism has been previously discussed.[4] Hormone substitution may affect either a ventilator response or structure of the thyroid gland with potential influence in airway patency. Nevertheless, studies in the field are few, restricted in size, and with variable results. Most recommendations favor CPAP in patients with OSA receiving supplementation therapy. Repeat sleep studies may be warranted once hypothyroidism has been fully substituted.

SUMMARY

There is an unmet need for a drug therapy in OSA. However, previous attempts to identify an omnipotent drug have generally been unsuccessful; there is currently no available pharmacologic alternative to the mechanical therapies generally applied in this condition. Although the general efficacy of a medication may be lower than, for instance, that seen after CPAP, it should be recognized that a poorer efficacy in comparative terms may be overcome by better compliance. In fact, the poor long-term compliance with, for example, CPAP, actually strengthens the incentive to explore novel drug candidates.

Systematic drug development is a time-consuming process; many currently available medications in the pharmacopeia have been developed from basic chemistry through early testing and larger-scale clinical trials. This process has not yet been applied in OSA because relevant experimental models of the disorder are lacking. However, we have recently seen an improved understanding of physiologic mechanisms that may accelerate the development of drugs in sleep apnea. These insights have also enabled a more differential approach to the disorder. Specific phenotypes of OSA have been described; because of better classification of the disorder, we might recognize responders to specific therapies. In brief, we may be able to develop tailored medication strategies, which recognize the pathophysiology of OSA in each specific patient.

REFERENCES

1. Dempsey JA, Veasey SC, Morgan BJ, et al. Pathophysiology of sleep apnea. Physiol Rev 2010;90(1): 47–112.
2. McNicholas WT, Bonsigore MR, Management Committee of ECAB. Sleep apnoea as an independent risk factor for cardiovascular disease: current evidence, basic mechanisms and research priorities. Eur Respir J 2007;29(1):156–78.
3. Javaheri S, Barbe F, Campos-Rodriguez F, et al. Sleep apnea: types, mechanisms, and clinical cardiovascular consequences. J Am Coll Cardiol 2017;69(7):841–58.
4. Hedner J, Grote L, Zou D. Pharmacological treatment of sleep apnea: current situation and future strategies. Sleep Med Rev 2008;12(1): 33–47.
5. Sullivan SS, Guilleminault C. Emerging drugs for common conditions of sleepiness: obstructive sleep apnea and narcolepsy. Expert Opin Emerg Drugs 2015;20(4):571–82.
6. Mason M, Welsh EJ, Smith I. Drug therapy for obstructive sleep apnoea in adults. Cochrane Database Syst Rev 2013;(5):CD003002.
7. White DP. Pharmacologic approaches to the treatment of obstructive sleep apnea. Sleep Med Clin 2016;11(2):203–12.
8. Eckert DJ. Phenotypic approaches to obstructive sleep apnoea - new pathways for targeted therapy. Sleep Med Rev 2018;37:45–59.
9. Weaver TE, Grunstein RR. Adherence to continuous positive airway pressure therapy: the challenge to effective treatment. Proc Am Thorac Soc 2008;5(2):173–8.
10. Grote L, Hedner J, Grunstein R, et al. Therapy with nCPAP: incomplete elimination of sleep related breathing disorder. Eur Respir J 2000;16(5):921–7.
11. Peker Y, Glantz H, Eulenburg C, et al. Effect of positive airway pressure on cardiovascular outcomes in coronary artery disease patients with nonsleepy obstructive sleep apnea. The RICCADSA randomized controlled trial. Am J Respir Crit Care Med 2016;194(5):613–20.
12. Kohler M, Bloch KE, Stradling JR. Pharmacological approaches to the treatment of obstructive sleep apnoea. Expert Opin Investig Drugs 2009;18(5): 647–56.
13. Tkacova R, McNicholas WT, Javorsky M, et al. Nocturnal intermittent hypoxia predicts prevalent hypertension in the European Sleep Apnoea Database cohort study. Eur Respir J 2014;44(4):931–41.
14. Eckert DJ, White DP, Jordan AS, et al. Defining phenotypic causes of obstructive sleep apnea. Identification of novel therapeutic targets. Am J Respir Crit Care Med 2013;188(8):996–1004.
15. Younes M. Role of arousals in the pathogenesis of obstructive sleep apnea. Am J Respir Crit Care Med 2004;169(5):623–33.
16. Eckert DJ, Younes MK. Arousal from sleep: implications for obstructive sleep apnea pathogenesis and treatment. J Appl Physiol (1985) 2014;116(3): 302–13.
17. Younes M, Ostrowski M, Thompson W, et al. Chemical control stability in patients with obstructive sleep apnea. Am J Respir Crit Care Med 2001; 163(5):1181–90.
18. Brownell LG, West P, Sweatman P, et al. Protriptyline in obstructive sleep apnea: a double-blind trial. N Engl J Med 1982;307(17):1037–42.
19. Smith PL, Haponik EF, Allen RP, et al. The effects of protriptyline in sleep-disordered breathing. Am Rev Respir Dis 1983;127(1):8–13.
20. Whyte KF, Gould GA, Airlie MA, et al. Role of protriptyline and acetazolamide in the sleep apnea/hypopnea syndrome. Sleep 1988;11(5):463–72.
21. Series F, Cormier Y. Effects of protriptyline on diurnal and nocturnal oxygenation in patients with chronic obstructive pulmonary disease. Ann Intern Med 1990;113(7):507–11.
22. Series F, Marc I, Cormier Y, et al. Long-term effects of protriptyline in patients with chronic obstructive pulmonary disease. Am Rev Respir Dis 1993; 147(6 Pt 1):1487–90.
23. Osanai S, Akiba Y, Fujiuchi S, et al. Depression of peripheral chemosensitivity by a dopaminergic mechanism in patients with obstructive sleep apnoea syndrome. Eur Respir J 1999;13(2):418–23.
24. Larrain A, Kapur VK, Gooley TA, et al. Pharmacological treatment of obstructive sleep apnea with

a combination of pseudoephedrine and domperidone. J Clin Sleep Med 2010;6(2):117–23.

25. Grace KP, Hughes SW, Horner RL. Identification of a pharmacological target for genioglossus reactivation throughout sleep. Sleep 2014;37(1):41–50.

26. Taranto-Montemurro L, Sands SA, Azarbarzin A, et al. Effect of 4-aminopyridine on genioglossus muscle activity during sleep in healthy adults. Ann Am Thorac Soc 2017;14(7):1177–83.

27. Wirth KJ, Steinmeyer K, Ruetten H. Sensitization of upper airway mechanoreceptors as a new pharmacologic principle to treat obstructive sleep apnea: investigations with AVE0118 in anesthetized pigs. Sleep 2013;36(5):699–708.

28. Christ T, Wettwer E, Voigt N, et al. Pathology-specific effects of the IKur/Ito/IK,ACh blocker AVE0118 on ion channels in human chronic atrial fibrillation. Br J Pharmacol 2008;154(8):1619–30.

29. Linz D, Schotten U, Neuberger HR, et al. Combined blockade of early and late activated atrial potassium currents suppresses atrial fibrillation in a pig model of obstructive apnea. Heart Rhythm 2011;8(12):1933–9.

30. Real C, Seif I, Adrien J, et al. Ondansetron and fluoxetine reduce sleep apnea in mice lacking monoamine oxidase A. Respir Physiol Neurobiol 2009;168(3):230–8.

31. Neuzeret PC, Sakai K, Gormand F, et al. Application of histamine or serotonin to the hypoglossal nucleus increases genioglossus muscle activity across the wake-sleep cycle. J Sleep Res 2009; 18(1):113–21.

32. Yue W, Liu H, Zhang J, et al. Association study of serotonin transporter gene polymorphisms with obstructive sleep apnea syndrome in Chinese Han population. Sleep 2008;31(11):1535–41.

33. Veasey SC. Serotonin agonists and antagonists in obstructive sleep apnea: therapeutic potential. Am J Respir Med 2003;2(1):21–9.

34. Veasey SC, Chachkes J, Fenik P, et al. The effects of ondansetron on sleep-disordered breathing in the English bulldog. Sleep 2001;24(2):155–60.

35. Stradling J, Smith D, Radulovacki M, et al. Effect of ondansetron on moderate obstructive sleep apnoea, a single night, placebo-controlled trial. J Sleep Res 2003;12(2):169–70.

36. Sood S, Morrison JL, Liu H, et al. Role of endogenous serotonin in modulating genioglossus muscle activity in awake and sleeping rats. Am J Respir Crit Care Med 2005;172(10):1338–47.

37. Hanzel DA, Proia NG, Hudgel DW. Response of obstructive sleep apnea to fluoxetine and protriptyline. Chest 1991;100(2):416–21.

38. Kraiczi H, Hedner J, Dahlof P, et al. Effect of serotonin uptake inhibition on breathing during sleep and daytime symptoms in obstructive sleep apnea. Sleep 1999;22(1):61–7.

39. Sunderram J, Parisi RA, Strobel RJ. Serotonergic stimulation of the genioglossus and the response to nasal continuous positive airway pressure. Am J Respir Crit Care Med 2000;162(3 Pt 1):925–9.

40. Berry RB, Yamaura EM, Gill K, et al. Acute effects of paroxetine on genioglossus activity in obstructive sleep apnea. Sleep 1999;22(8):1087–92.

41. Aslan S, Isik E, Cosar B. The effects of mirtazapine on sleep: a placebo controlled, double-blind study in young healthy volunteers. Sleep 2002;25(6): 677–9.

42. Berry RB, Koch GL, Hayward LF. Low-dose mirtazapine increases genioglossus activity in the anesthetized rat. Sleep 2005;28(1):78–84.

43. Carley DW, Radulovacki M. Mirtazapine, a mixed-profile serotonin agonist/antagonist, suppresses sleep apnea in the rat. Am J Respir Crit Care Med 1999;160(6):1824–9.

44. Carley DW, Olopade C, Ruigt GS, et al. Efficacy of mirtazapine in obstructive sleep apnea syndrome. Sleep 2007;30(1):35–41.

45. Marshall NS, Yee BJ, Desai AV, et al. Two randomized placebo-controlled trials to evaluate the efficacy and tolerability of mirtazapine for the treatment of obstructive sleep apnea. Sleep 2008;31(6):824–31.

46. Liu X, Sood S, Liu H, et al. Opposing muscarinic and nicotinic modulation of hypoglossal motor output to genioglossus muscle in rats in vivo. J Physiol 2005;565(Pt 3):965–80.

47. Gothe B, Strohl KP, Levin S, et al. Nicotine: a different approach to treatment of obstructive sleep apnea. Chest 1985;87(1):11–7.

48. Davila DG, Hurt RD, Offord KP, et al. Acute effects of transdermal nicotine on sleep architecture, snoring, and sleep-disordered breathing in nonsmokers. Am J Respir Crit Care Med 1994;150(2):469–74.

49. Zevin S, Swed E, Cahan C. Clinical effects of locally delivered nicotine in obstructive sleep apnea syndrome. Am J Ther 2003;10(3):170–5.

50. Slamowitz DI, Edwards JK, Chajek-Shaul T, et al. The influence of a transmucosal cholinergic agonist on pharyngeal muscle activity. Sleep 2000;23(4):543–50.

51. Gilman S, Chervin RD, Koeppe RA, et al. Obstructive sleep apnea is related to a thalamic cholinergic deficit in MSA. Neurology 2003;61(1):35–9.

52. Hedner J, Kraiczi H, Peker Y, et al. Reduction of sleep-disordered breathing after physostigmine. Am J Respir Crit Care Med 2003;168(10):1246–51.

53. Sukys-Claudino L, Moraes W, Guilleminault C, et al. Beneficial effect of donepezil on obstructive sleep apnea: a double-blind, placebo-controlled clinical trial. Sleep Med 2012;13(3):290–6.

54. Li Y, Owens RL, Sands S, et al. The effect of donepezil on arousal threshold and apnea-hypopnea index. A randomized, double-blind, cross-over study. Ann Am Thorac Soc 2016;13(11):2012–8.

55. Carley DW, Paviovic S, Janelidze M, et al. Functional role for cannabinoids in respiratory stability during sleep. Sleep 2002;25(4):391–8.
56. Prasad B, Radulovacki MG, Carley DW. Proof of concept trial of dronabinol in obstructive sleep apnea. Front Psychiatry 2013;4:1.
57. Carley DW, Prasad B, Reid KJ, et al. Pharmacotherapy of apnea by cannabimimetic enhancement, the PACE clinical trial: effects of dronabinol in obstructive sleep apnea. Sleep 2018;41(1).
58. Mulloy E, McNicholas WT. Theophylline in obstructive sleep apnea. A double-blind evaluation. Chest 1992;101(3):753–7.
59. Hein H, Behnke G, Jorres RA, et al. The therapeutic effect of theophylline in mild obstructive sleep apnea/hypopnea syndrome: results of repeated measurements with portable recording devices at home. Eur J Med Res 2000;5(9):391–9.
60. Saletu B, Oberndorfer S, Anderer P, et al. Efficiency of continuous positive airway pressure versus theophylline therapy in sleep apnea: comparative sleep laboratory studies on objective and subjective sleep and awakening quality. Neuropsychobiology 1999;39(3):151–9.
61. Orth MM, Grootoonk S, Duchna HW, et al. Short-term effects of oral theophylline in addition to CPAP in mild to moderate OSAS. Respir Med 2005;99(4):471–6.
62. Javaheri S, Parker TJ, Wexler L, et al. Effect of theophylline on sleep-disordered breathing in heart failure. N Engl J Med 1996;335(8):562–7.
63. Hu K, Li Q, Yang J, et al. The effect of theophylline on sleep-disordered breathing in patients with stable chronic congestive heart failure. Chin Med J (Engl) 2003;116(11):1711–6.
64. Andreas S, Reiter H, Luthje L, et al. Differential effects of theophylline on sympathetic excitation, hemodynamics, and breathing in congestive heart failure. Circulation 2004;110(15):2157–62.
65. Edwards BA, Sands SA, Eckert DJ, et al. Acetazolamide improves loop gain but not the other physiological traits causing obstructive sleep apnoea. J Physiol 2012;590(5):1199–211.
66. Fischer R, Lang SM, Leitl M, et al. Theophylline and acetazolamide reduce sleep-disordered breathing at high altitude. Eur Respir J 2004;23(1):47–52.
67. Nussbaumer-Ochsner Y, Latshang TD, Ulrich S, et al. Patients with obstructive sleep apnea syndrome benefit from acetazolamide during an altitude sojourn: a randomized, placebo-controlled, double-blind trial. Chest 2012;141(1):131–8.
68. Javaheri S. Acetazolamide improves central sleep apnea in heart failure: a double-blind, prospective study. Am J Respir Crit Care Med 2006;173(2):234–7.
69. Tojima H, Kunitomo F, Kimura H, et al. Effects of acetazolamide in patients with the sleep apnoea syndrome. Thorax 1988;43(2):113–9.
70. Wang T, Eskandari D, Zou D, et al. Increased carbonic anhydrase activity is associated with sleep apnea severity and related hypoxemia. Sleep 2015;38(7):1067–73.
71. Parati G, Revera M, Giuliano A, et al. Effects of acetazolamide on central blood pressure, peripheral blood pressure, and arterial distensibility at acute high altitude exposure. Eur Heart J 2013; 34(10):759–66.
72. Eskandari D, Zou D, Grote L, et al. Acetazolamide reduces blood pressure and sleep-disordered breathing in patients with hypertension and obstructive sleep apnea: a randomized controlled trial. J Clin Sleep Med 2018;14(3):309–17.
73. Weber MV. Topiramate for obstructive sleep apnea and snoring. Am J Psychiatry 2002;159(5):872–3.
74. Winslow DH, Bowden CH, DiDonato KP, et al. A randomized, double-blind, placebo-controlled study of an oral, extended-release formulation of phentermine/topiramate for the treatment of obstructive sleep apnea in obese adults. Sleep 2012;35(11):1529–39.
75. Eskandari D, Zou D, Karimi M, et al. Zonisamide reduces obstructive sleep apnoea: a randomised placebo-controlled study. Eur Respir J 2014; 44(1):140–9.
76. Gadde KM, Franciscy DM, Wagner HR 2nd, et al. Zonisamide for weight loss in obese adults: a randomized controlled trial. JAMA 2003;289(14): 1820–5.
77. Roy-Byrne PP. The GABA-benzodiazepine receptor complex: structure, function, and role in anxiety. J Clin Psychiatry 2005;66(Suppl 2):14–20.
78. Richter DW, Schmidt-Garcon P, Pierrefiche O, et al. Neurotransmitters and neuromodulators controlling the hypoxic respiratory response in anaesthetized cats. J Physiol 1999;514(Pt 2):567–78.
79. Carter SG, Berger MS, Carberry JC, et al. Zopiclone increases the arousal threshold without impairing genioglossus activity in obstructive sleep apnea. Sleep 2016;39(4):757–66.
80. Lofaso F, Goldenberg F, Thebault C, et al. Effect of zopiclone on sleep, night-time ventilation, and daytime vigilance in upper airway resistance syndrome. Eur Respir J 1997;10(11):2573–7.
81. Hoijer U, Hedner J, Ejnell H, et al. Nitrazepam in patients with sleep apnoea: a double-blind placebo-controlled study. Eur Respir J 1994;7(11): 2011–5.
82. Rosenberg R, Roach JM, Scharf M, et al. A pilot study evaluating acute use of eszopiclone in patients with mild to moderate obstructive sleep apnea syndrome. Sleep Med 2007;8(5):464–70.
83. Eckert DJ, Owens RL, Kehlmann GB, et al. Eszopiclone increases the respiratory arousal threshold and lowers the apnoea/hypopnoea index in obstructive sleep apnoea patients with a low

arousal threshold. Clin Sci (Lond) 2011;120(12): 505–14.

84. Chapman JL, Vakulin A, Hedner J, et al. Modafinil/armodafinil in obstructive sleep apnoea: a systematic review and meta-analysis. Eur Respir J 2016; 47(5):1420–8.

85. Avellar AB, Carvalho LB, Prado GF, et al. Pharmacotherapy for residual excessive sleepiness and cognition in CPAP-treated patients with obstructive sleep apnea syndrome: a systematic review and meta-analysis. Sleep Med Rev 2016;30: 97–107.

86. Williams SC, Marshall NS, Kennerson M, et al. Modafinil effects during acute continuous positive airway pressure withdrawal: a randomized crossover double-blind placebo-controlled trial. Am J Respir Crit Care Med 2010;181(8):825–31.

87. Roth T, White D, Schmidt-Nowara W, et al. Effects of armodafinil in the treatment of residual excessive sleepiness associated with obstructive sleep apnea/hypopnea syndrome: a 12-week, multicenter, double-blind, randomized, placebo-controlled study in nCPAP-adherent adults. Clin Ther 2006; 28(5):689–706.

88. Dauvilliers Y, Bassetti C, Lammers GJ, et al. Pitolisant versus placebo or modafinil in patients with narcolepsy: a double-blind, randomised trial. Lancet Neurol 2013;12(11):1068–75.

89. Ruoff C, Swick TJ, Doekel R, et al. Effect of oral JZP-110 (ADX-N05) on wakefulness and sleepiness in adults with narcolepsy: a phase 2b study. Sleep 2016;39(7):1379–87.

90. Strollo PJ, Redline S, Hedner J, et al. Treatment of excessive sleepiness in patients with obstructive sleep apnea: efficacy and safety results of a 6-week, double-blind, placebo-controlled, randomized-withdrawal trial of solriamfetol (JZP-110). Sleep Med 2017;40(Supplement 1):e316.

91. Young T, Palta M, Dempsey J, et al. The occurrence of sleep-disordered breathing among middle-aged adults. N Engl J Med 1993;328(17): 1230–5.

92. Young T, Peppard PE, Gottlieb DJ. Epidemiology of obstructive sleep apnea: a population health perspective. Am J Respir Crit Care Med 2002; 165(9):1217–39.

93. Yee BJ, Phillips CL, Banerjee D, et al. The effect of sibutramine-assisted weight loss in men with obstructive sleep apnoea. Int J Obes (Lond) 2007;31(1):161–8.

94. Phillips CL, Yee BJ, Trenell MI, et al. Changes in regional adiposity and cardio-metabolic function following a weight loss program with sibutramine in obese men with obstructive sleep apnea. J Clin Sleep Med 2009;5(5):416–21.

95. Ferland A, Poirier P, Series F. Sibutramine versus continuous positive airway pressure in obese obstructive sleep apnoea patients. Eur Respir J 2009;34(3):694–701.

96. Blackman A, Foster GD, Zammit G, et al. Effect of liraglutide 3.0 mg in individuals with obesity and moderate or severe obstructive sleep apnea: the SCALE Sleep Apnea randomized clinical trial. Int J Obes (Lond) 2016;40(8):1310–9.

97. Drager LF, Brunoni AR, Jenner R, et al. Effects of CPAP on body weight in patients with obstructive sleep apnoea: a meta-analysis of randomised trials. Thorax 2015;70(3):258–64.

98. Hedner J, Grote L, Bonsignore M, et al. The European Sleep Apnoea Database (ESADA): report from 22 European sleep laboratories. Eur Respir J 2011;38(3):635–42.

99. Logan AG, Perlikowski SM, Mente A, et al. High prevalence of unrecognized sleep apnoea in drug-resistant hypertension. J Hypertens 2001; 19(12):2271–7.

100. Garpestad E, Basner RC, Ringler J, et al. Phenylephrine-induced hypertension acutely decreases genioglossus EMG activity in awake humans. J Appl Physiol (1985) 1992;72(1):110–5.

101. Mayer J, Weichler U, Herres-Mayer B, et al. Influence of metoprolol and cilazapril on blood pressure and on sleep apnea activity. J Cardiovasc Pharmacol 1990;16(6):952–61.

102. Planes C, Foucher A, Leroy M, et al. Effect of celiprolol treatment in hypertensive patients with sleep apnea. Sleep 1999;22(4):507–13.

103. Grote L, Wutkewicz K, Knaack L, et al. Association between blood pressure reduction with antihypertensive treatment and sleep apnea activity. Am J Hypertens 2000;13(12):1280–7.

104. Pepin JL, Tamisier R, Barone-Rochette G, et al. Comparison of continuous positive airway pressure and valsartan in hypertensive patients with sleep apnea. Am J Respir Crit Care Med 2010;182(7): 954–60.

105. Kraiczi H, Hedner J, Peker Y, et al. Comparison of atenolol, amlodipine, enalapril, hydrochlorothiazide, and losartan for antihypertensive treatment in patients with obstructive sleep apnea. Am J Respir Crit Care Med 2000;161(5):1423–8.

106. Khurshid K, Yabes J, Weiss PM, et al. Effect of antihypertensive medications on the severity of obstructive sleep apnea: a systematic review and meta-analysis. J Clin Sleep Med 2016;12(8): 1143–51.

107. Kasai T, Bradley TD, Friedman O, et al. Effect of intensified diuretic therapy on overnight rostral fluid shift and obstructive sleep apnoea in patients with uncontrolled hypertension. J Hypertens 2014; 32(3):673–80.

108. Gaddam K, Pimenta E, Thomas SJ, et al. Spironolactone reduces severity of obstructive sleep apnoea in patients with resistant hypertension: a

preliminary report. J Hum Hypertens 2010;24(8): 532–7.

109. Xiao G, Wang Z, Ke M, et al. The relationship between obstructive sleep apnea and gastroesophageal reflux and the effect of antireflux therapy. Zhonghua Nei Ke Za Zhi 1999;38(1):33–6 [in Chinese].

110. Ing AJ, Ngu MC, Breslin AB. Obstructive sleep apnea and gastroesophageal reflux. Am J Med 2000; 108(Suppl 4a):120S–5S.

111. Senior BA, Khan M, Schwimmer C, et al. Gastroesophageal reflux and obstructive sleep apnea. Laryngoscope 2001;111(12):2144–6.

112. Orr WC, Robert JJ, Houck JR, et al. The effect of acid suppression on upper airway anatomy and obstruction in patients with sleep apnea and gastroesophageal reflux disease. J Clin Sleep Med 2009;5(4):330–4.

113. Jokic R, Klimaszewski A, Mink J, et al. Surface tension forces in sleep apnea: the role of a soft tissue lubricant: a randomized double-blind, placebo-controlled trial. Am J Respir Crit Care Med 1998; 157(5 Pt 1):1522–5.

114. Morrell MJ, Arabi Y, Zahn BR, et al. Effect of surfactant on pharyngeal mechanics in sleeping humans: implications for sleep apnoea. Eur Respir J 2002; 20(2):451–7.

115. Kirkness JP, Madronio M, Stavrinou R, et al. Relationship between surface tension of upper airway lining liquid and upper airway collapsibility during sleep in obstructive sleep apnea hypopnea syndrome. J Appl Physiol (1985) 2003;95(5): 1761–6.

116. Kiely JL, Nolan P, McNicholas WT. Intranasal corticosteroid therapy for obstructive sleep apnoea in patients with co-existing rhinitis. Thorax 2004; 59(1):50–5.

117. Braver HM, Block AJ. Effect of nasal spray, positional therapy, and the combination thereof in the asymptomatic snorer. Sleep 1994;17(6):516–21.

118. Popovic RM, White DP. Upper airway muscle activity in normal women: influence of hormonal status. J Appl Physiol (1985) 1998;84(3):1055–62.

119. Block AJ, Wynne JW, Boysen PG, et al. Menopause, medroxyprogesterone and breathing during sleep. Am J Med 1981;70(3):506–10.

120. Pickett CK, Regensteiner JG, Woodard WD, et al. Progestin and estrogen reduce sleep-disordered breathing in postmenopausal women. J Appl Physiol (1985) 1989;66(4):1656–61.

121. Cistulli PA, Barnes DJ, Grunstein RR, et al. Effect of short-term hormone replacement in the treatment of obstructive sleep apnoea in postmenopausal women. Thorax 1994;49(7):699–702.

122. Keefe DL, Watson R, Naftolin F. Hormone replacement therapy may alleviate sleep apnea in menopausal women: a pilot study. Menopause 1999; 6(3):196–200.

123. Manber R, Kuo TF, Cataldo N, et al. The effects of hormone replacement therapy on sleep-disordered breathing in postmenopausal women: a pilot study. Sleep 2003;26(2):163–8.

124. Wesstrom J, Ulfberg J, Nilsson S. Sleep apnea and hormone replacement therapy: a pilot study and a literature review. Acta Obstet Gynecol Scand 2005; 84(1):54–7.

125. Saaresranta T, Polo-Kantola P, Rauhala E, et al. Medroxyprogesterone in postmenopausal females with partial upper airway obstruction during sleep. Eur Respir J 2001;18(6):989–95.

Pharmacologic and Nonpharmacologic Treatment of Restless Legs Syndrome

Galia V. Anguelova, MD, MSc, Monique H.M. Vlak, MD, PhD,
Arthur G.Y. Kurvers, MD, Roselyne M. Rijsman, MD, PhD*

KEYWORDS

- Restless legs syndrome • Therapy • Treatment • Pharmacologic • Nonpharmacologic
- Augmentation

KEY POINTS

- There is limited evidence for nonpharmacologic treatment in primary restless legs syndrome (RLS): pneumatic compression, near-infrared light spectroscopy, and transcranial magnetic stimulation.
- In moderate to severe RLS, pharmacologic treatment may be considered, starting with iron suppletion if applicable.
- There is strong evidence for both $\alpha2\delta$ ligands and dopamine agonists in the therapy for RLS.
- When single-drug therapy with an $\alpha2\delta$ ligand or dopamine agonist is insufficient, a combination of both may be considered or oxycodone/naloxone.
- To treat augmentation, a low dose or longer-acting dopaminergic drug may be chosen, or a switch to an $\alpha2\delta$ ligand or oxycodone/naloxone may be considered.

INTRODUCTION

Restless legs syndrome (RLS) is a sleep-related disorder defined by an urgency to move the legs, usually combined with uncomfortable or unpleasant sensations, which occurs or worsens during rest, usually in the evening or at night, and disappears with movement of the legs.[1] It occurs in 5% to 15% of European and North American adults, 2% to 3% with moderate to severe symptoms, twice as often in women as in men, and has a mean onset age between 30 and 40 years.[1] RLS can be classified as idiopathic or primary, and secondary to comorbid conditions (eg, renal disease, polyneuropathy).[1] The pathophysiology of RLS is still unclear. However, dopaminergic dysfunction and iron deficiency have been suggested to play an essential role, possibly interacting with each other as well.[1] Glutamate, adenosine, and opiate systems are also considered to play a role in the pathophysiology.[1] This article provides an updated practical guide for the treatment of primary RLS in adults. Iron deficiency is included in our definition of primary RLS because of its essential role in the pathophysiology. Treatment of periodic limb movements was beyond the focus of this article. The available evidence is reviewed for pharmacologic as well as nonpharmacologic treatment options.

Disclosure: The authors declare that they have no conflict of interest. This research received no specific grant from any funding agency in the public, commercial, or not-for-profit sectors.
Center for Sleep and Wake Disorders, Haaglanden Medical Center, The Hague, The Netherlands
* Corresponding author. Center for Sleep and Wake disorders, Haaglanden Medical Center, PO 432, The Hague 2501 CK, The Netherlands.
E-mail address: r.rijsman@haaglandenmc.nl

Sleep Med Clin 13 (2018) 219–230
https://doi.org/10.1016/j.jsmc.2018.02.005
1556-407X/18/© 2018 Elsevier Inc. All rights reserved.

METHODS

This article was written in continuation of the 2016 RLS guidelines by the American Academy of Neurology (AAN).[2] The authors performed a PubMed search for articles on treatment of primary RLS using MeSH (Medical Subject Headings) terms and keywords with a start date of 1 January 2015, because the AAN guideline included articles published until the 15 July 2015.[2] Our search was last performed on 15 October 2017. Details on the search strategy are given in **Box 1**.

The titles and abstracts of the eligible articles were screened. The authors only included studies that met the following criteria: (1) original article; (2) on treatment of primary RLS (including iron deficiency–related RLS); (3) in humans; (4) published in English. Case reports were excluded. We focused primarily on the effect on RLS symptoms and periodic limb movements. A standardized tool to report RLS symptom severity is the International Restless Legs Syndrome Study Group rating scale (IRLS), which measures symptoms in the past week with 10 items each graded from 0 to 4 with increasing severity (with a maximum score of 40).[2] Because international guidelines no longer recommend the use of pergolide for RLS, we did not include new studies on pergolide alone. Acupuncture, Chinese herbs, meditation, music, and prayer were considered outside the scope of our review.

Additional articles found in the references of articles identified through our database search were also reviewed if considered relevant according to the criteria mentioned earlier. Relevant articles were classified according to their risk of bias (increasing from I to IV) and subsequent recommendations were made according to the criteria described by the AAN guideline (level A, B, C, and U in decreasing order of evidence level).[2] Studies published after the 2016 AAN guideline are discussed in detail. For studies already described in the 2016 AAN guideline, we refer to the AAN guideline.

RESULTS
Pharmacologic Treatment Options

Table 1 shows the pharmacologic agents effective in RLS treatment with at least evidence level C with their initial and usual daily dose, pharmacokinetics, specific considerations, and side effects.

Dopamine precursors
Levodopa Levodopa was one of the first drugs studied for treating RLS. There are 4 class III studies showing a benefit of levodopa (100–200 mg) on RLS severity (level C).[2] Also a possible effect on the periodic limb movement index (PLMI) was found based on 3 class III studies (level C).[2] Augmentation (discussed later) is a major problem with long-term daily use of levodopa in RLS. It occurs in 40% to 60% of patients after 6 months of follow-up, but augmentation rates as high as 71% have been reported.[3]

Non–ergot-derived dopamine agonists
Pramipexole Pramipexole is a dopamine agonist which is excreted by the kidney. There is level A evidence that pramipexole improves RLS symptoms based on 3 class I studies and 6 class II studies.[2] Improvement of PLMI was seen in 3 class II studies giving level B evidence.[2] Two open-label studies reported that efficacy on RLS symptoms continues up to 1 year.[4,5] A study comparing pramipexole with dual-release levodopa/benserazide found that both drugs are effective in reducing RLS symptoms and PLMI, but levodopa had a higher rate of augmentation (21%) compared with pramipexole (6%).[6]

Ropinirole Ropinirole was effective in improving RLS symptoms up to 6 months according to 2 class I studies and up to 1 year according to 2 class I studies (level B).[2] Ropinirole also improves PLMI according to 2 class I studies (level A).[2] Ropinirole is a dopamine agonist primarily metabolized by the liver, mainly via the cytochrome P (CYP) 1A2 enzyme but also via CYP3A. Substances that inhibit and promote those enzymes can interact with ropinirole.[7]

Rotigotine Rotigotine is a dopaminergic agonist delivered through a transdermal patch allowing a continuous release and thus maintaining stable concentrations that mimic physiologic striatal dopamine receptor function.[8–10] Because of the transdermal delivery, rotigotine is especially useful in patients with daytime symptoms, patients with swallowing difficulties, and patients undergoing surgery.[11] Rotigotine has been shown to reduce RLS symptoms up to 6 months in 2 class I and 3 class II studies (level A) and reduce PLMI in 1 class I study (level B).[2] Our search strategy identified 1 new class I study that has been published since the AAN guideline in 2016.[12] This study randomized 150 patients to receive an optimal dose of rotigotine (1–3 mg) or placebo (randomization 2:1). Although rotigotine was effective in improving IRLS scores at 4 weeks of treatment, there was no superiority compared with placebo (least square mean with 95% confidence intervals [CIs] from an ANCOVA [Analysis of Covariance] model −0.27, 95% CI, −3.0–2.4; $P = .8451$). Long-term efficacy was studied in 3 noncomparative

Box 1
PubMed search strategy

- Dopamine agonists ("Dopamine Agonists"[Mesh] OR "Dopamine Agonists" [Pharmacological Action] OR (dopamin* AND agonist*) OR "Levodopa"[Mesh] OR levodopa*[tiab] OR "pramipexole" [Supplementary Concept] OR pramipexol*[tiab] OR "ropinirole" [Supplementary Concept] OR ropinirol* [tiab] OR "rotigotine" [Supplementary Concept] OR Rotigotin*[tiab] OR "Pergolide"[Mesh] OR Pergolid*[tiab] OR "cabergoline" [Supplementary Concept] OR Cabergolin*[tiab]) AND ("Restless Legs Syndrome"[Mesh] OR "rls"[ti] OR rls'*[ti] OR (restles*[ti] AND leg*[ti]) OR restless leg*[tiab] OR ekbom*[tiab]) NOT ("Animals"[Mesh] NOT "Humans"[Mesh]) AND 2015/01:3000/01 [dp]

- α2δ ligands (alpha-2-delta[tiab] OR alpha2delta[tiab] OR α2δ[tiab] OR α-2-δ[tiab] OR "gabapentin" [Supplementary Concept] OR gabapentin*[tiab] OR "Pregabalin"[Mesh] OR pregabalin*[tiab] OR "1-(((alpha-isobutanoyloxyethoxy)carbonyl)aminomethyl)-1-cyclohexaneacetic acid" [Supplementary Concept] OR "Cyclohexanecarboxylic Acids"[Mesh] OR "gamma-Aminobutyric Acid"[Mesh]) AND ("Restless Legs Syndrome"[Mesh] OR "rls"[ti] OR rls'*[ti] OR (restles*[ti] AND leg*[ti]) OR restless leg*[tiab] OR ekbom*[tiab]) NOT ("Animals"[Mesh] NOT "Humans"[Mesh]) AND 2015/01:3000/01 [dp]

- Specific N-methyl-D-aspartate receptor agonists and drugs acting on AMPA-receptors ("traxoprodil mesylate" [Supplementary Concept] OR Traxoprodil*[tiab] OR "ifenprodil" [Supplementary Concept] OR Ifenprodil*[tiab] OR "aniracetam" [Supplementary Concept] OR Aniracetam*[tiab] OR "Kynurenic Acid"[Mesh] OR Kynurenic acid*[tiab] OR Kynurenate[tiab] OR "perampanel" [Supplementary Concept] OR Perampanel*[tiab] OR "tezampanel" [Supplementary Concept] OR Tezampanel*[tiab]) AND ("Restless Legs Syndrome"[Mesh] OR "rls"[ti] OR rls'*[ti] OR (restles*[ti] AND leg* [ti]) OR restless leg*[tiab] OR ekbom*[tiab]) NOT ("Animals"[Mesh] NOT "Humans"[Mesh]) AND 2015/01:3000/01 [dp]

- Opioids ("Analgesics, Opioid"[Mesh] OR "Analgesics, Opioid" [Pharmacological Action] OR "Narcotics" [Pharmacological Action] OR Opiate[tiab] OR opioid*[tiab] OR "Tramadol"[Mesh] OR tramadol[tiab] OR tramdol[tiab] OR "Morphine"[Mesh] OR morphin*[tiab] OR "Oxycodone"[Mesh] OR Oxycodon*[tiab] OR "Fentanyl"[Mesh] OR Fentanyl[tiab] OR "Naloxone"[Mesh] OR Naloxon*[tiab] OR "Methadone"[Mesh] OR Methadon*[tiab] OR "Ketamine"[Mesh] OR Ketamin*[tiab] OR "Tilidine"[Mesh] OR Tilidine[tiab]) AND ("Restless Legs Syndrome"[Mesh] OR "rls"[ti] OR rls'*[ti] OR (restles*[ti] AND leg*[ti]) OR restless leg*[tiab] OR ekbom*[tiab]) NOT ("Animals"[Mesh] NOT "Humans"[Mesh]) AND 2015/01:3000/01 [dp]

- Iron ("Iron"[Mesh] OR "ferric carboxymaltose" [Supplementary Concept] AND ferric carboxymaltose[tiab] OR iron carboxymaltose[tiab] OR "ferrous sulfate" [Supplementary Concept] OR ferrous sulfate[tiab] OR iron sulfate[tiab] OR ferric sulfate[tiab] OR ferrous sulphate[tiab] OR iron sulphate[tiab] OR ferric sulphate[tiab] OR "ferric oxide, saccharated" [Supplementary Concept] OR iron-saccharate[tiab] OR iron sucrose[tiab] OR "saccharated iron oxide"[tiab] OR ferric saccharate[tiab] OR ferri saccharate[tiab] OR "ferric gluconate" [Supplementary Concept] AND "Bioferrico" [Supplementary Concept] OR ferric gluconate[tiab] OR iron gluconate[tiab] OR ferrous gluconate[tiab] OR ferrigluconate[tiab] OR "Iron-Dextran Complex"[Mesh] OR Iron Dextran[tiab] OR ferridextran[tiab] OR "Ferrosoferric Oxide"[Mesh] OR Ferrosoferric Oxide[tiab] OR ferumoxytol[tiab] OR ferriferrous oxide[tiab] OR "iron isomaltoside 1000" [Supplementary Concept] OR iron isomaltoside[tiab]) AND ("Restless Legs Syndrome"[Mesh] OR "rls"[ti] OR rls'*[ti] OR (restles*[ti] AND leg*[ti]) OR restless leg*[tiab] OR ekbom*[tiab]) NOT ("Animals"[Mesh] NOT "Humans"[Mesh]) AND 2015/01:3000/01 [dp]

- Other medication ("Melatonin"[Mesh] OR melatonin*[tiab] OR "Glucosamine"[Mesh] OR Glucosamine[tiab] OR 2-Amino-2-Deoxyglucose[tiab] OR Hespercorbin[tiab] OR dona[tiab] OR xicil[tiab] OR "Magnesium"[Mesh] OR magnesium*[tiab] OR "Creatine"[Mesh] OR creatin*[tiab] OR "coenzyme Q10" [Supplementary Concept] OR coenzyme Q10[tiab] OR co-enzyme Q10[tiab] OR "CoQ 10"[tiab] OR "CoQ10"[tiab] OR ubidecarenone[tiab] OR ubiquinone[tiab] OR Bio-Quinone Q10 [tiab] OR ubisemiquinone radical[tiab] OR Q-ter[tiab] OR ubisemiquinone[tiab]) AND ("Restless Legs Syndrome"[Mesh] OR "rls"[ti] OR rls'*[ti] OR (restles*[ti] AND leg*[ti]) OR restless leg*[tiab] OR ekbom*[tiab]) NOT ("Animals"[Mesh] NOT "Humans"[Mesh]) AND 2015/01:3000/01 [dp]

  - Benzodiazepines ("Benzodiazepines"[Mesh] OR Benzodiazepin*[tiab] OR "Clonazepam"[Mesh] OR clonazepam*[tiab] OR "zolpidem" [Supplementary Concept] OR zolpidem*[tiab]) AND ("Restless Legs Syndrome"[Mesh] OR "rls"[ti] OR rls'*[ti] OR (restles*[ti] AND leg*[ti]) OR restless leg*[tiab] OR ekbom*[tiab]) NOT ("Animals"[Mesh] NOT "Humans"[Mesh]) AND 2015/ 01:3000/01 [dp]

○ Antiepileptics ("Anticonvulsants" [Pharmacological Action] OR "Anticonvulsants"[Mesh] OR anticonvuls*[tiab] OR anti-convuls*[tiab] OR antiepileptic*[tiab] OR anti-epileptic*[tiab] OR "Carbamazepine"[Mesh] OR Carbamazepin*[tiab] OR "etiracetam" [Supplementary Concept] OR etiracetam[tiab] OR Levetiracetam[tiab] OR "Valproic Acid"[Mesh] OR Valproic acid*[tiab] OR Tegretol[tiab] OR Carbazepin[tiab] OR Epitol[tiab] OR Finlepsin[tiab] OR Neurotol[tiab] OR Amizepine[tiab] OR keppla[tiab] OR Propylisopropylacetic Acid[tiab] OR 2 Propylpentanoic Acid[tiab] OR Divalproex[tiab] OR Depakene[tiab] OR Depakine[tiab] OR Convulsofin[tiab] OR Depakote[tiab] OR Vupral[tiab] OR Divalproex Sodium[tiab] OR Valproate[tiab] OR Ergenyl[tiab] OR Dipropyl Acetate[tiab]) AND ("Restless Legs Syndrome"[Mesh] OR "rls"[ti] OR rls'*[ti] OR (restles*[ti] AND leg*[ti]) OR restless leg*[tiab] OR ekbom* [tiab]) NOT ("Animals"[Mesh] NOT "Humans"[Mesh]) AND 2015/01:3000/01 [dp]

Nonpharmacologic treatment options

- Sleep hygiene ("Sleep Hygiene"[Mesh] OR sleep hygiene[tiab] OR sleep habit*[tiab]) AND ("Restless Legs Syndrome"[Mesh] OR "rls"[ti] OR rls'*[ti] OR (restles*[ti] AND leg*[ti]) OR restless leg*[tiab] OR ekbom*[tiab]) NOT ("Animals"[Mesh] NOT "Humans"[Mesh]) AND 2015/01:3000/01 [dp]

- Caffeine and alcohol intake and smoking ("coffee"[MeSH Terms] OR "Caffeine"[Mesh] OR coffee [tiab] OR Caffeine[tiab] OR "Alcohol Drinking"[Mesh] OR "alcoholic beverages"[MeSH Terms] OR alcohol*[tiab]) AND ("Restless Legs Syndrome"[Mesh] OR "rls"[ti] OR rls'*[ti] OR (restles*[ti] AND leg*[ti]) OR restless leg*[tiab] OR ekbom*[tiab]) NOT ("Animals"[Mesh] NOT "Humans"[Mesh]) AND 2015/01:3000/01 [dp]

- Mental activity ("Mental Processes"[Mesh] OR "mental activity"[tiab] OR "Reading"[Mesh] OR reading[tiab] OR read[tiab] OR card game*[tiab] OR brain teaser*[tiab] OR chess[tiab] OR computer work[tiab]) AND ("Restless Legs Syndrome"[Mesh] OR "rls"[ti] OR rls'*[ti] OR (restles*[ti] AND leg*[ti]) OR restless leg*[tiab] OR ekbom*[tiab]) NOT ("Animals"[Mesh] NOT "Humans"[Mesh]) AND 2015/01:3000/01 [dp]

- Physical activity (including yoga) (Aerobic*[tiab] OR "Exercise Therapy"[MeSH] OR "Exercise"[MeSH] OR exercise[tiab] OR "Yoga"[Mesh] OR yoga[tiab] OR "Resistance Training"[Mesh] OR resistance training[tiab] OR "Weight Lifting"[Mesh] OR Weight lifting[tiab] OR weight bearing[tiab] OR "Bicycling"[Mesh] OR bicycl*[tiab] OR cycling[tiab] OR cycle[tiab]) AND ("Restless Legs Syndrome"[Mesh] OR "rls"[ti] OR rls'*[ti] OR (restles*[ti] AND leg*[ti]) OR restless leg*[tiab] OR ekbom*[tiab]) NOT ("Animals"[Mesh] NOT "Humans"[Mesh]) AND 2015/01:3000/01 [dp]

- Pneumatic compression ("Intermittent Pneumatic Compression Devices"[Mesh] OR ((Pneumatic[tiab] OR mechanical[tiab]) AND compression[tiab]) OR IPC[tiab]) AND ("Restless Legs Syndrome"[Mesh] OR "rls"[ti] OR rls'*[ti] OR (restles*[ti] AND leg*[ti]) OR restless leg*[tiab] OR ekbom*[tiab]) NOT ("Animals"[Mesh] NOT "Humans"[Mesh]) AND 2015/01:3000/01 [dp]

- Tactile stimulus (including hot baths, massage and vibratory pads) ("Vibration"[Mesh] OR vibrat* [tiab] OR pad[tiab] OR pads[tiab] OR "Balneology"[Mesh] OR "Hydrotherapy"[Mesh] OR "Hot Temperature"[Mesh] OR "Hot Springs"[Mesh] OR bath*[tiab] OR "Massage"[Mesh] OR massage*[tiab] OR bodywork*[tiab]) AND ("Restless Legs Syndrome"[Mesh] OR "rls"[ti] OR rls'*[ti] OR (restles*[ti] AND leg*[ti]) OR restless leg*[tiab] OR ekbom*[tiab]) NOT ("Animals"[Mesh] NOT "Humans"[Mesh]) AND 2015/01:3000/01 [dp]

- Current or magnetic stimulus (("Transcranial Direct Current Stimulation"[Mesh] OR tsDCS*[tiab] OR tDCS*[tiab] OR ((transcranial[tiab] OR cathodal[tiab] OR anodal[tiab] OR electric*[tiab]) AND stimul*[tiab]) OR "Transcutaneous Electric Nerve Stimulation"[Mesh] OR TENS[tiab] OR tsDCS[tiab] OR ((Percutaneous[tiab] OR Transcutaneous[tiab] OR transdermal[tiab] OR cutaneous[tiab]) AND (Electric[tiab] OR electrical[tiab] OR electrostimulation[tiab] OR stimul*[tiab])) OR ("Transcranial Magnetic Stimulation"[Mesh] OR Transcranial Magnetic Stimulation*[tiab] OR rTMS[tiab] OR TMS [tiab] OR "Cortical Excitability"[Mesh] OR Cortical Excitability[tiab])) AND ("Restless Legs Syndrome"[Mesh] OR "rls"[ti] OR rls'*[ti] OR (restles*[ti] AND leg*[ti]) OR restless leg*[tiab] OR ekbom*[tiab]) NOT ("Animals"[Mesh] NOT "Humans"[Mesh]) AND ("2015/01/01"[PDAT]: "3000/12/31"[PDAT])

- Light stimulus ("Infrared Rays"[Mesh] OR near-infrared light[tiab] OR NIR[tiab] OR near-infrared ray* [tiab] OR "Phototherapy"[Mesh] OR phototherap*[tiab] OR light therap*[tiab] OR phototherap* [tiab] OR photoradiation therap*[tiab] OR heliotherap*[tiab] OR) AND ("Restless Legs Syndrome"[Mesh] OR "rls"[ti] OR rls'*[ti] OR (restles*[ti] AND leg*[ti]) OR restless leg*[tiab] OR ekbom*[tiab]) NOT ("Animals"[Mesh] NOT "Humans"[Mesh]) AND 2015/01:3000/01 [dp]

- Cognitive therapy ("Adaptation, Psychological"[Mesh] OR "Cognitive Therapy"[Mesh] OR (cogniti* [ti] AND therap*[ti]) OR psychotherap*[tiab] OR "Mindfulness"[Mesh] OR mindful*[tiab]) AND ("Restless Legs Syndrome"[Mesh] OR "rls"[ti] OR rls'*[ti] OR (restles*[ti] AND leg*[ti]) OR restless leg*[tiab] OR ekbom*[tiab]) NOT ("Animals"[Mesh] NOT "Humans"[Mesh]) AND 2015/01:3000/01 [dp]

Vitamins ("Vitamins"[Pharmacological Action] OR vitamin*[tiab] OR ascorbic acid[tiab] OR cholecal-ciferol[tiab] OR calcitriol[tiab] OR calciol[tiab] OR "Calcium"[Mesh] OR "Calcium Carbonate"[Mesh] OR calcium[tiab] OR tocopherol[tiab] OR alpha-tocopherol[tiab] OR beta-tocopherol[tiab] OR gamma-tocopherol[tiab] OR "Vitamin B 6"[Mesh] OR "Vitamin B 12"[Mesh] OR "Vitamin B Com-plex"[Mesh] OR "Vitamin B Complex" [Pharmacological Action] OR "Folic Acid"[Mesh] OR folic acid[tiab] OR folvite[tiab] OR folacin[tiab] OR folate[tiab]) AND ("Restless Legs Syndrome"[Mesh] OR "rls"[ti] OR rls'*[ti] OR (restles*[ti] AND leg*[ti]) OR restless leg*[tiab] OR ekbom*[tiab]) NOT ("An-imals"[Mesh] NOT "Humans"[Mesh]) AND 2015/01:3000/01 [dp]

extension studies that found continued efficacy up to 5 years.[13–15]

Piribedil There is insufficient evidence (level U) for the effectiveness of piribedil on RLS symptoms based on 1 open-label class IV study in which RLS symptoms improved in a group of 13 patients with a median dose of 50 mg of piribedil daily.[16]

Ergot-derived dopamine agonists
Both pergolide (1 class I study and 2 class II studies) and cabergoline (2 class I studies) have been shown to be effective in treating RLS (level A).[2] However, all ergot-derived dopamine agonists have been associated with severe life-threatening side effects, including fibrosis and valvulopathy. International guidelines do not recommend the use of pergolide, which is no longer available in the United States for RLS.[2,17,18] European RLS guidelines also no longer recommend cabergoline for treating patients with RLS.[18] In the United States, cabergoline is only suggested as an option when other recommended agents have been tried first and failed, and on the condition that close clin-ical follow-up is provided.[17]

α2δ Ligands
Gabapentin enacarbil Gabapentin enacarbil is a slow-release prodrug of gabapentin. It is absorbed by active transport in the gut and then converted to gabapentin. Four class I studies show that gabapentin enacarbil is effective in moderate to severe RLS in treating daytime symptoms (level A).[2] It is likely to be effective for at least 6 months (1 class II study).[2] The IRLS score had improved by 15.5 points at 24 weeks. Relapses were less com-mon in the active treatment arm compared with the placebo arm (9% vs 23%; P = .02). There is insufficient evidence based on 1 class III study (level U) for gabapentin enacarbil to have any sig-nificant effect on PLMI, although it is likely to improve other sleep measures based on 1 class I and 1 class III study.[2]

Pregabalin Pregabalin is effective in the treatment of moderate to severe primary RLS up to 1 year when dosed 150 to 450 mg/d (level B). This advice is based on 1 class I study: at 52 weeks pregabalin

significantly reduced IRLS scores compared with pramipexole.[2] Pregabalin is likely to improve PLMI (2 class II studies), also likely to improve some other sleep measures (1 class I study, 2 class II studies), and likely to improve subjective sleep (1 class I study, 3 class II studies).[1,2] Compared with pramipexole, pregabalin is more likely to improve subjective sleep outcomes (based on 2 class II studies).[2]

Gabapentin There is 1 class III study showing an effect of gabapentin at 6 weeks.[2] However, no long-term studies were performed (level U).[19] Un-like gabapentin enacarbil, the absorption of gaba-pentin is variable, which makes it more difficult to select the optimal dose.

Specific N-methyl-D-aspartate (NMDA) receptor agonists and drugs acting on α-amino-3-hydroxy-5-methyl-4-isoxazolepropionic acid (AMPA) re-ceptors α2δ Ligands reduce glutamatergic trans-mission. Therefore, other drugs with a similar effect are being studied, such as AMPA-type glutamate receptor antagonists. One class IV study showed that perampanel (a selective noncompetitive AMPA-type glutamate receptor antagonist) administered 2 to 4 mg orally daily significantly improves IRLS scores after 2 months (longer follow-up is currently investigated by the same study group) and decreases PLMI and the periodic limb movement arousal index.[20]

Opioids
In 1 class II study, prolonged-release oxycodone/naloxone improved, for example, IRLS scores compared with placebo after 12 weeks (level C).[2] One class III crossover study showed that oxyco-done improved RLS symptoms and PLMI compared with placebo (level C).[2] There is insuffi-cient evidence (level U) for both methadone (1 class III and 1 class IV study), tramadol (1 class IV study), and intrathecal morphine (1 class IV study).[2] There was also insufficient evidence (level U) for dihydrocodeine, propoxyphene, and tilidine (2 class IV studies).[2] Two studies have reported augmentation after RLS treatment with tramadol, whereas it has not been reported with other opioids.[21,22]

Table 1
Pharmacologic treatment options for primary restless legs syndrome with a focus on restless legs syndrome symptoms

Medication	Level of Evidence	Initial Daily Dose (mg)	Usual Dose Range	$T_{1/2}$ (h)	T_{max}	Specific Considerations	Side Effects
Carbidopa/levodopa	C	125	25/100 mg PO	1.5	10–30 min	Occasional use	Headache, muscle cramps, confusion, somnolence, dizziness, depression, palpitations, orthostatic hypotension, gastrointestinal symptoms
Pramipexole	B	0.125	0.125 mg PO up to 0.5–0.75 mg 2–3 h before bedtime Dose increasing every 4–7 d	8–12, regular; 24, extended release	1–3 h, regular; 6 h, extended release	Chronic therapy; can be used for patients with medications that affect hepatic enzymes	Nausea, sleepiness and insomnia, fatigue, vivid dreams, confusion, visual hallucinations, headache, postural hypotension, impulse control disorder
Ropinirole	B	0.25(–0.5)	0.25–0.5 mg PO in the evening during the first week up to 4 mg PO	1.5–2.5, regular; 6–10, extended release	1.5 h	Chronic therapy; can be used for patients with decreased renal function	Nausea, somnolence, fatigue, depression, impulse control disorder

Drug		Starting dose	Dose	T$_{max}$	T$_{1/2}$	Notes	Side effects
Rotigotine	A	1	1–3 mg/24 h transdermal Dose increasing every 7 d	5–7	1–3 h	Chronic therapy; round-the-clock symptoms or swallowing difficulties	Allergic reactions at the application site, nausea, headache, fatigue, orthostatic hypotension, sleepiness, impulse control disorders
Gabapentin enacarbil	A	600	600–1200 mg PO	5.1–6	5–7.3 h	—	Somnolence, dizziness
Pregabalin	B	75	150–450 mg PO	6	1 h	—	Unsteadiness, daytime sleepiness
Oxycodone/naloxone prolonged release	C	5/2.5	5/2.5–40/20 mg PO	4.1–17.2	1.3–5.3 h	To consider in refractory RLS	Fatigue, constipation, nausea, headache, hyperhidrosis, somnolence, dry mouth, pruritus, OSAS
Ferrous sulfate	C	325	325 mg PO twice daily with 100 mg vitamin C	6	4 h	—	Nausea, sickness, and constipation
Ferric carboxymaltose	A	—	1000 mg IV	7–12	15 min–1.2 h	—	Nausea, headache

Abbreviations: IV, intravenous; OSAS, obstructive sleep apnea syndrome; PO, medication administered orally; T$_{max}$, time to maximum plasma concentration; T$_{1/2}$, elimination half-life.

Iron

One class II study found that oral iron as ferrous sulfate 325 mg combined with vitamin C 100 mg twice a day was effective for treating RLS in patients with a serum ferritin level of less than or equal to 75 µg/L (level C).[23] Two class I studies found that ferric carboxymaltose 1000 mg is effective for the treatment of moderate to severe RLS in patients with a serum ferritin level less than 300 µg/L and a transferrin saturation of less than 45% (level A).[23] One class I study using iron sucrose 200 mg and 1 class II study using iron sucrose 500 mg found no effect on RLS symptoms or PLMI (level B).[23] Expert consensus considered iron sucrose to be effective for treatment of RLS but less so than ferric carboxymaltose or low-molecular-weight iron dextran.[23] There is insufficient evidence for the efficacy of low-molecular-weight iron dextran for the treatment of RLS (2 class IV studies, level U).[23] Expert consensus, however, points at substantial clinical experience that shows it to be effective. There is insufficient evidence for the efficacy of iron gluconate (1 class IV study, level U).[23] No studies were available to evaluate the efficacy of ferumoxytol or isomaltoside for the treatment of RLS. Expert consensus was that 1000 mg of these formulations given intravenously as a single dose or as 2 divided doses is possibly effective for RLS.[23] In a class III study, oral iron 150 mg was compared with bupropion 300 mg and ropinirole 0.25 to 0.5 mg. IRLS score reduction was seen in all groups, but most in the ropinirole group.[24]

Other medications

There is insufficient evidence (level U) for the use of clonidine (1 class III study),[2] selenium (1 class III study and 1 class IV study),[2,25] botulinum toxin A (1 class III study),[2] oxcarbazepine (1 class IV study),[26] carbamazepine (1 class III study),[2] valproic acid (1 class III study),[2] levetiracetam (1 class IV study),[27] and clonazepam (2 contradictory class III studies).[2]

Valerian (1 class II study) is possibly ineffective (level C).[2] Since the 2016 AAN guideline, a new class III study has supported bupropion efficacy, because it improved RLS symptoms significantly at 6 weeks compared with baseline. A group of 30 patients treated with 300 mg of bupropion (initial 5 days with a 150 mg dose) was also compared with 30 patients treated with ropinirole (0.25–0.5 mg), but there was no placebo group.[24] A lower than recommended ropinirole dose was used in this study and it is unclear how randomization, blinding, and allocation concealment were performed. Therefore, this class III study should be viewed as a noninferiority study

assuming ropinirole as the standard treatment, and bupropion was inferior to ropinirole. Based on this class III study and a class II study included in the AAN guideline, bupropion is possibly ineffective (level C).[2,24]

Augmentation

A well-known side effect of levodopa and dopamine agonist is augmentation. Augmentation is characterized by an advance of the RLS symptoms compared with the onset time before starting the medication, a shorter latency of symptoms at rest, a spread of symptoms to other parts of the body, or a greater intensity of the symptoms. Another key symptom of augmentation is the paradoxic effect on RLS symptoms after changing the dose: dose increase causes symptom worsening, and dose reduction improvement. The time of onset of the paradoxic effect after dose change is considered, by expert opinion, drug dependent: several days after change of levodopa and weeks to months after change of the longer-acting dopamine agonists. These characteristics were outlined by the Max Planck Institute (MPI) diagnostic criteria in 2007.[28] Because the MPI definition criteria have shown some shortcomings in the everyday clinical setting, the International RLS Task Force (IRLSTF) has established consensus-based recommendation for screening for augmentation in the clinical setting to facilitate the identification of augmentation (**Box 2**).[29]

Box 2
International Restless Legs Syndrome Study Group Task Force screening questions for augmentations in the clinical setting

1. Do RLS symptoms appear earlier than when the drug was first started?

2. Are higher doses of the drug now needed, or do you need to take the medicine earlier, to control the RLS symptoms, compared to the original effective dose?

3. Has the intensity of symptoms worsened since starting the medication?

4. Have symptoms spread to other parts of the body (eg, arms) since starting the medication?

From Garcia-Borreguero D, Silber MH, Winkelman JW, et al. Guidelines for the first-line treatment of restless legs syndrome/Willis-Ekbom disease, prevention and treatment of dopaminergic augmentation: a combined task force of the IRLSSG, EURLSSG, and the RLS-foundation. Sleep Med 2016;21:4; with permission.

Augmentation is seen in all dopaminergic drugs but is most prevalent in levodopa (up to 73%) and less in dopamine agonists. Prevalence rates for dopamine agonist–related augmentation vary from less than 10% in the short term to 42% to 68% after approximately 10 years of treatment.[29] Seventy-six percent of all patients treated with dopaminergic agents showed indications for partial or full augmentation, with a yearly incidence rate of approximately 8%.[30] The prevalence of augmentation seems to be lower in the longer-acting dopamine agonists (rotigotine and cabergoline) compared with the short-acting dopamine agonists (ropinirole and pramipexole). Other possible risk factors for the development of augmentation are low ferritin levels, having more frequent and more severe RLS symptoms pre-treatment, greater discomfort with RLS symptoms before treatment, comorbid asthma, older age, longer treatment duration, development of tolerance on dopaminergic medication, positive family history of RLS, fewer out-patient clinic visits, and lack of any neuropathy. Polysomnographic analysis does not seem useful to identify augmentation and immobilization tests might be promising.[29]

It is important to rule out augmentation mimics before diagnosing augmentation, such as the natural waxing and waning course of RLS. Other causes of RLS progression to distinguish from augmentation are iron deficiency, poor RLS medication adherence, lifestyle changes (eg, more immobile), use of RLS exacerbating medications (eg, antihistamines, selective serotonin reuptake inhibitors), and other physiologic or comorbid conditions (eg, pregnancy and renal failure). In addition, tolerance and end-of-dose exacerbation must be distinguished from augmentation, although tolerance is likely to precede augmentation and could therefore be recognized as a possible indicator to develop augmentation in the further course of the treatment. Several consensus-based measures are suggested to prevent and treat augmentation (**Fig. 1**).[29]

Nonpharmacologic Treatment Options

Evidence level B was found for the effectiveness of pneumatic compression (1 class I and 1 class IV study)[2,31] and near-infrared light spectroscopy (NIRS) (2 class II studies and 1 new class IV

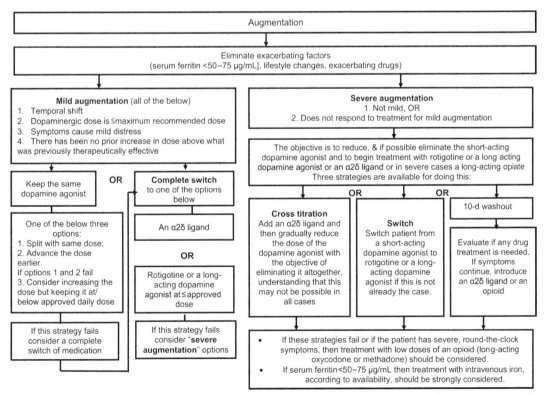

Fig. 1. Augmentation treatment algorithm. (*From* Garcia-Borreguero D, Silber MH, Winkelman JW, et al. Guidelines for the first-line treatment of restless legs syndrome/Willis-Ekbom disease, prevention and treatment of dopaminergic augmentation: a combined task force of the IRLSSG, EURLSSG, and the RLS-foundation. Sleep Med 2016;21:7; with permission.)

study).[2,32] Transcranial direct current stimulation (1 class I study)[2] is probably ineffective (level B). Repetitive transcranial magnetic stimulation is possibly effective based on 1 class II study and 2 new class IV studies[2,33,34] and vibratory treatment (2 class II studies and 1 class IV study)[2,35] possibly ineffective (level C). There is insufficient evidence (level U) for an effect on RLS symptoms of sleep hygiene improvement, change in caffeine or alcohol intake or smoking, mental activity, massage, hot baths, vitamins, aerobics/lower body training (1 class III study),[36] straight leg traction (1 class IV study),[37] yoga (1 class III study),[38] whole-body vibration (1 class III study),[39] transcutaneous spinal direct current stimulation (1 class III study),[40] posterior tibial nerve stimulation (1 class IV study),[41] enhanced external counterpulsation (1 class IV study),[42] and cognitive behavior therapy (1 class IV study).[43]

SUMMARY

For nonpharmacologic treatment options, there is some evidence for the effectiveness of pneumatic compression, NIRS, and possibly transcranial magnetic stimulation. For all other nonpharmacologic treatment options, including lifestyle changes, there is insufficient evidence.

In moderate to severe primary RLS, pharmacologic treatment can be considered (**Fig. 2**).[2] The first step of pharmacologic treatment is iron suppletion if applicable. Dopamine agonists and α2δ

ligands are both effective for the treatment of RLS.[2] Considering the risk of augmentation with dopaminergic treatment and clinical consensus,[2,19] an α2δ ligand may be preferred to a dopamine agonist as first-line treatment.[2] The choice of treatment may also depend on comorbidity, although recommendations are mainly based on clinical consensus.[19] In patients with comorbid insomnia, painful RLS, comorbid pain syndrome, history of impulse control disorder, and comorbid anxiety, an α2δ ligand can be preferred, whereas, in patients with excessive weight or comorbid depression, a dopamine agonist can be the preferred drug.[19] When prescribing dopaminergic drugs, a low dose or longer-acting version may reduce the risk of augmentation. Rotigotine could also be preferred for patients with round-the-clock symptoms or in case of swallowing difficulties. Levodopa can be considered only in patients who need occasional treatment during periods of prolonged forced immobilization or with intermittent or sporadic RLS. When single-drug therapy is insufficient, a combination of an α2δ ligand and a dopamine agonist may be considered, based on clinical consensus. In otherwise refractory primary RLS, oxycodone/naloxone may be considered.[2] If augmentation has already occurred, there are several consensus-based strategies to address, including reducing the dopamine agonist dose or switching to a longer-lasting version or an α2δ ligand.

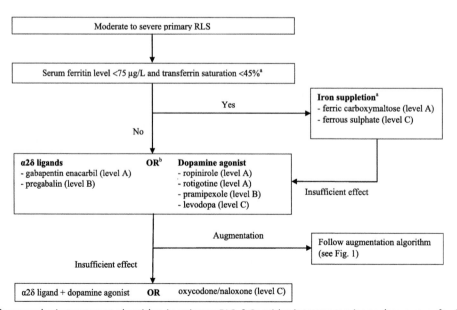

Fig. 2. Pharmacologic treatment algorithm in primary RLS. [a] Consider intravenous iron when serum ferritin level is less than 100 μg/L and transferrin saturation less than 45%. [b] The choice for an α2δ ligand or dopamine agonist may be based on considerations regarding patient characteristics (see **Table 1**), comorbidities, and the risk of augmentation with dopaminergic treatment.

Most new trials are now focusing on nondopaminergic treatment options, and future studies will include intravenous iron treatments and substances that act on adenosine and glutamate.[1]

ACKNOWLEDGMENTS

The authors thank T. Visser and A. van der Velden for their support with the PubMed search strategy.

REFERENCES

1. Garcia-Borreguero D, Cano-Pumarega I. New concepts in the management of restless legs syndrome. BMJ 2017;356:j104.
2. Winkelman JW, Armstrong MJ, Allen RP, et al. Practice guideline summary: treatment of restless legs syndrome in adults: report of the Guideline Development, Dissemination, and Implementation Subcommittee of the American Academy of Neurology. Neurology 2016;87(24):2585–93.
3. Garcia-Borreguero D, Benitez A, Kohnen R, et al. Augmentation of restless leg syndrome (Willis-Ekbom disease) during long-term dopaminergic treatment. Postgrad Med 2015;127(7):716–25.
4. Inoue Y, Kuroda K, Hirata K, et al. Long-term open-label study of pramipexole in patients with primary restless legs syndrome. J Neurol Sci 2010;294(1–2):62–6.
5. Partinen M, Hirvonen K, Jama L, et al. Open-label study of the long-term efficacy and safety of pramipexole in patients with restless legs syndrome (extension of the PRELUDE study). Sleep Med 2008;9(5):537–41.
6. Bassetti CL, Bornatico F, Fuhr P, et al. Pramipexole versus dual release levodopa in restless legs syndrome: a double blind, randomised, cross-over trial. Swiss Med Wkly 2011;141:w13274.
7. Kvernmo T, Hartter S, Burger E. A review of the receptor-binding and pharmacokinetic properties of dopamine agonists. Clin Ther 2006;28(8): 1065–78.
8. Boroojerdi B, Wolff HM, Braun M, et al. Rotigotine transdermal patch for the treatment of Parkinson's disease and restless legs syndrome. Drugs Today (Barc) 2010;46(7):483–505.
9. Elshoff JP, Braun M, Andreas JO, et al. Steady-state plasma concentration profile of transdermal rotigotine: an integrated analysis of three, open-label, randomized, phase I multiple dose studies. Clin Ther 2012;34(4):966–78.
10. Benitez A, Edens H, Fishman J, et al. Rotigotine transdermal system: developing continuous dopaminergic delivery to treat Parkinson's disease and restless legs syndrome. Ann N Y Acad Sci 2014; 1329:45–66.
11. Hogl B, Oertel WH, Schollmayer E, et al. Transdermal rotigotine for the perioperative management of restless legs syndrome. BMC Neurol 2012;12:106.
12. Garcia-Borreguero D, Allen R, Hudson J, et al. Effects of rotigotine on daytime symptoms in patients with primary restless legs syndrome: a randomized, placebo-controlled study. Curr Med Res Opin 2016; 32(1):77–85.
13. Oertel W, Trenkwalder C, Benes H, et al. Long-term safety and efficacy of rotigotine transdermal patch for moderate-to-severe idiopathic restless legs syndrome: a 5-year open-label extension study. Lancet Neurol 2011;10(8):710–20.
14. Oertel WH, Benes H, Garcia-Borreguero D, et al. One year open-label safety and efficacy trial with rotigotine transdermal patch in moderate to severe idiopathic restless legs syndrome. Sleep Med 2008;9(8):865–73.
15. Hogl B, Oertel WH, Stiasny-Kolster K, et al. Treatment of moderate to severe restless legs syndrome: 2-year safety and efficacy of rotigotine transdermal patch. BMC Neurol 2010;10:86.
16. Evidente VG. Piribedil for restless legs syndrome: a pilot study. Mov Disord 2001;16(3):579–81.
17. Aurora RN, Kristo DA, Bista SR, et al. The treatment of restless legs syndrome and periodic limb movement disorder in adults–an update for 2012: practice parameters with an evidence-based systematic review and meta-analyses: an American Academy of Sleep Medicine Clinical Practice Guideline. Sleep 2012;35(8):1039–62.
18. Garcia-Borreguero D, Ferini-Strambi L, Kohnen R, et al. European guidelines on management of restless legs syndrome: report of a joint task force by the European Federation of Neurological Societies, the European Neurological Society and the European Sleep Research Society. Eur J Neurol 2012; 19(11):1385–96.
19. Garcia-Borreguero D, Kohnen R, Silber MH, et al. The long-term treatment of restless legs syndrome/Willis-Ekbom disease: evidence-based guidelines and clinical consensus best practice guidance: a report from the International Restless Legs Syndrome Study Group. Sleep Med 2013; 14(7):675–84.
20. Garcia-Borreguero D, Cano I, Granizo JJ. Treatment of restless legs syndrome with the selective AMPA receptor antagonist perampanel. Sleep Med 2017; 34:105–8.
21. Vetrugno R, La Morgia C, D'Angelo R, et al. Augmentation of restless legs syndrome with long-term tramadol treatment. Mov Disord 2007;22(3): 424–7.
22. Earley CJ, Allen RP. Restless legs syndrome augmentation associated with tramadol. Sleep Med 2006;7(7):592–3.

23. Allen RP, Picchietti DL, Auerbach M, et al. Evidence-based and consensus clinical practice guidelines for the iron treatment of restless legs syndrome/Willis-Ekbom disease in adults and children: an IRLSSG task force report. Sleep Med 2018;41:27–44.

24. Vishwakarma K, Kalra J, Gupta R, et al. A double-blind, randomized, controlled trial to compare the efficacy and tolerability of fixed doses of ropinirole, bupropion, and iron in treatment of restless legs syndrome (Willis-Ekbom disease). Ann Indian Acad Neurol 2016;19(4):472–7.

25. Ulfberg J, Stehlik R, Mitchell U. Treatment of restless legs syndrome/Willis-Ekbom disease with selenium. Iran J Neurol 2016;15(4):235–6.

26. Jimenez-Trevino L. Oxcarbazepine treatment of restless legs syndrome: three case reports. Clin Neuropharmacol 2009;32(3):169–70.

27. Della Marca G, Vollono C, Mariotti P, et al. Levetiracetam can be effective in the treatment of restless legs syndrome with periodic limb movements in sleep: report of two cases. J Neurol Neurosurg Psychiatry 2006;77(4):566–7.

28. Garcia-Borreguero D, Allen RP, Kohnen R, et al. Diagnostic standards for dopaminergic augmentation of restless legs syndrome: report from a World Association of Sleep Medicine-International Restless Legs Syndrome Study Group consensus conference at the Max Planck Institute. Sleep Med 2007;8(5): 520–30.

29. Garcia-Borreguero D, Silber MH, Winkelman JW, et al. Guidelines for the first-line treatment of restless legs syndrome/Willis-Ekbom disease, prevention and treatment of dopaminergic augmentation: a combined task force of the IRLSSG, EURLSSG, and the RLS-foundation. Sleep Med 2016;21:1–11.

30. Allen RP, Ondo WG, Ball E, et al. Restless legs syndrome (RLS) augmentation associated with dopamine agonist and levodopa usage in a community sample. Sleep Med 2011;12(5):431–9.

31. Eliasson AH, Lettieri CJ. Sequential compression devices for treatment of restless legs syndrome. Medicine (Baltimore) 2007;86(6):317–23.

32. Guffey JS, Motts S, Barymon D, et al. Using near infrared light to manage symptoms associated with restless legs syndrome. Physiother Theory Pract 2016;32(1):34–44.

33. Liu C, Dai Z, Zhang R, et al. Mapping intrinsic functional brain changes and repetitive transcranial magnetic stimulation neuromodulation in idiopathic restless legs syndrome: a resting-state functional magnetic resonance imaging study. Sleep Med 2015;16(6):785–91.

34. Lin YC, Feng Y, Zhan SQ, et al. Repetitive transcranial magnetic stimulation for the treatment of restless legs syndrome. Chin Med J (Engl) 2015;128(13): 1728–31.

35. Montagna P, Sassoli de Bianchi L, Zucconi M, et al. Clonazepam and vibration in restless legs syndrome. Acta Neurol Scand 1984;69(6):428–30.

36. Aukerman MM, Aukerman D, Bayard M, et al. Exercise and restless legs syndrome: a randomized controlled trial. J Am Board Fam Med 2006;19(5): 487–93.

37. Dinkins EM, Stevens-Lapsley J. Management of symptoms of restless legs syndrome with use of a traction straight leg raise: a preliminary case series. Man Ther 2013;18(4):299–302.

38. Innes KE, Selfe TK, Agarwal P, et al. Efficacy of an eight-week yoga intervention on symptoms of restless legs syndrome (RLS): a pilot study. J Altern Complement Med 2013;19(6):527–35.

39. Mitchell UH, Hilton SC, Hunsaker E, et al. Decreased symptoms without augmented skin blood flow in subjects with RLS/WED after vibration treatment. J Clin Sleep Med 2016;12(7):947–52.

40. Heide AC, Winkler T, Helms HJ, et al. Effects of transcutaneous spinal direct current stimulation in idiopathic restless legs patients. Brain Stimul 2014; 7(5):636–42.

41. Rozeman AD, Ottolini T, Grootendorst DC, et al. Effect of sensory stimuli on restless legs syndrome: a randomized crossover study. J Clin Sleep Med 2014;10(8):893–6.

42. Rajaram SS, Rudzinskiy P, Walters AS. Enhanced external counter pulsation (EECP) for restless legs syndrome (RLS): preliminary negative results in a parallel double-blind study. Sleep Med 2006;7(4): 390–1.

43. Hornyak M, Grossmann C, Kohnen R, et al. Cognitive behavioural group therapy to improve patients' strategies for coping with restless legs syndrome: a proof-of-concept trial. J Neurol Neurosurg Psychiatry 2008;79(7):823–5.

Drugs Used in Circadian Sleep-Wake Rhythm Disturbances

Helen J. Burgess, PhD[a],*, Jonathan S. Emens, MD[b,c]

KEYWORDS

• Advance • Agonist • Circadian • Delay • Melatonin • Shift • Sleep

KEY POINTS

• Exogenous melatonin and other melatonin receptor agonists can be used to shift circadian timing and improve sleep in patients with sleep and circadian disturbances.
• Each medication varies in its circadian resetting and sleep-enhancing properties, and safety concerns.
• The latest exogenous melatonin treatment recommendations for circadian rhythm sleep-wake disorders are reviewed.

INTRODUCTION

The focus of this article is on the use of melatonin and other melatonin receptor agonists as chronobiotics; that is, drugs that shift central circadian timing (ie, reset the 24-hour biological clock) and that also have potential to improve sleep. The aim is to provide a relevant update from a recent review of melatonin and other melatonin receptor agonists[1] and highlight the practical use of these drugs. The authors recognize that other drugs have the potential to act as chronobiotics and that different medications, including hypnotics and alerting medications, may have potential for treating circadian rhythm sleep-wake disorders, but these are not addressed here because they remain to be tested in clinical trials examining circadian rhythm sleep-wake disorders.

This article provides a brief review of the circadian system and circadian rhythm sleep-wake disorders, followed by a summary of the relevant agents available and the safety concerns surrounding their use. The circadian phase shifting and sleep-enhancing properties of these particular chronobiotics are reviewed, along with the latest American Academy of Sleep Medicine (AASM) clinical practice guidelines regarding the use of exogenous melatonin for treating intrinsic circadian rhythm disorders.[2] The article concludes with a discussion of the use of these medications in clinical practice.

THE CIRCADIAN SYSTEM AND CIRCADIAN RHYTHM SLEEP-WAKE DISORDERS

The circadian system orchestrates the near-24-hour endogenous rhythms seen in a wide variety of physiologic variables. The molecular "gears" of the clock exist in most organ systems and these disparate clocks are internally synchronized by a central pacemaker in the suprachiasmatic nuclei (SCN) of the hypothalamus, which is itself

Disclosure: H.J. Burgess is a consultant for Natrol, LLC. J.S. Emens has nothing to disclose.
[a] Biological Rhythms Research Laboratory, Department of Behavioral Sciences, Rush University Medical Center, 1645 West Jackson Boulevard, Suite 425, Chicago, IL 60612, USA; [b] Department of Psychiatry, Oregon Health & Science University, VA Portland Health Care System, 3710 Southwest US Veterans Hospital, Road P3-PULM, Portland, OR 97239, USA; [c] Department of Medicine, Oregon Health & Science University, VA Portland Health Care System, 3710 Southwest US Veterans Hospital, Road P3-PULM, Portland, OR 97239, USA
* Corresponding author.
E-mail address: Helen_J_Burgess@rush.edu

Sleep Med Clin 13 (2018) 231–241
https://doi.org/10.1016/j.jsmc.2018.02.006
1556-407X/18/© 2018 Elsevier Inc. All rights reserved.

synchronized (reset) by external time cues, primarily the light/dark cycle.[3] The timing of the clock (circadian phase) can be shifted to an earlier or later time (phase advances and phase delays, respectively) depending on when during the biological day or night a resetting stimulus is given. Circadian timing and sleep have a profound influence on mental and physical health (eg, see Refs.[4–7]), and circadian rhythm sleep-wake disorders result when wakefulness and sleep are scheduled in opposition to the timing of the biological clock (eg, attempting to sleep during the biological day). A key to understanding circadian rhythm sleep-wake disorders, and their treatment, is appreciating this difference between internal biological timing and external clock time.

The third edition of the International Classification of Sleep Disorders describes 6 circadian rhythm sleep-wake disorders that have been reviewed in depth previously.[2,8] These include the extrinsic circadian rhythm sleep-wake disorders (jet lag disorder and shift work disorder) and also the intrinsic circadian rhythm sleep-wake disorders (delayed sleep-wake phase disorder), advanced sleep-wake phase disorder, irregular sleep-wake rhythm disorder, and non-24-hour sleep-wake rhythm disorder (non-24). Their primary features and possible causes are summarized in **Table 1**.

MELATONIN AND OTHER MELATONIN RECEPTOR AGONISTS

The circadian resetting effects of melatonin are well documented[9–12] and both receptor subtypes have been shown to contribute to this effect.[13,14] Melatonin is available without a prescription in the United States both alone and in combination with other supplements, and in multiple formulations. It is estimated that 2% of US adults use exogenous melatonin, most commonly to improve sleep.[15,16] There are also melatonin formulations and other melatonin receptor agonists available via prescription in various countries, including Circadin, Tasimelteon, Ramelteon, and Agomelatine, which are summarized in **Table 2**.

TREATMENT SAFETY CONSIDERATIONS

Side effects are infrequent with exogenous melatonin, with the exception of sleepiness, but the side effects discussed in several meta-analyses are listed in **Table 2**. Because of the sleepiness side effect, patients should not drive or operate machinery after ingesting melatonin, and should test their individual response to particular doses and formulations in safe environments.

Bioavailability of melatonin can vary (eg, 1%–37%).[17] Meta-analyses have reported potential for melatonin to adversely affect people with epilepsy,[18] and for melatonin to interact with warfarin and potentially other oral anticoagulants.[18] There have also been concerns about potential effects of melatonin on development in children,[19] and so caution is advised in the administration of melatonin to prepubertal children unless the demonstrated benefits outweigh the potential risks (eg, in children with significant developmental delay or children with non-24-hour sleep-wake schedule disorder). It is also generally recommended that women who are pregnant, trying to get pregnant, or breastfeeding do not take exogenous melatonin.[20] Exogenous melatonin (5 mg) has been found to acutely impair glucose tolerance when administered with food[21] and further research on the effects of exogenous melatonin on glucose metabolism, and on which patients might be vulnerable to these effects,[22] is warranted. In general, large-scale randomized controlled trials are needed to evaluate the long-term safety of melatonin in children and adults.[20] Other prescription-based melatonin receptor agonists also carry their own potential side effect profiles, which are summarized in **Table 2**.

USING MELATONIN AND OTHER MELATONIN RECEPTOR AGONISTS TO SHIFT CIRCADIAN TIMING

As described in detail in our previous review,[1] both the dose and timing of exogenous melatonin administration need to be considered when attempting to reset the biological clock. The timing of melatonin administration simultaneously determines the direction and magnitude of the resulting circadian phase shift. Melatonin phase response curves (PRCs; eg, see Refs.[11,12]) are plots of average data that are similar to dose response curves, but instead of describing the effect of a drug at different doses, they describe the effect of a drug administered at different biological times. Biological timing can be determined by measuring a convenient marker of the biological clock, such as the onset of endogenous melatonin secretion assayed in plasma or saliva samples collected under dim light conditions (the dim light melatonin onset [DLMO]).[23–25] These PRCs indicate that exogenous melatonin typically causes phase advances when administered in the late biological afternoon and early evening (peaking about 5–7 hours before habitual bedtime), phase delays when administered late in the biological night and early morning (peaking around habitual wake

Table 1
International Classification of Sleep Disorders, Third Edition classification of circadian rhythm sleep-wake disorders

Disorder	Jet Lag Disorder	Shift Work Disorder	Delayed Sleep-Wake Phase Disorder	Advanced Sleep-Wake Phase Disorder	Irregular Sleep-Wake Rhythm Disorder	Non-24-h Sleep-Wake Rhythm Disorder
Primary Features	Insomnia and/or hypersomnolence with decreased total sleep time associated with transmeridian travel across ≥2 time zones	Insomnia and/or hypersomnolence with decreased total sleep time associated with work times during habitual sleep times	Sleep-wake timing is shifted ≥2 h later, sleep onset insomnia, morning somnolence, and an absence of difficulty when sleep timing is delayed	Sleep-wake timing is shifted ≥2 h earlier, evening somnolence, early morning insomnia, and an absence of difficulty when sleep timing is advanced	Irregular sleep/wake schedule with insomnia during scheduled sleep and somnolence during scheduled wake times	Sleep/wake timing that drifts progressively later (or earlier) across the 24-h day. In the blind: relapsing/remitting insomnia and somnolence while keeping a consistent sleep/wake schedule
Cause	Scheduling of sleep and wakefulness during the biological day and night, respectively, as a result of rapid transmeridian travel	Scheduling of work during the biological night with corresponding scheduling of sleep during the biological day	Altered circadian resetting (increased response to delaying evening light or decreased response to advancing morning light), altered exposure to resetting agents (eg, increased evening light exposure), and/or a long biological day (long circadian period)	Altered circadian resetting (increased response to advancing morning light or decreased response to delaying evening light), altered exposure to resetting agents (eg, increased morning light exposure), and/or a short biological day (short circadian period)	Seen in individuals with neurodegenerative or neurodevelopmental disorders	In the blind: a lack of light input to the circadian pacemaker In the sighted: possible self-selected light/dark schedule in conjunction with factors seen in delayed sleep-wake phase disorder

Data from American Academy of Sleep Medicine. Classification of Circadian Rhythm Sleep-Wake Disorders. In: International Classification of Sleep Disorders. 3rd ed. Darien, IL; 2014:191–224.

Table 2
A summary of the circadian, sleep, and possible side effects of melatonin and other melatonin receptor agonists

Drug	Approved for	Mechanism of Action	Circadian Phase Shifting Effects	Sleep Effects	Possible Side Effects
Melatonin	Available over the counter in the United States, via prescription in most other countries	MT1 and MT2 receptor agonist	Can phase advance and phase delay[11,12]	Decreases latency to sleep onset[32–34]; may increase total sleep time, sleep quality[33] Effects may be larger when endogenous melatonin levels are low[36]	Sleepiness, dizziness, headache, blood pressure changes, gastrointestinal upset[18,20,32]
Circadin	Insomnia in adults ≥55 y old	MT1 and MT2 receptor agonist	Not clear as a prolonged release melatonin formulation	Decreases latency to sleep onset, improves sleep quality[54]	Similar to exogenous melatonin[55]
Tasimelteon	Non–24-h sleep-wake rhythm disorder	MT1 and MT2 receptor agonist	Can phase advance[56,57]	Decreases latency to sleep onset; increases sleep efficiency when administered to enhance sleep 5 h before habitual bedtime[57]	Headache, increased liver enzyme levels, cardiac conduction changes, upper respiratory and urinary tract infections, nightmares[58]
Ramelteon	Insomnia in adults	MT1 and MT2 receptor agonist	Can phase advance[59]	Decreases latency to sleep onset; increases total sleep time, sleep efficiency, sleep quality[60]	Sleepiness, dizziness, headache, gastrointestinal upset, upper respiratory tract infections, dysmenorrhea[60]
Agomelatine	Depression	MT1 and MT2 receptor agonist, serotonin 5-HT2c receptor antagonist	Can phase advance[61,62]	Decreases latency to sleep onset in patients with major depressive disorder[63]	Liver injury[64,65]

Abbreviations: MT1, melatonin receptor 1; MT2, melatonin receptor 2.

time), and shifts from causing phase advances to phase delays in the biological evening (**Fig. 1**). It is therefore important to point out that exogenous melatonin causes the largest phase shifts when patients are likely to be awake (assuming they are maintaining a conventional sleep/wake schedule), and so low doses that will not result in somnolence are preferred, as discussed later.

The dose of melatonin can also affect the resulting phase shift. A wide range of doses have been examined for circadian resetting[11,12,26,27] and there is evidence that a therapeutic window exists for melatonin's chronobiotic effects: at lower doses of 0.02 to 0.30 mg, a dose response relationship has been shown,[27] whereas 0.5-mg and 3.0-mg doses cause similar resetting[12] and higher doses of 10 mg or more have smaller resetting effects.[26,28] This therapeutic window likely exists because increasing the dose of exogenous melatonin also increases the duration of time that circulating levels of melatonin are increased. Within the lower part of this dose range, increasing doses simply result in increased resetting effects,[27] but with higher doses more and more of the melatonin PRC is stimulated until the opposite zone begins to be stimulated and less net circadian resetting occurs. This phenomenon of exogenous melatonin

"spilling over"[28] onto the opposite zone of the melatonin PRC occurs, despite a half-life of 30 to 45 minutes,[17] because even doses of 0.5 to 1.0 mg of melatonin can produce supraphysiologic levels over several hours or more.[11,29] As reviewed later, melatonin also has soporific effects and therefore care should be taken to use the lowest dose possible when exogenous melatonin is taken during the habitual waking hours, as is often necessary for maximal circadian resetting effects.

The latest AASM clinical practice guidelines for the treatment of intrinsic circadian rhythm disorders with exogenous melatonin[2] are shown in **Table 3**. Details of the studies that formed the basis of the recommendations, including exogenous melatonin dose and timing of administration, are also summarized. Other reviews address how exogenous melatonin can be used to reduce jet lag and improve adaptation to shift work.[30,31]

USING MELATONIN AND OTHER MELATONIN RECEPTOR AGONISTS TO IMPROVE SLEEP

Melatonin is well recognized to reduce the time taken to fall asleep (sleep onset latency).[32–34]

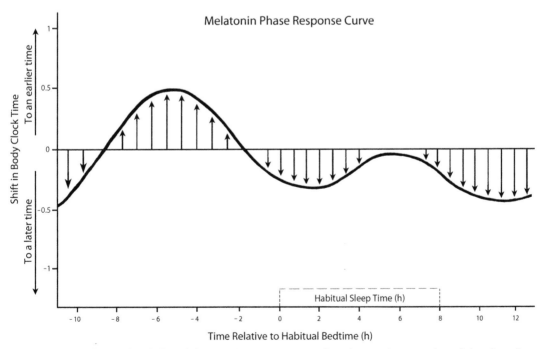

Fig. 1. A PRC rereferenced to habitual sleep timing. PRCs are usually referenced to a marker of circadian phase, but, for ease of use, the authors have rereferenced this PRC to habitual sleep timing. The melatonin phase response curve is adapted from a phase response curve generated to 3 days of a daily dose of 0.5 mg of exogenous melatonin.[12] Accordingly, we have reduced the amplitude of the melatonin phase response curve by a factor of 3, to better estimate the effects of a single dose. Any resulting phase shift will be a combined effect of exogenous melatonin plus concomitant light exposure.

Table 3
Melatonin treatment recommendations from the 2015 clinical practice guideline for treatment of intrinsic circadian rhythm sleep-wake disorders

Disorder	Number of Studies That Formed Guideline	Effective Doses and Timing Tested	Treatment Guideline
Delayed sleep-wake phase disorder	3 Adult studies 3 Children studies	Adults: 0.3 mg or 3 mg fast release, 1.5–6.5 h before baseline DLMO, time pill taken advanced by 1 h after 2 wk[66] 5 mg fast release between 7 and 9 PM, treatment advanced by ~1 h after first week[67,68] Children: 0.15 mg/kg fast release 1.5–2.0 h before habitual bedtime[69] 3 or 5 mg fast release 6 or 7 PM[70,71]	Use strategically timed melatonin or other melatonin receptor agonists
Advanced sleep-wake phase disorder	No studies	NA	No recommendation
Irregular sleep-wake rhythm disorder (elderly with dementia)	1 Adult study	Null effects[72]	Do not use melatonin or other melatonin receptor agonists
Irregular sleep-wake rhythm disorder (children/adolescents with neurologic disorders)	1 Child study	2–10 mg fast release, ~30 min before planned bedtime[73]	Use strategically timed melatonin or other melatonin receptor agonists
Non–24-h sleep-wake rhythm disorder	3 Adult blind studies in patients whose circadian phase drifts later in time	10 mg 1 h before preferred bedtime[26] 0.5 mg[74] or 5 mg[75] at 9 PM	Use strategically timed melatonin or other melatonin receptor agonists

Note that a lack of recommendation does not indicate melatonin should not be used in those disorders but that the available evidence was insufficient to make a recommendation for or against treatment with melatonin and other melatonin receptor agonists.[76]

Abbreviation: NA, not available.

Data from refs[2,48,68–76].

The reports on whether melatonin can increase sleep duration and/or consolidation (eg, sleep efficiency) are mixed,[32–34] and it may not be soporific when administered during the biological night when endogenous melatonin levels are increased.[35] The soporific effects of exogenous melatonin can be larger in populations with lower levels of endogenous melatonin (eg, in hypertensive patients treated with β-blockers[36]). Nonetheless, the sleep-enhancing effects of exogenous melatonin are usually smaller than those associated with hypnotics, and sometimes are not considered clinically meaningful.[37] The sleep-enhancing effects of melatonin may in part be mediated via binding to melatonin receptors in the periphery, which can induce thermoregulatory changes that induce sleepiness and sleep.[38] Melatonin may also reduce circadian alerting signals by binding to melatonin receptors on the SCN.[39]

PRACTICAL ASPECTS OF MELATONIN AND OTHER MELATONIN AGONIST TREATMENTS
Melatonin Preparations

The first practical consideration for clinicians is related to exogenous melatonin's classification as a dietary supplement by the US Food and

Drug Administration (FDA): the purity and dose accuracy of different formulations is not necessarily assured.[40,41] In recent years, individual manufacturers have adopted improved testing procedures,[42] but ultimately clinicians may need to choose from among those formulations that have been subject to some type of outside review.[43,44] An important consideration for therapy with melatonin is the low cost (often <10 cents per pill[44]).

Melatonin Administration

As described earlier, the potential interactions between exogenous melatonin and prescription medications and/or other dietary supplements should be considered before recommending melatonin treatment. In addition, drugs metabolized by cytochrome P450 1A2 liver enzymes, including some antidepressants, caffeine, and oral contraceptives, can inadvertently increase levels of plasma melatonin after exogenous melatonin administration.[19,20] Clinicians should note that less than half of the general population are estimated to consult with their physicians about their use of supplements.[16]

Before beginning treatment, clinicians should first make sure the patient is maintaining a consistent light/dark schedule. This schedule is critical for ensuring that a correct biological time of administration is chosen and hence the desired circadian resetting effect is achieved. This schedule may also offer some benefit all on its own, because it minimizes the circadian misalignment associated with rapidly changing sleep/wake opportunities. Clinicians should be aware that exogenous melatonin, on its own, cannot overcome the resetting effect of a patient's self-selected light/dark cycle, and that it is important that the timing of melatonin and light act in concert to achieve the desired resetting effect. Evidence of this potential competition between melatonin and light can be seen in the larger resetting effects observed with exogenous melatonin administered in the laboratory (where light levels are controlled),[12] compared with administration at home.[11]

Once a patient is successfully maintaining a consistent light/dark schedule, the clinician should then administer melatonin about 5 to 6 hours before habitual bedtime to shift circadian timing to an earlier hour or at habitual wake time to shift circadian timing later. These administration times can be slowly moved an hour or less earlier or later, respectively, every few days,[45] if insomnia or somnolence symptoms have improved but sleep timing is still delayed or

advanced. Just as consistent light/dark timing is critical to success, so is consistently timed administration of melatonin, and the use of alarms, such as on mobile phones, can help in this respect. In all cases, the aim is to achieve a normal and consistent relationship between the timing of sleep and the timing of the biological clock.

Non-24 in the blind is unique among the intrinsic circadian rhythm sleep-wake disorders, because the cause is clear but the treatment is more complex (for review of treatment see Ref.[46]). Non-24 arises in blind individuals because the biological clock is no longer reset by light. Most commonly, this results in circadian timing shifting ~20 minutes later every day.[47] Melatonin can arrest this drift,[26] but experiments have shown that the drift in circadian timing often does not immediately cease, nor does the eventual timing of the clock necessarily correspond with the timing of melatonin administration. As a result, clinicians should initially administer melatonin 6 hours before the desired bedtime and, as discussed earlier, slowly shift the administration time earlier or later if there are remaining symptoms that indicate a phase delay or phase advance, respectively. Less frequently, circadian timing shifts earlier each day[47] and melatonin should be administered at the desired wake time[48] (note that this is more likely to be the case in female patients[47,49]).

Melatonin and Light Combination Treatment

Apart from the case of blind patients, patients generally receive exogenous melatonin or other melatonin receptor agonists while exposed to a light-dark cycle, which is, as noted earlier, the strongest circadian resetting agent.[1] In general, light has opposite phase shifting effects to melatonin, such that evening light phase delays and morning light phase advances.[1] Consequently, when administering melatonin or other melatonin receptor agonists, phase shifting effects can be altered depending on whether the concomitant light exposure is facilitating or opposing the melatonin agonist phase shift.[50–52] Thus, in the case of sighted patients, concomitant light exposure and/or light avoidance should also be included in the treatment plan.

EVALUATION OF OUTCOME

A continued limitation in the diagnosis and treatment of circadian rhythm sleep-wake disorders is the lack of an FDA approved test of circadian timing. Although some progress has been made in this regard[53] since our last review,[1] clinicians should still use symptom improvement to gauge treatment response. This approach is similar to the treatment of most insomnias, in which the use of sleep diaries and rating scales can be useful. Wrist actigraphy offers a more objective measure, although, in clinical practice, the authors find it is more useful in determining the consistency of rest/activity and light/dark timing (discussed earlier).

SUMMARY

This article focuses on melatonin and other melatonin receptor agonists and summarizes their circadian phase shifting and sleep-enhancing properties, along with their associated possible safety concerns. The circadian system and circadian rhythm sleep-wake disorders are described, along with the latest AASM recommendations for the use of exogenous melatonin in treating them. In addition, the practical aspects of using exogenous melatonin obtainable over the counter in the United States, consideration of the effects of concomitant light exposure, and assessing treatment response are discussed.

ACKNOWLEDGMENTS

The authors thank Muneer Rizvydeen for his assistance in creating the figure. H.J. Burgess and J.S. Emens are supported by grants from the National Center for Complementary and Integrative Health (R34AT008347); National Heart, Lung, and Blood Institute (R01HL125893), (R01HL140577); National Institute of Nursing Research (R21NR014377); and National Institute on Alcohol Abuse and Alcoholism (R01AA023839). The content is solely the responsibility of the authors and does not necessarily represent the official views of the National Institutes of Health.

REFERENCES

1. Emens J, Burgess HJ. Effect of light and melatonin and other melatonin receptor agonists on human circadian physiology. Sleep Med Clin 2015;10: 435–53.
2. Auger RR, Burgess HJ, Emens JS, et al. Clinical practice guideline for the treatment of intrinsic circadian rhythm sleep-wake disorders: advanced sleep-wake phase disorder (ASWPD), delayed sleep-wake phase disorder (DSWPD), non-24-hour sleep-wake rhythm disorder (N24SWD), and irregular sleep-wake rhythm disorder (ISWRD). An update for 2015: an American Academy of Sleep Medicine clinical practice guideline. J Clin Sleep Med 2015; 11(10):1199–236.
3. Buhr ED, Takahashi JS. Molecular components of the mammalian circadian clock. Handb Exp Pharmacol 2013;217:3–27.
4. Wright KP, Hull JT, Hughes RJ, et al. Sleep and wakefulness out of phase with internal biological time impairs learning in humans. J Cogn Neurosci 2006;18(4):508–21.
5. Scheer FA, Hilton MF, Mantzoros CS, et al. Adverse metabolic and cardiovascular consequences of circadian misalignment. Proc Natl Acad Sci U S A 2009;106(11):4453–8.
6. Levandovski R, Dantas G, Fernandes LC, et al. Depression scores associate with chronotype and social jetlag in a rural population. Chronobiol Int 2011;28(9):771–8.
7. Watson NF, Badr MS, Belenky G, et al. Recommended amount of sleep for a healthy adult: a joint consensus statement of the American Academy of Sleep Medicine and Sleep Research Society. Sleep 2015;38(6):843–4.
8. Reid KJ, Burgess HJ. Circadian rhythm sleep disorders. Prim Care 2005;32:449–73.
9. Redman J, Armstrong S, Ng KT. Free-running activity rhythms in the rat: entrainment by melatonin. Science 1983;219(4588):1089–91.
10. Arendt J, Bojkowski C, Folkard S, et al. Some effects of melatonin and the control of its secretion in humans. In: Evered D, Clark S, editors. Photoperiodism, melatonin, and the pineal. London: Pitman; 1985. p. 266–83.
11. Lewy AJ, Bauer VK, Ahmed S, et al. The human phase response curve (PRC) to melatonin is about 12 hours out of phase with the PRC to light. Chronobiol Int 1998;15:71–83.
12. Burgess HJ, Revell VL, Molina TA, et al. Human phase response curves to three days of daily melatonin: 0.5 mg versus 3.0 mg. J Clin Endocrinol Metab 2010;95(7):3325–31.
13. Reppert SM, Weaver DR, Godson C. Melatonin receptors step into the light: cloning and classification of subtypes. Trends Pharmacol Sci 1996;17: 100–2.
14. Dubocovich ML. Melatonin receptors: role on sleep and circadian rhythm regulation. Sleep Med 2007; 8(Suppl 3):34–42.
15. National Sleep Foundation. 2005 Sleep in America Poll. Available at: https://sleepfoundation.org/sleep-polls-data/sleep-in-america-poll/2005-adult-sleep-habits-and-styles. Accessed Jan 2, 2018.
16. Bliwise DL, Ansari FP. Insomnia associated with valerian and melatonin usage in the 2002 National Health Interview Survey. Sleep 2007;30(7): 881–4.
17. Fourtillan JB, Brisson AM, Gobin P, et al. Bioavailability of melatonin in humans after day-time administration of D(7) melatonin. Biopharm Drug Dispos 2000;21(1):15–22.

18. Herxheimer A, Petrie KJ. Melatonin for the prevention and treatment of jet lag. Cochrane Database Syst Rev 2002;2:CD001520.

19. Kennaway DJ. Potential safety issues in the use of the hormone melatonin in paediatrics. J Paediatr Child Health 2015;51(6):584–9.

20. Andersen LP, Gogenur I, Rosenberg J, et al. The safety of melatonin in humans. Clin Drug Investig 2016;36(3):169–75.

21. Rubio-Sastre P, Scheer FA, Gomez-Abellan P, et al. Acute melatonin administration in humans impairs glucose tolerance in both the morning and evening. Sleep 2014;37(10):1715–9.

22. Garaulet M, Gomez-Abellan P, Rubio-Sastre P, et al. Common type 2 diabetes risk variant in MTNR1B worsens the deleterious effect of melatonin on glucose tolerance in humans. Metabolism 2015; 64(12):1650–7.

23. Lewy AJ, Cutler NL, Sack RL. The endogenous melatonin profile as a marker of circadian phase position. J Biol Rhythms 1999;14(3):227–36.

24. Klerman EB, Gershengorn HB, Duffy JF, et al. Comparisons of the variability of three markers of the human circadian pacemaker. J Biol Rhythms 2002; 17(2):181–93.

25. Burgess HJ, Wyatt JK, Park M, et al. Home circadian phase assessments with measures of compliance yield accurate dim light melatonin onsets. Sleep 2015;38(6):889–97.

26. Sack RL, Brandes RW, Kendall AR, et al. Entrainment of free-running circadian rhythms by melatonin in blind people. N Engl J Med 2000;343(15): 1070–7.

27. Lewy AJ, Emens JS, Lefler BJ, et al. Melatonin entrains free-running blind people according to a physiological dose-response curve. Chronobiol Int 2005;22(6):1093–106.

28. Lewy AJ, Emens JS, Sack RL, et al. Low, but not high, doses of melatonin entrained a free-running blind person with long circadian period. Chronobiol Int 2002;19(3):649–58.

29. Dollins AB, Zhdanova IV, Wurtman RJ, et al. Effect of inducing nocturnal serum melatonin concentrations in daytime on sleep, mood, body temperature, and performance. Proc Natl Acad Sci USA 1994;91(5): 1824–8.

30. Burgess HJ. Using bright light and melatonin to reduce jet lag. In: Perlis M, Aloia M, Kuhn B, editors. Behavioral treatments for sleep disorders: a comprehensive primer of behavioral sleep medicine treatment protocols. Burlington (New Jersey): Elsevier; 2011. p. 151–7.

31. Burgess HJ. Using bright light and melatonin to adjust to night work. In: Perlis M, Aloia M, Kuhn B, editors. Behavioral treatments for sleep disorders: a comprehensive primer of behavioral sleep medicine treatment protocols. Burlington (New Jersey): Elsevier; 2011. p. 159–65.

32. Buscemi N, Vandermeer B, Hooton N, et al. The efficacy and safety of exogenous melatonin for primary sleep disorders. A meta-analysis. J Gen Int Med 2005;20:1151–8.

33. Ferracioli-Oda E, Qawasmi A, Bloch MH. Meta-analysis: melatonin for the treatment of primary sleep disorders. PLoS One 2013;8(5):e63773.

34. Auld F, Maschauer EL, Morrison I, et al. Evidence for the efficacy of melatonin in the treatment of primary adult sleep disorders. Sleep Med Rev 2017;34: 10–22.

35. Wyatt JK, Dijk DJ, Ritz-de Cecco A, et al. Sleep-facilitating effect of exogenous melatonin in healthy young men and women is circadian-phase dependent. Sleep 2006;29(5):609–18.

36. Scheer FA, Morris CJ, Garcia JI, et al. Repeated melatonin supplementation improves sleep in hypertensive patients treated with beta-blockers: a randomized controlled trial. Sleep 2012;35(10): 1395–402.

37. Sateia MJ, Buysse DJ, Krystal AD, et al. Clinical practice guideline for the pharmacologic treatment of chronic insomnia in adults: an American Academy of Sleep Medicine clinical practice guideline. J Clin Sleep Med 2017;13(2):307–49.

38. Krauchi K, Cajochen C, Pache M, et al. Thermoregulatory effects of melatonin in relation to sleepiness. Chronobiol Int 2006;23:475–84.

39. Reppert SM, Weaver DR, Rivkees SA, et al. Putative melatonin receptors in a human biological clock. Science 1988;242:78–81.

40. Erland LA, Saxena PK. Melatonin natural health products and supplements: presence of serotonin and significant variability of melatonin content. J Clin Sleep Med 2017;13(2):275–81.

41. Hahm H, Kujawa J, Augsburger L. Comparison of melatonin products against USP's nutritional supplements standards and other criteria. J Am Pharm Assoc (Wash) 1999;39(1):27–31.

42. Available at: http://well.blogs.nytimes.com/2015/03/30/gnc-to-strengthen-supplement-quality-controls. Accessed Jan 2, 2018.

43. Available at: http://www.usp.org/verification-services/program-participants. Accessed Jan 2, 2018.

44. ConsumerLab.com. Product review: melatonin supplements. Available at: www.consumerlab.com/results/melatonin.asp. Accessed Jan 2, 2018.

45. Crowley SJ, Eastman CI. Melatonin in the afternoons of a gradually advancing sleep schedule enhances the circadian rhythm phase advance. Psychopharmacol (Berl) 2013;225(4):825–37.

46. Emens JS, Eastman CI. Diagnosis and treatment of non-24-h sleep-wake disorder in the blind. Drugs 2017;77:637–50.

47. Emens JS, Laurie AL, Songer JB, et al. Non-24-hour disorder in blind individuals revisited: variability and the influence of environmental time cues. Sleep 2013;36(07):1091–100.

48. Emens J, Lewy A, Yuhas K, et al. Melatonin entrains free-running blind individuals with circadian periods less than 24 hours. Sleep 2006;29(Suppl):A62.

49. Duffy JF, Cain SW, Chang AM, et al. Sex difference in the near-24-hour intrinsic period of the human circadian timing system. Proc Natl Acad Sci USA 2011;108(Suppl 3):15602–8.

50. Revell VL, Burgess HJ, Gazda CJ, et al. Advancing human circadian rhythms with afternoon melatonin and morning intermittent bright light. J Clin Endocr Metab 2006;91:54–9.

51. Paul MA, Gray GW, Lieberman HR, et al. Phase advance with separate and combined melatonin and light treatment. Psychopharmacology (Berl) 2011;214(2):515–23.

52. Burke TM, Markwald RR, Chinoy ED, et al. Combination of light and melatonin time cues for phase advancing the human circadian clock. Sleep 2013;36(11):1617–24.

53. Burgess HJ, Park M, Wyatt JK, et al. Home dim light melatonin onsets with measures of compliance in delayed sleep phase disorder. J Sleep Res 2016;25(3):314–7.

54. Wade A, Ford I, Crawford G, et al. Efficacy of prolonged release melatonin in insomnia patients aged 55-80 years: quality of sleep and next-day alertness outcomes. Curr Med Res Opin 2007;23(10):2597–605.

55. Available at: http://www.ema.europa.eu/docs/en_GB/document_library/EPAR_-_Summary_for_the_public/human/000695/WC500026805.pdf. Accessed Jan 2, 2018.

56. Lockley SW, Dressman MA, Licamele L, et al. Tasimelteon for non-24-hour sleep-wake disorder in totally blind people (SET and RESET): two multicentre, randomised, double-masked, placebo-controlled phase 3 trials. Lancet 2015;386:1754–64.

57. Rajaratnam SM, Polymeropoulos MH, Fisher DM, et al. Melatonin agonist tasimelteon (VEC-162) for transient insomnia after sleep-time shift: two randomised controlled multicentre trials. Lancet 2009;373(9662):482–91.

58. Available at: https://wayback.archive-it.org/7993/20170405224953/https://www.fda.gov/downloads/AdvisoryCommittees/CommitteesMeetingMaterials/Drugs/PeripheralandCentralNervousSystemDrugsAdvisoryCommittee/UCM374388.pdf. Accessed Jan 2, 2018.

59. Richardson GS, Zee PC, Wang-Weigand S, et al. Circadian phase-shifting effects of repeated ramelteon administration in healthy adults. J Clin Sleep Med 2008;4(5):456–61.

60. Kuriyama A, Honda M, Hayashino Y. Ramelteon for the treatment of insomnia in adults: a systematic review and meta-analysis. Sleep Med 2014;15(4):385–92.

61. Krauchi K, Cajochen C, Mori D, et al. Early evening melatonin and S-20098 advance circadian phase and nocturnal regulation of core body temperature. Am J Physiol 1997;272:R1178–88.

62. Leproult R, Onderbergen AV, L'Hermite-Baleriaux M, et al. Phase-shifts of 24-h rhythms of hormonal release and body temperature following early evening administration of the melatonin agonist agomelatine in healthy older men. Clin Endocrinol 2005;63:298–304.

63. Quera-Salva MA, Hajak G, Philip P, et al. Comparison of agomelatine and escitalopram on nighttime sleep and daytime condition and efficacy in major depressive disorder patients. Int Clin Psychopharmacol 2011;26(5):252–62.

64. Freiesleben SD, Furczyk K. A systematic review of agomelatine-induced liver injury. J Mol Psychiatry 2015;3(1):4.

65. Taylor D, Sparshatt A, Varma S, et al. Antidepressant efficacy of agomelatine: meta-analysis of published and unpublished studies. BMJ 2014;348:g1888.

66. Mundey K, Benloucif S, Harsanyi K, et al. Phase-dependent treatment of delayed sleep phase syndrome with melatonin. Sleep 2005;28:1271–8.

67. Kayumov L, Brown G, Jindal R, et al. A randomized, double-blind, placebo-controlled crossover study of the effect of exogenous melatonin on delayed sleep phase syndrome. Psychosom Med 2001;63:40–8.

68. Rahman SA, Kayumov L, Shapiro CM. Antidepressant action of melatonin in the treatment of delayed sleep phase syndrome. Sleep Med 2010;11(2):131–6.

69. van Geijlswijk IM, van der Heijden KB, Egberts AC, et al. Dose finding of melatonin for chronic idiopathic childhood sleep onset insomnia: an RCT. Psychopharmacology (Berl) 2010;212(3):379–91.

70. Smits MG, Nagtegaal EE, van der Heijden J, et al. Melatonin for chronic sleep onset insomnia in children: a randomized placebo-controlled trial. J Child Neurol 2001;16(2):86–92.

71. Van der Heijden KB, Smits MG, Van Someren EJ, et al. Effect of melatonin on sleep, behavior, and cognition in ADHD and chronic sleep-onset insomnia. J Am Acad Child Adolesc Psychiatry 2007;46(2):233–41.

72. Serfaty M, Kennell-Webb S, Warner J, et al. Double blind randomised placebo controlled trial of low dose melatonin for sleep disorders in dementia. Int J Geriatr Psychiatry 2002;17(12):1120–7.

73. Wright B, Sims D, Smart S, et al. Melatonin versus placebo in children with autism spectrum conditions

and severe sleep problems not amenable to behaviour management strategies: a randomised controlled crossover trial. J Autism Dev Disord 2011;41(2):175–84.

74. Hack LM, Lockley SW, Arendt J, et al. The effects of low-dose 0.5-mg melatonin on the free-running circadian rhythms of blind subjects. J Biol Rhythms 2003;18:420–9.

75. Lockley SW, Skene DJ, James K, et al. Melatonin administration can entrain the free-running circadian system of blind subjects. J Endocrinol 2000;164:R1–6.

76. Auger RR, Burgess HJ, Emens J, et al. Do evidence-based treatments for circadian rhythm sleep-wake disorders make the GRADE? Updated guidelines point to need for more clinical research. J Clin Sleep Med 2015;11(10):1079–80.

Pharmacologic Treatment of Sleep Disorders in Pregnancy

Laura P. McLafferty, MD[a],*, Meredith Spada, MD[b],
Priya Gopalan, MD[b]

KEYWORDS

• Pregnancy • Sleep disorders • Sleep aids • Insomnia • Restless legs syndrome • Narcolepsy

KEY POINTS

- Sleep disorders during pregnancy have adverse effects on both mother and fetus that may necessitate pharmacologic treatment.
- In addition to general side effects, sleep medications in pregnancy may affect fetal development, timing and duration of delivery, and postnatal outcomes.
- Pharmacologic treatment of sleep disorders in pregnancy must include an individualized assessment of benefit and risk for both the patient and her unborn child.

INTRODUCTION

Pregnancy is a unique physiologic state whose characteristics often predispose women to new-onset sleep disturbances or exacerbations of pre-existing sleep disorders. Pregnancy-related factors that can disrupt sleep include heartburn, nocturnal oxytocin secretion, nocturia, and fetal movement. Sleep disorders in pregnancy include insomnia (primary and secondary), restless legs syndrome (RLS), and narcolepsy.[1]

Primary and Secondary Insomnia

Sleep duration decreases during the later phases of pregnancy.[2] Factors associated with shorter sleep duration include nulliparity, younger maternal age, advanced gestational age, and elevated blood pressure.[3] Excessive sleep disruption places pregnant and postpartum women at risk of new-onset and recurrent mood disturbance,[4] and is associated with increased risk of longer labor duration and need for caesarean delivery in nulliparous women,[5] as well as risk of preterm birth.[6] For primary insomnia, treatment strategies include cognitive behavioral and pharmacologic therapies.[1] For secondary insomnia, therapeutic management should include treatment of the underlying psychiatric and/or medical disorder.

Restless Legs Syndrome

Patients with RLS describe an unpleasant sensation that causes an overwhelming urge to move their legs. This sensation tends to worsen at night and during periods of rest. RLS is found in more than one-fourth of pregnant women[7,8] and almost two-thirds have no symptoms before pregnancy.[9] For most women, symptoms resolve

Disclosure Statement: None of the authors have any relationship with a commercial company that has a direct financial interest in subject matter or materials discussed in the article or with a company making a competing product.
[a] Department of Psychiatry and Human Behavior, Thomas Jefferson University, Thompson Building, Suite 1652, 1020 Sansom Street, Philadelphia, PA 19107, USA; [b] Department of Psychiatry, Western Psychiatric Institute and Clinic, University of Pittsburgh Medical Center, 3811 O'Hara St., Pittsburgh, PA 15213, USA
* Corresponding author.
E-mail address: laura.mclafferty@jefferson.edu

Sleep Med Clin 13 (2018) 243–250
https://doi.org/10.1016/j.jsmc.2018.02.004
1556-407X/18/© 2018 Elsevier Inc. All rights reserved.

postdelivery.[10] RLS is linked to dopamine metabolism dysfunction in the central nervous system,[1] which, in pregnancy, may be linked to serum iron deficiency due to increased iron requirements,[8] folate deficiency,[11] and hormones such as estradiol.[12] Management strategies include pharmacologic therapy and reducing exposure to known triggers such as caffeine, smoking, and certain drugs.[1]

Narcolepsy

It is a clinical syndrome of daytime sleepiness caused by dysfunctional transition between sleep stages and is often accompanied by cataplexy, hypnagogic hallucinations, and sleep paralysis.[13] Given the peak incidence of narcolepsy from adolescence to early in the third decade of life, afflicted women are likely to have a pregnancy affected by the condition, and 40% report worsening symptoms in pregnancy.[1,14] Pregnant women with narcolepsy have higher rates of anemia and glucose intolerance, although there is no significant difference in mean weight and gestational age at birth.[14] Labor may be a trigger for cataplexy.[1]

SLEEP MEDICATIONS IN PREGNANCY

The goals of treating sleep disorders in pregnancy include the promotion of restorative sleep and the benefits it brings to both mother and fetus. Pregnancy is unique, however, in the presence of a fetus, who is also affected by any medication the patient takes. The prescribing of any sleep aid in pregnancy must include consideration of the risks and benefits of that medication for both mother and fetus.[15] The following pharmacologic agents and their perinatal effects are organized according to the sleep disorders they are intended to treat.

Primary and Secondary Insomnia

Benzodiazepines
Benzodiazepines function at the limbic, thalamic, and hypothalamic levels of the central nervous system to enhance neurotransmission of gamma-aminobutyric acid (GABA). They work via a modulatory site on the $GABA_A$ receptor complex to produce their sedative, anxiolytic, and antiepileptic effects are, used for the treatment of insomnia, anxiety, and seizures.[16,17] Although better suited for the short-term treatment of insomnia and anxiety, long-term use for these purposes is common and is associated with significant morbidity, including dependence and withdrawal, drowsiness and cognitive

dulling, falls, and fractures.[18,19] They are commonly prescribed for the treatment of perinatal insomnia[16] and, because half of pregnancies are unplanned, there is the potential for accidental early fetal exposure.[20]

Benzodiazepines readily cross the placenta. However, despite access to fetal tissues as a result of placental transfer, studies indicate that benzodiazepines are not teratogenic.[21,22] Although early case-control investigations reported increased incidence of cleft lip or palate with benzodiazepines,[23,24] these findings have not been replicated in subsequent research.[21,25–27] Evidence does suggest, however, that benzodiazepines may contribute to increased rates of preterm birth and low birthweight.[28]

Hypnotic benzodiazepine receptor agonists
Medications in the hypnotic benzodiazepine receptor agonist (HBRA) class, also known as Z-drugs, include the imidazopyridine zolpidem; the pyrazolopyrimidine zaleplon; and the cyclopyrrolone, zopiclone (not commercially available on the market in the United States); and eszopiclone (the active enantiomer of zopiclone). HBRAs are now the most commonly prescribed hypnotics worldwide, including among pregnant women. Although not chemically related to benzodiazepines, they are agonists at the $GABA_A$ receptor, reducing sleep latency and improving sleep quality,[29,30] and they are thought to have minimal disruption of sleep architecture. Many potential adverse reactions have been noted, including memory loss, daytime fatigue, hallucinations, and tolerance or physiologic dependence.[31,32] HBRAs, like benzodiazepines, cross the human placenta and rapidly clear the fetal circulation.[33,34] HBRAs do not seem to increase risk for congenital malformations at usual clinical doses.[28,34–37] There is a case report, however, of neural tube defects occurring with high-dose exposure to zolpidem in the first trimester of pregnancy.[38] HBRAs may increase rates of preterm birth, low birthweight, and/or small-for-gestational-age infants[34,39]; however, studies were small and results showed statistical but likely no clinical significance.

Antidepressants
Regardless of class, all currently available antidepressants are thought to work through the modulation of the monoamine neurotransmitters, serotonin, norepinephrine, and dopamine, for the treatment of depression and anxiety. Given the sedating nature of some antidepressants, including tricyclic antidepressants (TCAs); the piperazinoazepine agent mirtazapine; and the serotonin-2 receptor antagonist and serotonin

reuptake inhibitor (SARI), trazodone, it comes as no surprise that these medications are sometimes used off-label for the treatment of perinatal insomnia.[40] Doxepin and amitriptyline are TCAs that are often used as sleep aids at low doses. Their hypnotic effects are thought to be related to their antihistaminergic properties. TCAs carry the risk of significant morbidity given their action at multiple receptor sites; side effects include confusion, constipation, blurred vision, weight gain, tachycardia, cardiac arrhythmias, and death in overdose. Low-dose doxepin for insomnia seems to be relatively well tolerated in the general adult population.[41] Treatment providers often take advantage of the main side effects of mirtazapine, namely drowsiness, increased appetite, and weight gain, for the treatment of depression with concomitant insomnia and poor appetite.[42] Originally developed as an antidepressant, trazodone is now almost exclusively used for the treatment of insomnia,[43] is generally well tolerated, and has been shown to improve sleep efficacy and shorten sleep onset latency.[44]

In contemporary studies, antidepressant use in the perinatal period does not seem to confer an increased risk for congenital malformations.[45,46] Studies do seem to support a small but increased risk for low birthweight and preterm birth,[46,47] although this is significantly confounded by underlying illness state. When used in late pregnancy, studies show a small but increased risk for respiratory symptoms, including persistent pulmonary hypertension of the newborn. However, the absolute risk is extremely low.[46,48] A systematic review of mirtazapine use in pregnant women found a possible increased risk of spontaneous abortion. However, this may have been related to underlying psychiatric disease. No association was found between prenatal mirtazapine use and congenital malformations.[49] The only study evaluating the effects of trazodone on the neonate was by Khazaie and colleagues,[50] which compared trazodone with other treatments of perinatal insomnia.

Antidepressant use in pregnancy has been associated with a constellation of adverse neurobehavioral effects in newborns (irritability, tremors, jitteriness, and sleep disturbances), known as neonatal adaptation syndrome, though these symptoms are generally transient and short-lived.[51,52] Additional neurologic effects noted in the neonate include abnormal general movements.[51] However, these results must be interpreted carefully because untreated depression has been implicated in many of the same processes.[53]

Antipsychotics

Antipsychotic medications work primarily as antagonists at dopamine receptors, though there is considerable variability in their receptor profiles. Although the first-generation antipsychotics are largely uniform in their D2 receptor antagonism (though to varying potencies), the second-generation antipsychotics do not uniformly have this effect and are largely known for serotonin antagonism. Although the off-label use of these medications for insomnia has become a widespread practice, their side-effect profile should preclude their use in pregnancy for the primary indication of insomnia. However, the sedating effects of many of the antipsychotics may be helpful in the treatment of psychosis and mood disorders. Sedating second-generation antipsychotics include clozapine, olanzapine, quetiapine, and risperidone, the latter 3 having the largest number of studies. Of these, olanzapine and clozapine cross the placenta at higher rates than quetiapine and risperidone due to the level of protein-binding. In vivo studies of antipsychotic levels during pregnancy suggest a decrease in maternal serum levels during the third trimester, consistent with other classes of medications and in line with the pharmacokinetic changes that occur during pregnancy.[54]

Second-generation antipsychotics have an emerging body of research that validates their safety profile during the perinatal period. Recent studies have found no association with congenital malformations[55,56] or gestational diabetes.[57] Sørensen and colleagues[58] found no difference in spontaneous abortion rates between pregnant women who stayed on their antipsychotic medications versus those who discontinued them; however, they did find a 2-fold increase in the risk of stillbirth, with an absolute risk difference of 1.2% versus 0.6%. Both medication-exposed groups had higher rates of stillbirths and spontaneous abortions compared with unexposed women but absolute numbers remained low in all groups.[58] The US Federal Drug Administration issued a class warning in 2011 for withdrawal symptoms and extrapyramidal symptoms in neonates born to mothers on antipsychotics.[59]

Melatonin and melatonin receptor agonists

Melatonin is a naturally produced neurotransmitter that modulates circadian rhythms in all mammals. It is known to have effects on sexual maturation and elevated secretion of endogenous melatonin during pregnancy.[60] Endogenous melatonin is also produced in the placenta, and protects against molecular damage and cellular dysfunction arising from oxidative stress.[61] However, only limited data are available for the use of exogenous melatonin in pregnancy. Studies investigating the neonatal effects of melatonin are primarily in mice. They show conflicted results, with some showing evidence of neuroprotection in the setting of toxin exposure,[62] whereas others have shown disruption to reproductive hormone development[63] and postpartum circadian rhythm.[64]

Antihistamines

Diphenhydramine and hydroxyzine are widely accepted for use during pregnancy, yet there are few studies in humans to confirm their safety profiles. Khazaie and colleagues[50] evaluated the effect of insomnia treatment during the third trimester of pregnancy on postpartum depression symptoms in 54 pregnant women who were randomly assigned to trazodone 50 mg per day, diphenhydramine 25 mg per day, or placebo treatment. Trazodone and diphenhydramine significantly improved sleep duration and sleep efficiency compared with placebo at 2 and 6 weeks of treatment ($P<.0001$), and both medications improved depressive symptoms. Doxylamine is present in numerous over-the-counter sleep aids and has been investigated almost exclusively in the context of treatment of nausea and vomiting.

Einarson and colleagues[65] prospectively compared 53 pregnant women on hydroxyzine with 23 women on cetirizine and a control group, and found no differences in rates of livebirths, spontaneous or therapeutic abortion, or stillbirth. A case report of a neonatal withdrawal syndrome with 150 mg (mg) of hydroxyzine was reported in 2005.[66] The Israel Teratogen Information Service followed 37 pregnancies with exposure to hydroxyzine and found no increased risk of congenital malformations.[67] A study by Li and colleagues[68] showed no significant associations between diphenhydramine and doxylamine and congenital malformations. Diphenhydramine was investigated in the setting of hyperemesis gravidarum and showed no effects on perinatal outcomes.[69] Another study found a possible association between diphenhydramine, doxylamine, and birth defects, but was significantly confounded by recall bias and limited by relatively small numbers.[70]

Restless Legs Syndrome

Dopamine agonists

The nonergot dopamine agonists, including pramipexole, ropinirole, and rotigotine, are considered first-line medications for the treatment of RLS in nonpregnant adults. Additionally, carbidopa-levodopa can be used for RLS symptoms that occur intermittently in the evening, at bedtime, on waking during the night, or for symptoms associated with specific activities, such as long car rides.[71] Ergot agonists, such as bromocriptine and cabergoline, as well as pergolide, should be avoided for the treatment of RLS because they have been associated with cardiac valvular fibrosis and other fibrotic reactions.[72,73] Minor potential side effects of the nonergot dopamine agonists include nausea and lightheadedness (which generally resolve within 10–14 days), and less common adverse reactions include nasal stuffiness, constipation, insomnia, and leg edema (which are reversible with discontinuation of treatment). At higher doses, hypersomnia may occur.[71] Treatment-limiting adverse reactions include the development of augmentation (ie, a worsening of RLS symptoms earlier in the day after an evening dose of medication) and impulse control disorders.[74,75]

The literature regarding the pharmacologic treatment of RLS in pregnancy is scarce. As such, a task force of 9 experts was chosen by the International RLS Study Group (IRLSSG) to develop guidelines for the diagnosis and treatment of RLS during pregnancy and lactation.[76] In 2015, the IRLSSG task force outlined nonpharmacologic treatment approaches; a rationale for iron supplementation; and, finally, pharmacologic treatment approaches for perinatal RLS. As with other medications, the task force called for a risk-benefit approach regarding the use of dopamine agonists for the treatment of RLS in pregnancy.[76]

Although there is more evidence for the effectiveness of the nonergot dopamine agonists for the treatment of RLS compared with carbidopa-levodopa, there are more safety data for carbidopa-levodopa in pregnancy.[76] Carbidopa-levodopa use during pregnancy has been reported in 38 cases of RLS in pregnancy without evidence for major malformations or other adverse outcomes.[77] However, the combination of levodopa with benserazide should be avoided owing to a possible adverse effect on bone development.[76] Due to limited data regarding the safety of nonergot dopamine agonists in pregnancy, the IRLSSG task force rated these medications as "insufficient evidence to reach consensus" for use in the treatment of RLS during pregnancy.[76] Task force recommendations include avoiding the ergot dopamine agonists for the treatment of RLS in pregnancy, given their potential for fibrotic reactions.[76,78]

Narcolepsy

Stimulants

Although stimulant use for the treatment of perinatal sleep disorders has not been systematically researched, clinical outcomes from studies on the treatment of attention-deficit hyperactivity disorder (ADHD) may guide the risk-benefit discussion of stimulant use for the management of narcolepsy in patients who require these medications. Animal studies on the use of stimulants in pregnancy have suggested structural and behavioral teratogenicity.[79,80] A Danish case-control study of 480 women taking methylphenidate, modafinil, or atomoxetine during pregnancy found a 2-fold increase in the risk of induced abortion and miscarriage in pregnancies exposed to these medications. However, in a case-crossover subanalysis of pregnant women with ADHD with and without medication exposure, the relative risk decreased, suggesting confounding by indication.[81] A multicenter prospective study comparing 382 women exposed to methylphenidate during pregnancy with a matched unexposed sample found a similar increased adjusted hazard ratio of 1.35, also confounded by indication.[82] The investigators did not find any associations with congenital or cardiovascular defects with perinatal use of methylphenidate.[82] A case-control study by Newport and colleagues[83] looking at the relationship between stimulants and hypertensive disorders of pregnancy is limited by a sample size (n = 12) that is too small to draw any meaningful conclusions.

Wake-promoting agents

In a retrospective case-control study of 25 women with narcolepsy with cataplexy, 6 pregnancies were determined to have occurred in which modafinil and methylphenidate were prescribed, and pregnancy outcomes were similar to controls.[84,85] There are no studies of armodafinil in pregnancy.

Sodium oxybate, gamma hydroxybutyrate, and other medications

There are no human studies on the use of sodium oxybate or gamma hydroxybutyrate during pregnancy. The management of narcolepsy in nonpregnant patients reports use of such medications as opioids, carbamazepine, valproic acid, clonidine, gabapentin, pregabalin, bromocriptine, and cabergoline.[1] Of these, opioids are not a first-line treatment and should not be used in this setting. Valproic acid and carbamazepine should not be used during pregnancy owing to known teratogenicity. Studies on gabapentin and pregabalin are limited to seizure indication and not studied for a narcolepsy indication. Bromocriptine and cabergoline are not recommended for use in pregnancy.[1]

SUMMARY

Sleep disorders, such as primary and secondary insomnia and RLS, have increased prevalence in pregnancy, whereas others, such as narcolepsy, have unique relationships with certain aspects of pregnancy, including delivery.[1] The roles of both mother and fetus in pregnancy affect provider consideration of sleep disorder outcome as well as treatment choice. Providers must keep in mind that literature on the use of sleep medications in pregnancy is often sparse or nonexistent.[15] Therefore, pharmacologic treatment of sleep disorders in pregnancy must include an individualized assessment of the potential risk of untreated disease for both mother and infant compared with the risks and benefits of maternal and fetal pharmacologic exposure.

REFERENCES

1. Oyiengo D, Louis M, Hott B, et al. Sleep disorders in pregnancy. Clin Chest Med 2014;35:571–87.
2. Hertz G, Fast A, Feinsilver SH, et al. Sleep in normal late pregnancy. Sleep 1992;14:246–51.
3. Fernandez-Alonso AM, Trabalon-Pastor M, Chedraui P, et al. Factors related to insomnia and sleepiness in the late third trimester of pregnancy. Arch Gynecol Obstet 2012;286:55–61.
4. Okun ML, Hanusa BJ, Hall M, et al. Sleep complaints in late pregnancy and the recurrence of postpartum depression. Behav Sleep Med 2009;7:106–17.
5. Lee KA, Gay CL. Sleep in late pregnancy predicts length of labor and type of delivery. Am J Obstet Gynecol 2004;191:2041–6.
6. Okun ML, Schetter CD, Glynn LM. Poor sleep quality is associated with preterm birth. Sleep 2011;34:1493–8.
7. Chen PH, Liou KC, Chen CP, et al. Risk factors and prevalence rate of restless legs syndrome among pregnant women in Taiwan. Sleep Med 2012;13:1153–7.
8. Manconi M, Govoni V, De Vito A, et al. Pregnancy as a risk factor for restless legs syndrome. Sleep Med 2004;5:305–8.
9. Manconi M, Govoni V, De Vito A, et al. Restless legs syndrome in pregnancy. Neurology 2004;63:1065–9.
10. Uglane MT, Westad S, Backe B. Restless legs syndrome in pregnancy is a frequent disorder with a good prognosis. Acta Obstet Gynecol Scand 2011;90(9):1046–8.
11. Lee KA, Zaffke ME, Baratte-Beebe K. Restless legs syndrome and sleep disturbance during pregnancy: the role of folate and iron. J Womens Health Gend Based Med 2001;10:335–41.
12. Djaza A, Wehrle R, Lancel M, et al. Elevated estradiol plasma levels in women with restless legs during pregnancy. Sleep 2009;32:169–74.
13. Scammell TE. The neurobiology, diagnosis, and treatment of narcolepsy. Ann Neurol 2003;53:154–66.
14. Maurovat-Horvich E, Kemlink D, Hogl B, et al. Narcolepsy and pregnancy: a retrospective European

evaluation of 249 pregnancies. J Sleep Res 2013;22: 496–512.

15. McAllister-Williams RH, Baldwin DS, Cantwell R, et al. British Association for Psychopharmacology consensus guidance on the use of psychotropic medication preconception, in pregnancy and postpartum 2017. J Psychopharmacol 2017; 31(5):519–52.

16. Iqbal MM, Sobhan T, Ryals T. Effects of commonly used benzodiazepines on the fetus, the neonate, and the nursing infant. Psychiatr Serv 2002;53(1): 39–49.

17. Hood SD, Norman A, Hince DA, et al. Benzodiazepine dependence and its treatment with low dose flumazenil. Br J Clin Pharmacol 2014;77(2):285–94.

18. Ballinger BR. New drugs. Hypnotics and anxiolytics. BMJ 1990;300(6722):456–8.

19. Pollmann AS, Murphy AL, Bergman JC, et al. Deprescribing benzodiazepines and Z-drugs in community-dwelling adults: a scoping review. BMC Pharmacol Toxicol 2015;16:19.

20. Koren G, Pastuszak A, Ito S. Drugs in pregnancy. N Engl J Med 1998;338:1128–37.

21. Ban L, West J, Gibson JE, et al. First trimester exposure to anxiolytic and hypnotic drugs and the risks of major congenital anomalies: a United Kingdom population-based cohort study. PLoS One 2014; 9(6):e100996.

22. Enato E, Moretti M, Koren G. The fetal safety of benzodiazepines: an updated meta-analysis. J Obstet Gynaecol Can 2011;33(1):46–8.

23. Saxén I. Associations between oral clefts and drugs taken during pregnancy. Int J Epidemiol 1975;4(1): 37–44.

24. Safra MJ, Oakley GP. Association between cleft lip with or without cleft palate and prenatal exposure to diazepam. Lancet 1975;2(7933):478–80.

25. Cates C. Benzodiazepine use in pregnancy and major malformations or oral clefts. Pooled results are sensitive to zero transformation used. BMJ 1999; 319(7214):918–9.

26. Czeizel A. Lack of evidence of teratogenicity of benzodiazepine drugs in Hungary. Reprod Toxicol 1987;1(3):183–8.

27. Rosenberg L, Mitchell AA, Parsells JL, et al. Lack of relation of oral clefts to diazepam use during pregnancy. N Engl J Med 1983;309(21):1282–5.

28. Wikner BN, Källén B. Are hypnotic benzodiazepine receptor agonists teratogenic in humans? J Clin Psychopharmacol 2011;31(3):356–9.

29. Sullivan SS, Guilleminault C. Emerging drugs for insomnia: new frontiers for old and novel targets. Expert Opin Emerg Drugs 2009;14(3):411–22.

30. Gunja N. The clinical and forensic toxicology of Z-drugs. J Med Toxicol 2013;9(2):155–62.

31. Siriwardena AN, Qureshi MZ, Dyas JV, et al. Magic bullets for insomnia? Patients' use and experiences of newer (Z drugs) versus older (benzodiazepine) hypnotics for sleep problems in primary care. Br J Gen Pract 2008;58(551):417–22.

32. Huedo-medina TB, Kirsch I, Middlemass J, et al. Effectiveness of non-benzodiazepine hypnotics in treatment of adult insomnia: meta-analysis of data submitted to the Food and Drug Administration. BMJ 2012;345:e8343.

33. Askew JP. Zolpidem addiction in a pregnant woman with a history of second-trimester bleeding. Pharmacotherapy 2007;27(2):306–8.

34. Juric S, Newport DJ, Ritchie JC, et al. Zolpidem (Ambien) in pregnancy: placental passage and outcome. Arch Womens Ment Health 2009;12(6): 441–6.

35. Diav-citrin O, Okotore B, Lucarelli K, et al. Pregnancy outcome following first-trimester exposure to zopiclone: a prospective controlled cohort study. Am J Perinatol 1999;16(4):157–60.

36. Wilton LV, Pearce GL, Martin RM, et al. The outcomes of pregnancy in women exposed to newly marketed drugs in general practice in England. Br J Obstet Gynaecol 1998;105(8):882–9.

37. Wikner BN, Stiller CO, Bergman U, et al. Use of benzodiazepines and benzodiazepine receptor agonists during pregnancy: neonatal outcome and congenital malformations. Pharmacoepidemiol Drug Saf 2007;16(11):1203–10.

38. Sharma A, Sayeed N, Khees CR, et al. High dose zolpidem induced fetal neural tube defects. Curr Drug Saf 2011;6(2):128–9.

39. Wang LH, Lin HC, Lin CC, et al. Increased risk of adverse pregnancy outcomes in women receiving zolpidem during pregnancy. Clin Pharmacol Ther 2010;88(3):369–74.

40. Winokur A, Gary KA, Rodner S, et al. Depression, sleep physiology, and antidepressant drugs. Depress Anxiety 2001;14(1):19–28.

41. Wilt TJ, Macdonald R, Brasure M, et al. Pharmacologic treatment of insomnia disorder: an evidence report for a clinical practice guideline by the American College of Physicians. Ann Intern Med 2016; 165(2):103–12.

42. Djulus J, Koren G, Einarson TR, et al. Exposure to mirtazapine during pregnancy: a prospective, comparative study of birth outcomes. J Clin Psychiatry 2006;67(8):1280–4.

43. Wong J, Motulsky A, Abrahamowicz M, et al. Off-label indications for antidepressants in primary care: descriptive study of prescriptions from an indication based electronic prescribing system. BMJ 2017; 356:j603.

44. Mashiko H, Niwa S, Kumashiro H, et al. Effect of trazodone in a single dose before bedtime for sleep disorders accompanied by a depressive state: dose-finding study with no concomitant use of hypnotic agent. Psychiatry Clin Neurosci 1999;53(2):193–4.

45. Einarson TR, Einarson A. Newer antidepressants in pregnancy and rates of major malformations: a meta-analysis of prospective comparative studies. Pharmacoepidemiol Drug Saf 2005;14(12):823–7.

46. Tak CR, Job KM, Schoen-gentry K, et al. The impact of exposure to antidepressant medications during pregnancy on neonatal outcomes: a review of retrospective database cohort studies. Eur J Clin Pharmacol 2017;73(9):1055–69.

47. Huang H, Coleman S, Bridge JA, et al. A meta-analysis of the relationship between antidepressant use in pregnancy and the risk of preterm birth and low birth weight. Gen Hosp Psychiatry 2014;36(1):13–8.

48. Huybrechts KF, Bateman BT, Palmsten K, et al. Antidepressant use late in pregnancy and risk of persistent pulmonary hypertension of the newborn. JAMA 2015;313(21):2142–51.

49. Smit M, Dolman KM, Honig A. Mirtazapine in pregnancy and lactation - a systematic review. Eur Neuropsychopharmacol 2016;26(1):126–35.

50. Khazaie H, Ghadami MR, Knight DC, et al. Insomnia treatment in the third trimester of pregnancy reduces postpartum depression symptoms: a randomized clinical trial. Psychiatry Res 2013;210(3):901–5.

51. De vries NK, Van der veere CN, Reijneveld SA, et al. Early neurological outcome of young infants exposed to selective serotonin reuptake inhibitors during pregnancy: results from the observational SMOK study. PLoS One 2013;8(5):e64654.

52. Grigoriadis S, Vonderporten EH, Mamisashvili L, et al. The effect of prenatal antidepressant exposure on neonatal adaptation: a systematic review and meta-analysis. J Clin Psychiatry 2013;74(4):e309–20.

53. Wisner KL, Sit DK, Hanusa BH, et al. Major depression and antidepressant treatment: impact on pregnancy and neonatal outcomes. Am J Psychiatry 2009;166(5):557–66.

54. Westin AA, Brekke M, Molden E, et al. Treatment with antipsychotics in pregnancy: changes in drug disposition. Clin Pharmacol Ther 2018;103(3):477–84.

55. Huybrechts KF, Hernández-Díaz S, Patorno E. Antipsychotic use in pregnancy and the risk for congenital malformations. JAMA Psychiatry 2016;73(9):938–46.

56. Cohen LS, Viguera AC, McInerney KA. Reproductive safety of second-generation antipsychotics: current data from the Massachusetts General Hospital National Pregnancy registry for atypical antipsychotics. Am J Psychiatry 2016;173(3):263–70.

57. Panchaud A, Hernandez-Diaz S, Freeman MP, et al. Use of atypical antipsychotics in pregnancy and maternal gestational diabetes. J Psychiatr Res 2017;95:84–90.

58. Sørensen MJ, Kjaersgaard MI, Pedersen HS, et al. Risk of fetal death after treatment with antipsychotic medications during pregnancy. PLoS One 2015;10(7):e0132280.

59. FDA. FDA drug safety communication: antipsychotic drug labels updated on use during pregnancy and risk of abnormal muscle movements and withdrawal symptoms in newborns. In: FDA Drug Safety and Availability. Available at: http://www.fda.gov/Drugs/DrugSafety/ucm243903.htm. Accessed October 1, 2017.

60. Tamura H, Takasaki A, Taketani T, et al. Melatonin and female reproduction. J Obstet Gynaecol Res 2014;40(1):1–11.

61. Soliman A, Lacasse AA, Lanoix D, et al. Placental melatonin system is present throughout pregnancy and regulates villous trophoblast differentiation. J Pineal Res 2015;59(1):38–46.

62. Dubovický M, Ujházy E, Kovacovský P, et al. Effect of melatonin on neurobehavioral dysfunctions induced by intrauterine hypoxia in rats. Cent Eur J Public Health 2004;12(Suppl):S23–5.

63. Domínguez Rubio AP, Correa F, Aisemberg J, et al. Maternal administration of melatonin exerts short- and long-term neuroprotective effects on the offspring from lipopolysaccharide-treated mice. J Pineal Res 2017. https://doi.org/10.1111/jpi.12439.

64. Davis FC. Melatonin: role in development. J Biol Rhythms 1997;12(6):498–508.

65. Einarson A, Bailey B, Jung G, et al. Prospective controlled study of hydroxyzine and cetirizine in pregnancy. Ann Allergy Asthma Immunol 1997;78(2):183–6.

66. Serreau R, Komiha M, Blanc F, et al. Neonatal seizures associated with maternal hydroxyzine hydrochloride in late pregnancy. Reprod Toxicol 2005;20(4):573–4.

67. Diav-Citrin O, Shechtman S, Aharonovich A. Pregnancy outcome after gestational exposure to loratadine or antihistamines: a prospective controlled cohort study. J Allergy Clin Immunol 2003;111(6):1239–43.

68. Li Q, Mitchell AA, Werler MM, et al. Assessment of antihistamine use in early pregnancy and birth defects. J Allergy Clin Immunol Pract 2013;1(6):666–74.

69. Nageotte MP, Briggs GG, Towers CV, et al. Droperidol and diphenhydramine in the management of hyperemesis gravidarum. Am J Obstet Gynecol 1996;174(6):1801–5.

70. Gilboa SM, Strickland MJ, Olshan AF, et al. Use of antihistamine medications during early pregnancy and isolated major malformations. Birth Defects Res A Clin Mol Teratol 2009;85(2):137–50.

71. Silber MH, Becker PM, Earley C, et al. Willis-Ekbom Disease Foundation revised consensus statement on the management of restless legs syndrome. Mayo Clin Proc 2013;88(9):977–86.

72. Andersohn F, Garbe E. Cardiac and noncardiac fibrotic reactions caused by ergot-and nonergot-derived dopamine agonists. Mov Disord 2009; 24(1):129–33.

73. Garcia-Borreguero D, Ferini-strambi L, Kohnen R, et al. European guidelines on management of restless legs syndrome: report of a joint task force by the European Federation of Neurological Societies, the European Neurological Society and the European Sleep Research Society. Eur J Neurol 2012; 19(11):1385–96.

74. Lipford MC, Silber MH. Long-term use of pramipexole in the management of restless legs syndrome. Sleep Med 2012;13(10):1280–5.

75. Cornelius JR, Tippmann-Peikert M, Slocumb NL, et al. Impulse control disorders with the use of dopaminergic agents in restless legs syndrome: a case-control study. Sleep 2010;33(1):81–7.

76. Picchietti DL, Hensley JG, Bainbridge JL, et al. Consensus clinical practice guidelines for the diagnosis and treatment of restless legs syndrome/Willis-Ekbom disease during pregnancy and lactation. Sleep Med Rev 2015;22:64–77.

77. Dostal M, Weber-schoendorfer C, Sobesky J, et al. Pregnancy outcome following use of levodopa, pramipexole, ropinirole, and rotigotine for restless legs syndrome during pregnancy: a case series. Eur J Neurol 2013;20(9):1241–6.

78. Araujo B, Belo S, Carvalho D. Pregnancy and tumor outcomes in women with prolactinoma. Exp Clin Endocrinol Diabetes 2017;125(10):642–8.

79. Costa Gdr A, Galvao TC, Bacchi AD, et al. Investigation of possible teratogenic effects in the offspring of mice exposed to methylphenidate during pregnancy. Reprod Biomed Online 2016;32(2): 170–7.

80. Peters HT, Strange LG, Brown SSD, et al. The pharmacokinetic profile of methylphenidate use in pregnancy: a study in mice. Neurotoxicol Teratol 2016; 54:1–4.

81. Haervig KB, Mortensen LH, Hansen AV, et al. Use of ADHD medication during pregnancy from 1999 to 2010: a Danish register-based study. Pharmacoepidemiol Drug Saf 2014;23(5):526–33.

82. Diav-Citrin O, Shechtman S, Arnon J, et al. Methylphenidate in pregnancy: a multicenter, prospective, comparative, observational Study. J Clin Psychiatry 2016;77(9):1176–81.

83. Newport DJ, Hostetter AL, Juul SH, et al. Prenatal psychostimulant and antidepressant exposure and risk of hypertensive disorders of pregnancy. J Clin Psychiatry 2016;77(11):1538–45.

84. Calvo-Ferrandiz E, Peraita-Adrados R. Narcolepsy with cataplexy and pregnancy: a case-control study. J Sleep Res 2017. https://doi.org/10.1111/jsr.12567.

85. Kuczkowski KM. Liquid ecstasy during pregnancy. Anaesthesia 2004;59(9):926.

Sleep-Related Drug Therapy in Special Conditions: Children

Nicholas-Tiberio Economou, MD, PhD[a,b],
Luigi Ferini-Strambi, MD, PhD[c],
Paschalis Steiropoulos, MD, PhD, FCCP[d],*

KEYWORDS

- Pediatric obstructive sleep apnea • Pediatric insomnia • Pediatric narcolepsy
- Pediatric parasomnias • Pediatric restless legs syndrome

KEY POINTS

- Early detection of sleep disorders in childhood is of great importance in order to proceed to treatment and prevent neurodevelopmental, neurocognitive, and other consequences.
- Insomnia and parasomnia in children present with various complaints, depending on the child's age, and are treated pharmacologically only after nonpharmacologic treatment has failed.
- Sleep apnea in children can be managed with nonpharmacologic, pharmacologic, or surgical treatment, based on specific indications and severity.
- Narcolepsy in children is frequently addressed with stimulants; however, behavioral and lifestyle modifications are still important.
- Restless legs syndrome in children can be treated with pharmacologic and nonpharmacologic options. Iron and ferritin levels should always be evaluated.

INTRODUCTION

There is a continuously growing body of evidence pointing out the importance of detecting and consequently assessing sleep disorders in children, resulting from the bimodal association between sleep and neurodevelopment, cognition, and behavior. Thus, poor sleep quality and/or quantity, especially in the presence of sleep disorders, is related to neurodevelopmental and neurocognitive deficits; reduced learning and social skills; and difficulties in adaptation, behavior, and emotion.[1,2]

Numerous reasons can be found to emphasize the importance of focusing on pediatric sleep medicine and on pediatric sleep (pharmaco)therapy. First, symptoms of sleep disorders in children are not only different compared with those of adults but also heterogeneous among children of different age. Obstructive sleep apnea (OSA) in children, for example, is related neither to body mass index nor to male sex, in contrast with adults. Moreover, the cardinal daytime symptom of OSA in adults is excessive daytime sleepiness (EDS), whereas children are more often characterized by attention or behavior disorders (such as irritability, overactivity and inattentiveness), instead of full-blown sleepiness.[3–5] Furthermore, there is variance in clinical manifestation

Conflicts of Interest: All authors declare no conflict of interest related to this publication.
[a] Sleep Study Unit, Department of Psychiatry, University of Athens, 74 Vas Sofias Avenue, 11528 Athens, Greece; [b] Enypnion Sleep-Epilepsy Center, Bioclinic Hospital Athens, 15 M. Geroulanou Street, 11524 Athens, Greece; [c] Division of Neuroscience, University Vita-Salute San Raffaele, Via Stamira d'Ancona 20, Milan 20127, Italy; [d] Sleep Unit, Department of Pulmomonolgy, Medical School, Democritus University of Thrace, University Campus, Dragana, Alexandroupolis 68100, Greece
* Corresponding author.
E-mail address: pstirop@med.duth.gr

Sleep Med Clin 13 (2018) 251–262
https://doi.org/10.1016/j.jsmc.2018.02.007
1556-407X/18/© 2018 Elsevier Inc. All rights reserved.

according to age. For example, during the first years of life, insomnia (sleep-onset difficulty or frequent awakenings during the night), parasomnia, and sleep disordered breathing are the most prevalent sleep disorders. Later, among school-aged children and mostly among teenagers, suboptimal sleep hygiene, sleep deprivation, delayed sleep phase syndrome, and other circadian disorders are the most prominent abnormalities.[1,6] Another issue, which makes sleep disorder assessment in children even more complicated, is the overall lack of training in pediatric sleep medicine worldwide. Thus, hesitancy of use or improper prescription of drugs (erroneous choice, underdosing, or overdosing) is observed. Moreover, there is also a lack of evidence-based guidelines and of officially approved pediatric sleep pharmacotherapy.[6,7] For example, pediatric insomnia is often treated in an empiric way with clonidine, a drug that is not used and approved for insomnia in adults.[8,9]

This article summarizes the current therapeutic management of sleep disorders in children, bearing in mind the absence of evidence-based guidelines on this topic.

Management of Insomnia in Children

Insomnia is defined as a difficulty to fall asleep, or difficulty in maintaining sleep (nocturnal awakenings), or as waking up earlier than desired. The last phenomena are related to daytime functioning.[10]

In children, insomnia has mainly behavioral features (commonly called behavioral insomnias of childhood [BIC]) and is classified in 2 main categories: sleep-onset association disorder (SOAD) and limit-setting sleep disorder, whereas there is a third subtype, which represents a mixture of the 2 types of behavioral insomnia.[11,12] SOAD occurs when a child needs special settings or objects (ie, a pacifier) in order to get to sleep or to return to sleep once awakened. In the BIC limit-setting type, delayed sleep onset is observed with or without awakenings and is caused by inappropriate limit-setting by parents, with the child refusing to go to bed or asking repeatedly for attention (eg, for a beverage or to use the bathroom).[12] As age advances, other types of insomnia may occur. Adolescents may have insomnia caused by poor sleep hygiene, delayed sleep phase syndrome, or by psychophysiologic conditioning. It is very common among adolescents to adopt bad sleep habits (ie, use of electronic devices in bed; having huge variation in sleep-wake schedule between weekdays and weekends; consuming considerable amounts of alcohol, caffeine [energy drinks],

or stimulating substances), or going to bed late at night and consequently waking up late in the morning. In addition, psychophysiologic insomnia is defined as hypervigilance and learned sleep-preventing associations. Therefore, there is an overall preoccupation regarding sleep in adolescents (going to sleep, falling asleep, time spent asleep, possible presence of nonrefreshing sleep, and consequent daytime fatigue, sleepiness, and low performance).[12–15]

The prevalence of insomnia in children is variable because of different classification criteria and its variation with age. It is thought that insomnia prevalence is up to 30% when referring to infants, toddlers, and preschoolers, whereas it is reduced to approximately 15% in later ages.[12,16] The causes of pediatric insomnia are also age related. In infants and toddlers, except for SOAD, medical issues are mostly involved (food allergies, gastroesophageal reflux, colic, chronic or acute infectious diseases). In preschoolers, nightmares, fear, parental separation, and anxiety may be more likely to be the insomnia aggravating factors. In addition, in adolescents, bad sleep hygiene practices, other sleep disorders such as circadian burdens (delayed sleep-wake phase disorder) or sleep-related movement disorders, in combination with psychiatric comorbidities (attention-deficit/hyperactivity disorder, depression, anxiety) are the main insomnia triggering factors.[12,17–19]

INSOMNIA TREATMENT
Pharmacologic Treatment

As previously mentioned, guidelines are lacking, such as US Food and Drug Administration (FDA) approvals/indications regarding pediatric sleep pharmacotherapy. Moreover, relevant literature is scarce. Pharmacotherapy in pediatric insomnia should be introduced if conservative measures, such as sleep hygiene and behavioral therapies, are not sufficient or efficacious.[20,21] Before opting for drug therapy in insomnia, as recommended for adults, comorbidities (medical, psychiatric, and other sleep disorders; ie, restless legs syndrome [RLS]) should be thoroughly assessed.

Melatonin

Melatonin has been mostly used in the treatment of insomnia in the context of autism spectrum disorder and in ADHD, whereas it has also been shown beneficial in other developmental disorders, such as Angelman syndrome and fragile X syndrome. Melatonin is a sleep-promoting hormone, produced in the pineal gland, with a peak secretion between 2 and 4 AM. It has an impact on sleep-onset latency and frequency of awakenings. The effective dose is 0.05 mg/kg taken 1 to 2 hours before bedtime, although it has also been proposed that melatonin should be taken 9 to 10 hours after the child wakes up.[22,23] Melatonin has a safe pharmacokinetic profile, with mild and rare side effects (mostly sedation). Moreover, melatonin does not interfere with antiepileptic drugs, it does not affect the developmental process, and is not linked with addiction.[24–26]

Antihistaminergic drugs

Antihistaminergic drugs (ie, diphenhydramine, promethazine, hydroxyzine) are widely used in the treatment of insomnia. Histamine is one of the main wake-promoting neurotransmitters. Antihistaminergic drugs act via blocking histamine H1 receptors, which results in a sleep-promoting effect (shown by reduced sleep-onset latency and less awakenings) but can cause sedation. Sedation, which may last until the next morning, together with dizziness, is the major side effect of these drugs. Anticholinergic side effects may also be present (dry mouth, blurred vision, constipation, urinary retention, tachycardia). Moreover, tolerance develops with habitual use.[27–29] The duration of the hypnotic effect lasts approximately 4 to 6 hours (peak circulation level is reached 2 hours after ingestion), and recommended dose is 0.5 to 20 mg/kg and 1 mg/kg for diphenhydramine and hydroxyzine, respectively.[12,28,29]

Alpha-adrenergic receptor agonists (α-agonists)

Alpha-adrenergic receptor agonists (α-agonists; basically clonidine and guanfacine) may promote sleep via a pathophysiologic mechanism that is still unclear.[30] They act as central α2-agonists with onset of action less than 1 hour after ingestion, with peak blood levels 2 to 4 hours later.[8] The off-label daily recommended dose for clonidine starts from 0.05 mg and goes up to 0.1 mg and 0.5 up to 4 mg for guanafacine.[8,30] Common side effects may be hypotension, bradycardia, and anticholinergic effects, whereas rapid discontinuation of clonidine can lead to tachycardia, hypertension, and shortness of breath. Other common indications for these α-agonists are ADHD and ADHD-related sleep problems. Clonidine is also used to treat posttraumatic stress disorder and nightmares.[30–32]

Benzodiazepines hypnotics

Benzodiazepines hypnotics (eg, estazolam, triazolam), which act on gamma-aminobutyric acid (GABA) receptors, although commonly used for insomnia in adults, are much less prescribed in children (with the exception of clonazepam, which is extremely often used, especially in sleep motor phenomena and is discussed later). Thus, the trend is to substitute typical hypnagogic benzodiazepines with other drugs (ie, nonbenzodiazepine receptor agonists [nBZRAs]) because of a better pharmacologic profile (they do not induce muscle relaxation, hence avoiding aggravation of possible comorbid sleep apnea).[24,33] As far as the effect of the benzodiazepines on sleep architecture is concerned, they reduce sleep latency and slow wave sleep (SWS), whereas, in contrast, they increase sleep stage 2 and the amplitude and total number of sleep spindles.

Nonbenzodiazepine receptor agonists

nBZRAs (zolpidem, zaleplon) have no indication in children; further, their use in children less than 12 year old is contraindicated. Nevertheless, because of their few side effects, they are used as off-label hypnotic drugs at doses of 5 mg or 0.25 mg/kg (for zolpidem) at bedtime.[24,27] Zolpidem and zaleplon have half-lives of 1.5 to 2.4 hours and 1 hour respectively, explaining their different clinical impacts: zolpidem is indicated for sleep-onset insomnia and sometimes for maintenance insomnia, whereas zaleplon only for sleep-onset insomnia.

Antidepressants

Antidepressants (trazodone, mirtazapine) and tricyclic antidepressants (ie, imipramine, amitriptyline, doxepin) are commonly used in adult insomnia but not as much in pediatric insomnia. Trazodone is a 5-HT2 receptor antagonist that blocks histamine receptors, and is the most commonly prescribed insomnia drug for children with mood and anxiety disorders.[34] Its dosage is up to 50 mg/d. Tricyclic antidepressants are typically used to treat non–rapid eye movement (NREM) parasomnias because of their suppressive effect on SWS. In cases of insomnia, they are usually indicated for maintenance insomnia, but have considerable side effects (sedation, anticholinergic activity and so forth). In pediatric insomnia, amitriptyline is used at a starting dose of 5 mg at bedtime (maximum 50 mg), whereas imipramine is used at a dose of 0.5 mg/kg.[7,24]

L-5-Hydroxytryptophan

L-5-Hydroxytryptophan is a serotonin precursor and a precursor of melatonin as well. It has some use in parasomnia (1–2 mg/kg at bedtime) because of an overall stabilizing impact on sleep. It may also be used for insomnia given its safe drug profile.[27]

Chloral hydrate

Chloral hydrate (CH) is used frequently as a hypnotic agent for both adults and children. It results in drowsiness and sedation within 1 hour after ingestion, whereas its half-life is 8 to 12 hours for toddlers and 3 to 4 hours more for neonates and infants. Dose regimen is 25 to 50 mg/kg. CH interferes with respiratory and cardiovascular function (respiratory suppression and cardiovascular instability if overdosed).[35]

NONPHARMACOLOGIC TREATMENT

As stated previously, insomnia treatment should be started with a nonpharmacologic approach that encompasses sleep hygiene routines and behavioral strategy. In short, sleep hygiene rules are the following: (1) maintenance of consistent sleep schedules (bedtime and wake-up time), (2) avoidance of caffeine (and other wake-promoting substances like tea and chocolate), (3) regular physical activity (preferably until afternoon), (4) sleep-promoting nocturnal atmosphere (relaxing activities at evening before sleep, appropriate sleep environment [bedroom]).

In adults, the behavioral approach targets the elimination of negative associations/thoughts about sleep, which lead to insomnia. This approach has been proved to be efficacious in children as well, and should be started after the age of 6 months. Relaxation techniques, sleep restriction, and stimulus control can be applied in children and in the pediatric setting are called planned bedtime and programmed awakening. Moreover, extinction and gradual extinction (which consist of ignoring, totally or partially respectively, the child's agitated nocturnal behavior) are further behavior techniques used in children.[21,36]

Management of Obstructive Sleep Apnea in Children

Obstructive sleep apnea syndrome (OSAS) can occur at any age in children and its prevalence is estimated between 2% and 5%.[37] The choice of treatment is made on an individual basis and depends on the following factors: child's age, polysomnographic pattern, comorbidities, and complications related to OSAS.[38] Surgical treatment, including tonsillectomy and adenoidectomy, is the first choice of treatment in children with adenotonsillar hypertrophy and OSAS. However, nasal continuous positive airway pressure (nCPAP) application remains a viable option for children not eligible for surgery, or in cases of residual disease.[39] Pharmacologic interventions for the treatment of OSAS in pediatric populations are very limited.

Pharmacologic treatment

Intranasal corticosteroids have been suggested as treatment of children with mild OSAS, to whom adenotonsillectomy is contraindicated or for mild postoperative OSAS.[38] Brouillette and colleagues[40] examined the effect of nasal corticosteroids on frequency of mixed and obstructive apneas and hypopneas in 25 children with OSAS. More specifically, nasal fluticasone propionate was administered in 13 children versus 12 children receiving placebo, for a period of 6 weeks. The mixed obstructive apnea/hypopnea index (AHI) decreased in the treatment group and increased in children receiving placebo (from 10.7 ± 2.6 to 5.8 ± 2.2/h in the fluticasone group and from 10.9 ± 2.3 to 13.1 ± 3.6/h in the placebo group; $P = .04$). The rates of oxyhemoglobin desaturation and arousals significantly improved in the fluticasone group compared with controls, whereas there were no changes in tonsillar size, adenoidal size, or symptom score. In another randomized placebo-controlled trial, intranasal mometasone furoate and placebo were administered, respectively, in 24 and 26 children with mild OSAS, for a total period of 4 months. The obstructive AHI decreased in the treatment group (from 2.7 ± 0.2/h to 1.7 ± 0.3/h) but increased in the placebo group (from 2.5 ± 0.2/h to 2.9 ± 0.6/h; $P = .039$).[41] In the same study, oxygen desaturation index also significantly decreased in the study group compared with controls (-0.6 ± 0.5/h vs 0.7 ± 0.4/h respectively; $P = .037$). In conclusion, intranasal corticosteroids can reduce the severity of the syndrome in children with mild OSAS. However, data on the minimum duration of therapy for sustained benefit are still lacking.

Leukotriene modifiers have also been studied in pediatric OSAS. In a double-blind, randomized, placebo-controlled trial, Kheirandish-Gozal and colleagues[42] showed a decrease in AHI in the montelukast-treated children, compared with children receiving placebo (from 9.2 ± 4.1/h to 4.2 ± 2.8/h and from 8.2 ± 5.0/h to 8.7 ± 4.9/h respectively; $P<.0001$).[42] Similar results were observed in another double-blind, placebo-controlled study by Goldbart and colleagues.[43] In another study with children with OSAS, 12 weeks of treatment with montelukast, after tonsillectomy and/or adenoidectomy, significantly improved AHI, nadir oxyhemoglobin saturation, and OSAS symptoms ($P<.001$).[44] In summary, leukotriene modifiers represent a valid option in the therapeutic approach of pediatric OSAS. In addition, as a complementary therapy, montelukast can improve sleep disturbances in children with OSAS after adenotonsillectomy. However, further research is necessary in order to better establish which pediatric patients with OSAS are most likely to benefit from montelukast therapy.

Recently, the combination of a leukotriene receptor antagonist with intranasal corticosteroids was evaluated in children with OSAS. A total of 183 children with OSAS were divided in 3 groups: group A received oral montelukast, group B received a nasal spray of mometasone furoate, and group C received a combination of montelukast plus mometasone furoate. After 12 weeks of treatment, OSAS symptoms such as snoring ($P<.01$), buccal respiration ($P<.05$), restless sleep ($P<.05$), hyperhidrosis ($P<.05$), and apnea ($P<.01$) improved in all groups compared with before treatment.[45] In addition, AHI decreased ($P<.05$) and minimum oxyhemoglobin saturation increased ($P<.05$) in all groups, whereas the adenoidal/nasopharyngeal ratio, assessed radiographically, decreased ($P<.05$).[45] Compared with the other groups, children belonging to group C showed shorter response duration regarding snoring, apnea, and restless sleep ($P<.05$).[45] The total effective rate was higher in group C than in A and B ($P<.05$).[45] Kheirandish and colleagues[46] studied children with residual OSAS after tonsillectomy and adenoidectomy who received treatment with montelukast and intranasal budesonide for a period of 12 weeks. Compared with children not receiving any therapy, the treatment group showed a significant improvement in AHI (0.3 ± 0.3/h; $P<.001$), nadir oxyhemoglobin saturation ($92.5 \pm 3.0\%$; $P<.01$), and arousal index (0.8 ± 0.7/h; $P<.001$).[46]

Several studies evaluated the role of antibiotic treatment in pediatric OSAS. Antibiotics act by reducing the size of the tonsils and adenoids in some children, thus temporarily alleviating OSAS symptoms. In a prospective randomized trial comparing azithromycin versus placebo, 22 children aged 2 to 12 years were randomly assigned to receive azithromycin or placebo for a 30-day period. A trend towards reduction in AHI in the azithromycin group and an increase in AHI in the placebo group were observed (0.97 ± 2.09 vs 3.41 ± 3.01/h; $P = .23$).[47] This study showed that even though antibiotics decrease OSAS severity, they do not provide persistent relief or prevent surgical therapy.

In addition, results from a meta-analysis comparing the therapeutic effects of pharmacologic therapy on pediatric OSAS revealed that therapeutic effect of placebo was significantly poorer than that of intranasal mometasone furoate, montelukast, budesonide, and fluticasone concerning syndrome severity and, additionally, fluticasone was better than placebo concerning sleep efficiency.[48]

In conclusion, there are pharmacologic options for the treatment of OSAS in pediatric populations.

However, further research is needed to support the role of prescribed medication in improving breathing function during sleep in children with OSAS.

Nonpharmacologic treatment

Nocturnal supplemental oxygen therapy can be used to treat children with recurrent oxygen desaturations during sleep, related to OSAS.[49] Marcus and colleagues[50] studied the effect of oxygen therapy in 23 children with OSAS aged 5 ± 3 years. In their randomized, double-blind study, oxygen was administered via nasal cannula at 1 L/min for 4 hours. Average and lowest oxygen saturation were higher when breathing supplemental oxygen. However, there was no difference in terms of number (AHI 10.9 ± 20.6/h on oxygen therapy vs 13.5 ± 19.3 on room air; $P>.05$) and duration (14 ± 7 s on oxygen therapy vs 13 ± 5 s on room air; $P>.05$) of obstructive apneas.[50] In the same study, 2 children showed a significant increase in end-tidal carbon dioxide pressure.[50] Thus, it was concluded that supplemental oxygen does not affect obstructive events during sleep and can be suggested as a temporary solution, in view of definitive therapy, in children with hypoxemia who cannot tolerate continuous positive airway pressure, or in those cases in which surgical treatment has not been shown to be curative.[50,51] The risk of hypercapnia emphasizes the need for strict monitoring during the initiation of treatment with nocturnal supplemental oxygen in children with OSAS.

Surgical treatment

As mentioned previously, adenotonsillectomy remains the treatment of choice, because adenotonsillar hypertrophy represents the principal cause of OSAS in children.[38] However, the procedure is not free of risks and complications. Moreover, there is no consensus on the cutoff of OSAS severity for adenotonsillectomy, and it is usually reserved for children with moderate to severe disease.[38]

Management of Parasomnias in Children

Parasomnias are defined as undesirable physical events or experiences that occur during entry into sleep, within sleep, or during arousal from sleep. Basically, they are a temporary unstable state of dissociation. Parasomnias are divided into 2 main categories: those arising from NREM sleep (mainly confusion arousal, sleep tremor, and sleepwalking) and those of rapid eye movement (REM) sleep (mainly nightmares, sleep paralysis, and REM sleep behavior disorder) At times, NREM and REM parasomnias coexist (overlap parasomnia).[10] Arousal parasomnias are very frequent in childhood. In a large population study, the prevalence of any kind of parasomnia occurring at least once in children between 2 and 6 years old was 84%.[52] NREM parasomnias affect 1% to 4% of the adult population.[53,54] They have characteristics of both sleep and wake states, and they usually occur in deep sleep (NREM stage 3). NREM parasomnias are more prominent during the first half of the night, because of the prominence of NREM 3, whereas REM parasomnias are more frequent during the second half of the night (more REM sleep). Sleepwalking, for example, therefore usually occurs early in the night, whereas nightmares more often at the end of the night. During an event, children may have a varied and complex clinical phenomenology, and, if they get awakened, they seem confused and disorientated.[55] There are several triggers for arousal disorders: sleep deprivation, sleep disturbing stimuli (either external [ie, noises] or internal [ie, OSAS, RLS]), and stress (emotional and/or physical). As far as the treatment is concerned, usually nonpharmacologic approaches are sufficient, but, if not, drug therapy is provided in order to avoid mainly hazardous consequences.

Pharmacologic treatment

As mentioned before, in pediatric parasomnias, medication is prescribed in cases of frequent and possibly hazardous episodes, unresponsive to conservative measures. As for insomnia, no FDA drug approval exists for pediatric parasomnias.[10,56] Given that NREM parasomnias occur mainly during deep sleep (SWS or N3), SWS suppressants are recommended, such as benzodiazepines or tricyclic antidepressants.[56,57] More specifically, the recommended tricyclic antidepressant is imipramine (in a low dose), and recommended benzodiazepine is clonazepam (0.125–0.5 at bedtime).[56,57] Therapy is indicated for a short period (3–6 months) and slow tapering should follow. Clonazepam's maximum plasma concentration is 1 to 4 hours after ingestion and its half-life is 30 to 40 hours (half-life is longer in adults).[27]

Nonpharmacologic treatment

This is the first-line treatment, and comprises reassurance and keeping the child and surrounding individuals (eg, siblings) safe. Moreover, safety measures should also be implemented in the sleep environment (alarms on doors, windows, removal of sharp or breakable objects from the child's room or from its common pathways).

Parasomnia triggers, which may be other primary sleep disorders (OSAS, RLS) should be, if present, addressed first. Other behavioral strategies include scheduled awakenings, but these are not recommended if the child is already in N3, because they may act as parasomnia triggers.[58,59] Management of nightmares should also comprise avoiding TV a couple of hours before bedtime, having a dim light in the room, and other cognitive-behavioral techniques.[55,60,61]

Management of Narcolepsy in Children

Narcolepsy is a chronic neurologic disorder characterized by a tetrad of clinical symptoms: EDS and 3 symptoms related to REM sleep; hypnagogic/hypnopompic hallucinations, sleep paralysis, and cataplexy. Cataplexy is found in more than half of patients with narcolepsy, and helps distinguishing between narcolepsy type 1 (narcolepsy with cataplexy) and narcolepsy type 2 (narcolepsy without cataplexy).[10] Other symptoms of narcolepsy (especially in children) may include disrupted nocturnal sleep, obesity, automatic behavior (ie, sloppy handwriting in children) and complex movement disorders (ie, chorea).[62–65] Narcolepsy is rare. Its prevalence in the general population is 0.025% to 0.05%, with a major incidence between 10 and 19 years.[66,67] All major symptoms of the narcoleptic tetrad, except EDS, result from intrusion of fragments of REM sleep into wakefulness. The deficiency of hypocretin (orexin), which is a wake-promoting/stabilizing neuropeptide, plays a cardinal role in the phenomenon mentioned earlier.[68,69] Narcolepsy may also present secondary to lesions of the posterior hypothalamus provoked by stroke, tumor, head injury, neuroinflammatory processes, and so forth.[70–73] In practice, the management of narcolepsy is symptomatic. The treatment should first address the most troublesome symptom, and then address less disturbing symptoms, because some patients describe mostly EDS whereas others cataplexy. There are both behavioral and lifestyle changes along with drug treatment.

Pharmacologic treatment

Excessive daytime sleepiness At present there are no approved drugs for treating EDS in the pediatric population, thus the common pharmacotherapy is off label. Treatment options for EDS include mainly central nervous system stimulants (salts of amphetamines and methylphenidate) and wake-promoting agents, such as modafinil or armodafinil[7,74]; a selective norepinephrine reuptake inhibitor (SNRI; atomoxetine) may be an adjuvant therapy, whereas lately a histamine H3 receptor antagonist (pitolisant) has been approved in the European Union with an orphan drug designation in the United States.[75–78] Amphetamines and methylphenidate have similar mechanisms of action, because they are both dopamine and norepinephrine agonists. Amphetamines have a long half-life (11–30 hours), but nevertheless drug administration twice a day is preferable (dextro-amphetamine 5–30 mg, dextroamphetamine-amphetamine 2.5–20 mg). Methylphenidate has a much shorter half-life (3 hours) and is again recommended twice a day (10–40 mg). Common side effects of stimulants include headache, anorexia, nervosity, insomnia, tics, and weight loss, whereas a red flag warning is heart failure.[79,80] In addition, prolonged use of amphetamines has a high risk of tolerance and addiction (FDA warning).[80,81] Modafinil and armodafinil have an unknown mechanism of action, which acts by enhancing the aminergic system (histamines and catecholamines) in the hypothalamus. Therefore, cortical arousal is promoted.[82] Both drugs are neither FDA nor European Medicines Agency approved for children younger than 17 years.[83] Half-life is 4 hours and 15 hours for modafinil and armodafinil (which is more potent), respectively.[84] Recommended dosages are 50 to 400 mg/d divided in 2. Common side effects include nausea, vomiting, headache, and (more rarely) Stevens-Johnson syndrome. Atomoxetine may help in the management of EDS and its potential side effects include headache, increase of blood pressure, tachycardia, and weight loss.[75,76] Pitolisant is a histaminergic H3-receptor antagonist. The histaminergic neurons project widely to the cerebral cortex and facilitate arousal. H3 receptors have an inhibiting role on the histamine secreting neurons, thus promoting sleep. Pitolisant blocks this loop and consequently promotes wakefulness by enhancing the histaminergic system, in an efficient way, but still less powerful than modafinil. However, pitolisant has not been approved for children.[77,78,85]

Cataplexy No drug has been formally approved by the FDA for treatment of cataplexy in children. Given that REM sleep and consequently REM intrusions, which play an important role in the cataplexy mechanism, are cholinergic driven, tricyclic antidepressants with their potent anticholinergic action have been used historically for treating cataplexy, although their action is modest.[86] Tricyclic agents used are imipramine and clomipramine, but, as mentioned in the earlier, these drugs have serious side effects. Dosages are 10 to 100 mg/d and 10 to 150 mg/d for imipramine and clomipramine, respectively. Except for tricyclic agents, other antidepressants (selective serotonin reuptake inhibitors [SSRIs]; eg, fluoxetine 10–30 mg/d) and SNRIs (venlafaxine 37.5–75 mg/d)] have been used for cataplexy treatment.[87,88] Sodium oxybate (gamma-hydroxybutyrate) has an FDA indication for the treatment of narcolepsy with cataplexy, for both EDS and cataplexy. Its mechanism of action (it has GABA type B receptor agonist properties) is not clear, but it is considered to consolidate the sleep architecture by reducing awakenings and by increasing SWS. Thus, there is a benefit to daytime alertness with fewer REM intrusion episodes.[89–92] Sodium oxybate is an oral solution (0.5 g/mL) with a short half-life. So, the first dose is taken at bedtime and a second one approximately 2.5 to 3 hours later. The recommended dose is 2 to 8 g twice a day. Its side effects include somnambulism and enuresis, aggravation of sleep disordered breathing, constipation, and tremor. Retrospective data on case series studies showed significant improvement of EDS and cataplexy with the use of sodium oxybate.[75,93,94]

Nonpharmacologic treatment
Behavioral and lifestyle changes are also important in the management of narcolepsy. Good sleep hygiene with regular and sufficient sleep and wake times are necessary. Scheduled brief naps are highly recommended for EDS. Sleep benefits also from exercise.[95] As far as cataplexy is concerned, patient and parental education about the triggers and the nature of the episodes is important.

Management of Restless Legs Syndrome/ Periodic Leg Movements in Children

RLS, also known as Willis-Ekbom disease, is a common neurologic sleep disorder. It is characterized by an urge to move the legs, usually accompanied by uncomfortable or unpleasant sensations. The symptoms begin or worsen during rest or inactivity, are relieved by movement, and occur exclusively or predominantly in the evening or night.[10] Consensus diagnostic criteria for children were updated recently.[96,97] Periodic limb movement disorder (PLMD) is characterized by clinical sleep disturbance and by repetitive limb jerking during sleep (known as periodic limb movements of sleep) that is not better explained by another condition, medication use, or substance use.[10] Diagnosis of PLM is set by using specific polysomnographic criteria. In children, PLMD seems to be closely related to RLS, although they are distinct diagnostic entities. Nevertheless, both diseases are related to iron deficiency and have a genetic predisposition. Comorbidities commonly associated with RLS and PLMD are ADHD, anxiety, and depression.[98,99] The prevalence of RLS in the pediatric population is between 2% and 4%, whereas the moderate to severe type occurs in between 0.5% and 1%. The known predominance of female gender in adults occurs only in the midteens to late teens.[100–102] As far as the pathophysiology of RLS/PLMD is concerned, this seems to be multifactorial, comprising genetics and iron and dopamine deficiency.[103,104]

Pharmacologic treatment

For mild cases of pediatric RLS, nonpharmacologic interventions are preferred, whereas drug therapy is reserved for chronic, moderate to severe cases. The FDA has approved no medications for pediatric RLS or PLMD.[105] For children with iron deficiency and RLS or PLMD, oral iron supplementation should be tried if ferritin levels are less than 50 μg/L, or are between 50 and 75 μg/L according to newer evidence.[106,107] Besides iron supplementation, there is limited knowledge regarding other drugs in children. Case series with benzodiazepines are the most consistent in the literature on this topic; thus, clonazepam (0.25–0.5 mg) or temazepam (7.5–22.5 mg according to age) are recommended.[99,108] In adults, dopaminergic agents or alpha-2-delta calcium channel ligands (gabapentin and pregabalin) are the treatment of choice for RLS. However, in children, these drugs must be used with skepticism. The known dopamine agonists used for RLS and for PLMD are pramipexole (0.125–0.375 mg/d) and ropinirole (0.25–0.75 mg/d). Dosages are increased in line with child's age, so these drugs should be administered 1 to 2 hours before the symptoms start. Rotigotine has no recommendation for ages less than 18 years.[99,108,109] In addition, alpha-2-delta calcium channel ligands (mainly gabapentin and pregabalin), although they do not have a specific indication for pediatric RLS pharmacotherapy, have performed well in pediatric epilepsy, which makes them safe to use.[7]

Nonpharmacologic treatment

Before introducing drug therapy, iron and ferritin levels should be measured. Moreover, RLS or PLMD triggers, such as caffeine, nicotine, medication (SSRIs, antihistamines, dopamine blockers), insufficient and irregular sleep, or sleep apnea, should be addressed. Physical exercise has also been proved to be efficient.

DISCUSSION

Sleep disorders in children should be a matter of special attention, because they are associated with developmental and cognitive deficits and with reduced learning or social skills. Of note, symptoms differ from those of the adult population and vary according to a child's age. In addition, assessment is further complicated by insufficient training in pediatric sleep medicine and the lack of guidelines and official approvals regarding pharmacotherapy.

In children, insomnia has mainly behavioral features, and pharmacotherapy should be introduced if conservative measures, such as sleep hygiene and behavioral therapies, are not sufficient. A variety of pharmaceutical agents, including melatonin, antihistaminic drugs, α-agonists, benzodiazepines and nonbenzodiazepine receptor agonists, antidepressants, L5-hydroxytryptophan, and CH have been proposed. However, the lack of specific guidelines, as well as the limited amount of available data in the literature, dictates caution in the selection of drug therapy.

As mentioned previously, OSAS can occur at any age in children and the choice of treatment depends on several factors, including the child's age, polysomnogram pattern, comorbidities, and complications related to OSAS. Surgery remains the first choice, whereas nCPAP application is a valid alternative for children not eligible for surgery or in case of residual disease. Pharmacologic options are limited. Intranasal corticosteroids, leukotriene modifiers, and their combination have been proposed and are shown to reduce severity in children with mild OSAS, to whom adenotonsillectomy is contraindicated, or for mild postoperative OSAS. However, important data, such as the minimum duration of therapy for sustained benefit, are still lacking. Antibiotics, which can reduce the size of the tonsils and adenoids, do not provide persistent relief or prevent surgical therapy. In addition, nocturnal supplemental oxygen therapy does not affect obstructive events during sleep and can be suggested only as a temporary solution, in view of definitive therapy.

Pharmacologic therapy for parasomnias is necessary only when nonpharmacologic approaches, such as reassurance, safety measures, and avoidance of possible triggers, are not sufficient, in order to avoid hazardous consequences. SWS suppressants, such as benzodiazepines or tricyclic antidepressants, given for a short period followed by slow tapering, are suggested for NREM parasomnias.

For narcolepsy, treatment targets symptom relief. Central nervous system stimulants and wake-promoting agents are used for the treatment of EDS, whereas norepinephrine reuptake inhibitors and histamine H3 receptor antagonists may represent an adjuvant therapy. Tricyclic antidepressants, SSRIs, and SNRIs have also been used for cataplexy treatment. However, none of the aforementioned agents have received approval. In contrast, sodium oxybate has an indication for the treatment of narcolepsy with cataplexy, showing significant improvement of both EDS and cataplexy. Regarding nonpharmacologic therapy, good sleep hygiene combined with frequent naps is highly recommended for EDS, and education about the triggers and the nature of the episodes is important for the management of cataplexy.

In addition, for mild cases of pediatric RLS, non-pharmacologic interventions are preferred, such as physical exercise together with good sleep hygiene and trigger control, whereas drug therapy is reserved for chronic, moderate to severe cases. For children with iron deficiency and RLS or PLMD, oral iron supplementation is suggested. Limited data indicate benzodiazepines as an alternative therapy. Dopaminergic agents or alpha-2-delta calcium channel ligands should be used with caution in pediatric populations.

In conclusion, pharmacologic treatment of the most common pediatric sleep disorders lacks evidence, and alternative methods, which have been proved to alleviate the symptoms, are preferred in most cases. The implementation of specific guidelines is of great importance, because sleep disorders in children are not rare and they can negatively affect children's development and their cognitive and social skills.

REFERENCES

1. Dillon JE, Chervin RD. Attention deficit, hyperactivity, and sleep disorders. In: Sheldon SH, Ferber R, Kryger MH, et al, editors. Principles and practice of pediatric sleep medicine. 2nd edition. New York: Elsevier Saunders; 2014. p. 111.

2. Gringras P. Sleep and its disturbances in autism spectrum disorder. In: Sheldon SH, Ferber R, Kryger MH, et al, editors. Principles and practice of pediatric sleep medicine. 2nd edition. New York: Elsevier Saunders; 2014. p. 125.

3. Chervin RD, Dillon JE, Bassetti C, et al. Symptoms of sleep disorders, inattention, and hyperactivity in children. Sleep 1997;20:1185–92.

4. Owens JA, Rosen CL, Mindell JA. Medication use in the treatment of pediatric insomnia: results of a survey of community-based pediatricians. Pediatrics 2003;111:e628–35.

5. Sheldon SH, Spire JP, Levy HB. Disorders of excessive somnolence. In: Sheldon SH, Spire JP, Levy HB, editors. Pediatric sleep medicine. Philadelphia: WB Saunders; 1992. p. 91.

6. Pelayo R, Dubik M. Pediatric sleep pharmacology. Semin Pediatr Neurol 2008;15(2):79–90.

7. Troester MM, Pelayo R. Pediatric sleep pharmacology: a primer. Semin Pediatr Neurol 2015; 22(2):135–47.

8. Schnoes CJ, Kuhn BR, Workman EF, et al. Pediatric prescribing practices for clonidine and other pharmacologic agents for children with sleep disturbance. Clin Pediatr (Phila) 2006;45:229–38.

9. Stojanovski SD, Rasu RS, Balkrishnan R, et al. Trends in medication prescribing for pediatric sleep difficulties in US outpatient settings. Sleep 2007;30:1013–7.

10. International classification of sleep disorders. 3rd edition. Darien (IL): American Academy of Sleep Medicine; 2014.

11. American Psychiatric Association. Diagnostic and Statistical Manual of Mental Disorders (Fifth ed.). Arlington (VA): American Psychiatric Publishing; 2013.

12. Owens JA, Mindell JA. Pediatric insomnia. Pediatr Clin North Am 2011;58:555–69.

13. Fossum IN, Nordnes LT, Storemark SS, et al. The association between use of electronic media in bed before going to sleep and insomnia symptoms, daytime sleepiness, morning- ness, and chronotype. Behav Sleep Med 2014;12:343–57.

14. Shochat T, Cohen-Zion M, Tzischinsky O. Functional consequences of inadequate sleep in adolescents: a systematic review. Sleep Med Rev 2014;18:75–87.

15. Jan JE, Bax MC, Owens JA, et al. Neurophysiology of circadian rhythm sleep disorders of children with neurodevelopmental disabilities. Eur J Paediatr Neurol 2012;16(5):403–12.

16. Honaker SM, Meltzer LJ. Bedtime problems and night wakings in young children: an update of the evidence. Paediatr Respir Rev 2014;15(4):333–9.

17. Sheldon SH, Spire JP, Levy HB. Pediatric sleep medicine. Philadelphia: WB Saunders; 1992.

18. Sivertsen B, Harvey AG, Lundervold AJ, et al. Sleep problems and depression in adolescence: results from a large population-based study of Norwegian adolescents aged 16-18 years. Eur Child Adolesc Psychiatry 2014;23:681–9.

19. Miano S, Parisi P, Villa MP. The sleep phenotypes of attention deficit disorder, the role of arousal during sleep and implications for treatment. Med Hypotheses 2012;79:147–53.

20. Owens JA. Update in pediatric sleep medicine. Curr Opin Pulm Med 2012;17(6):425–30.

21. Mindell JA, Owens JA. Sleep and medication. A clinical guide to pediatric sleep: diagnosis and management of sleep problems. sleep and medication. Philadelphia: Lippincott Williams & Wilkins; 2003. p. 226–8.

22. van Geijlswijk IM, van der Heijden KB, Egberts AC, et al. Dose finding of melatonin for chronic idiopathic childhood sleep onset insomnia: an RCT. Psychopharmacology 2010;212:379–91.

23. Zee PC. Shedding light on the effectiveness of melatonin for circadian rhythm sleep disorders. Sleep 2010;33:1581–2.

24. Bruni O, Alonso-Alconada D, Besag F, et al. Current role of melatonin in pediatric neurology: clinical recommendations. Eur J Paediatr Neurol 2015;19:122–33.

25. Andersen IM, Kaczmarska J, McGrew SG, et al. Melatonin for insomnia in children with autism spectrum disorders. J Child Neurol 2008;23(5): 482–5.

26. Schwichtenberg AJ, Malow BA. Melatonin treatment in children with developmental disabilities. Sleep Med Clin 2015;10(2):181–7.

27. Pelayo R, Yuen K. Pediatric sleep pharmacology. Child Adolesc Psychiatr Clin N Am 2012;21: 861–83.

28. Haydon RC 3rd. Are second-generation antihistamines appropriate for most children and adults? Arch Otolaryngol Head Neck Surg 2001;127: 1510–3.

29. Richardson GS, Roehrs TA, Rosenthal L, et al. Tolerance to daytime sedative effects of H1 antihistamines. J Clin Psychopharmacol 2002;22:511–5.

30. Ingrassia A, Turk J. The use of clonidine for severe and intractable sleep problems in children with neurodevelopmental disorders—A case series. Eur Child Adolesc Psychiatry 2005;14:34–40.

31. Wilens TE, Biederman J, Spencer T. Clonidine for sleep disturbances associated with attention-deficit hyperactivity disorder. J Am Acad Child Adolesc Psychiatry 1994;33:424–6.

32. Newcorn JH, Stein MA, Childress AC, et al. Randomized, double-blind trial of guanfacine extended release in children with attention-deficit/ hyperactivity disorder: morning or evening administration. J Am Acad Child Adolesc Psychiatry 2013;52:921–30.

33. Ashton H. Guidelines for the rational use of benzodiazepines. When and what to use. Drugs 1994;48: 25–40.

34. Owens JA, Rosen CL, Mindell JA, et al. Use of pharmacotherapy for insomnia in child psychiatry practice: a national survey. Sleep Med 2010;11: 692–700.

35. Pershad J, Palmisano P, Nichols M. Chloral hydrate: the good and the bad. Pediatr Emerg Care 1999;15:432–5.

36. Halal CS, Nunes ML. Education in children's sleep hygiene: which approaches are effective? A systematic review. J Pediatr (Rio J) 2014;90:449–56.

37. Rosen CL, Storfer-Isser A, Taylor HG, et al. Increased behavioral morbidity in school-aged children with sleep-disordered breathing. Pediatrics 2004;114:1640–8.

38. Marcus CL, Brooks LJ, Draper KA, et al. Diagnosis and management of childhood obstructive sleep apnea syndrome. Pediatrics 2012;130:576–84.

39. Marcus CL. Sleep-disordered breathing in children. Am J Respir Crit Care Med 2001;164:16–30.

40. Brouillette RT, Manoukian JJ, Ducharme FM, et al. Efficacy of fluticasone nasal spray for pediatric obstructive sleep apnea. J Pediatr 2001;138: 838–44.

41. Chan CC, Au CT, Lam HS, et al. Intranasal corticosteroids for mild childhood obstructive sleep apnea–a randomized, placebo-controlled study. Sleep Med 2015;16:358–63.

42. Kheirandish-Gozal L, Bandla HP, Gozal D. Montelukast for children with obstructive sleep apnea: results of a double-blind, randomized, placebo-controlled trial. Ann Am Thorac Soc 2016;13: 1736–41.

43. Goldbart AD, Greenberg-Dotan S, Tal A. Montelukast for children with obstructive sleep apnea: a double-blind, placebo-controlled study. Pediatrics 2012;130:e575–80.

44. Wang B, Liang J. The effect of montelukast on mild persistent OSA after adenotonsillectomy in children: a preliminary study. Otolaryngol Head Neck Surg 2017;156:952–4.

45. Yang DZ, Liang J, Zhang F, et al. Clinical effect of montelukast sodium combined with inhaled corticosteroids in the treatment of OSAS children. Medicine (Baltimore) 2017;96:e6628.

46. Kheirandish L, Goldbart AD, Gozal D. Intranasal steroids and oral leukotriene modifier therapy in residual sleep-disordered breathing after tonsillectomy and adenoidectomy in children. Pediatrics 2006;117:e61–6.

47. Don DM, Goldstein NA, Crockett DM, et al. Antimicrobial therapy for children with adenotonsillar hypertrophy and obstructive sleep apnea: a prospective randomized trial comparing azithromycin vs placebo. Otolaryngol Head Neck Surg 2005; 133:562–8.

48. Zhang J, Chen J, Yin Y, et al. Therapeutic effects of different drugs on obstructive sleep apnea/hypopnea syndrome in children. World J Pediatr 2017; 13:537–43.

49. Hudgel DW, Thanakitcharu S. Pharmacologic treatment of sleep-disordered breathing. Am J Respir Crit Care Med 1998;158:691–9.

50. Marcus CL, Carroll JL, Bamford O, et al. Supplemental oxygen during sleep in children with sleep-disordered breathing. Am J Respir Crit Care Med 1995;152:1297–301.

51. Aljadeff G, Gozal D, Bailey-Wahl SL, et al. Effects of overnight supplemental oxygen in obstructive sleep apnea in children. Am J Respir Crit Care Med 1996;153:51–5.

52. Petit D, Touchette E, Tremblay RE, et al. Dyssomnias and parasomnias in early childhood. Pediatrics 2007;119:e1016–25.

53. Bjorvatn B, Gronli J, Pallesen S. Prevalence of different parasomnias in the general population. Sleep Med 2010;11:1031–4.

54. Ohayon MM, Mahowald MW, Dauvilliers Y, et al. Prevalence and comorbidity of nocturnal wandering in the U.S. adult general population. Neurology 2012;78:1583–9.

55. Kotagal S. Parasomnias in childhood. Sleep Med Rev 2009;13:157–68.
56. Attarian H, Zhu L. Treatment options for disorders of arousal: a case series. Int J Neurosci 2013;123:3.
57. Provini F, Tinuper P, Bisulli F, et al. Arousal disorders. Sleep Med 2011;12(Suppl 2):S22–6.
58. Wills L, Garcia J. Parasomnias: epidemiology and management. CNS Drugs 2002;16:803–10.
59. Frank NC, Spirito A, Stark L, et al. The use of scheduled awakenings to eliminate childhood sleepwalking. J Pediatr Psychol 1997;22:345–53.
60. Sadeh A. Cognitive behavioral treatment for childhood sleep disorders. Clin Psychol Rev 2005;25:L612–28.
61. Hauri PJ, Silber MH, Boeve BF. The treatment of parasomnias with hypnosis: a 5-year follow up study. J Clin Sleep Med 2007;3:369–73.
62. Peterson PC, Husain AM. Pediatric narcolepsy. Brain Development 2008;30:609–23.
63. Serra L, Montagna P, Mignot E, et al. Cataplexy features in childhood narcolepsy. Mov Disord 2008;23:858–65.
64. Kotagal S, Krahn LE, Slocumb N. A putative link between childhood narcolepsy and obesity. Sleep Med 2004;5:147–50.
65. Plazzi G, Pizza F, Palaia V, et al. Complex movement disorders at disease onset in childhood narcolepsy with cataplexy. Brain 2011;134:3480–92.
66. Silber MH, Krahn LE, Olson EJ, et al. The epidemiology of narcolepsy in Olmsted County, Minnesota: a population-based study. Sleep 2002;25:197–202.
67. Longstreth WT Jr, Koepsell TD, Ton TG, et al. The epidemiology of narcolepsy. Sleep 2007;30:13–26.
68. Nishino S, Ripley B, Overeem S, et al. Hypocretin (orexin) deficiency in human narcolepsy. Lancet 2000;355:39.
69. Thannickal TC, Moore RY, Nienhuis R, et al. Reduced number of hypocretin neurons in human narcolepsy. Neuron 2000;27:469.
70. Arii J, Kanbayashi T, Tanabe Y, et al. A hypersomnolent girl with decreased CSF hypocretin level after removal of a hypothalamic tumor. Neurology 2001;56:1775–6.
71. Scammell TE, Nishino S, Mignot E, et al. Narcolepsy and low CSF orexin (hypocretin) concentration after a diencephalic stroke. Neurology 2001;56:1751–3.
72. Malik S, Boeve BF, Krahn LE, et al. Narcolepsy associated with other central nervous system disorders. Neurology 2001;57:539–41.
73. Gledhill RF, Bartel PR, Yoshida Y, et al. Narcolepsy caused by acute disseminated encephalomyelitis. Arch Neurol 2004;61:758–60.
74. Babiker MO, Prasad M. Narcolepsy in children: a diagnostic and management approach. Pediatr Neurol 2015;52(6):557–65.
75. Aran A, Einen M, Lin L, et al. Clinical and therapeutic aspects of childhood narcolepsy-cataplexy: a retrospective study of 51 children. Sleep 2010;33:1457–64.
76. Billiard M, Bassetti C, Dauvilliers Y, et al. EFNS guidelines on management of narcolepsy. Eur J Neurol 2006;13:1035–48.
77. Syed YY. Pitolisant: first global approval. Drugs 2016;76(13):1313–8.
78. Szakacs Z, Dauvilliers Y, Mikhaylov V, et al. Safety and efficacy of pitolisant on cataplexy in patients with narcolepsy: a randomized, double-blind, placebo-controlled trial. Lancet Neurol 2017;16(3):200–7.
79. Product information: dextroamphetamine sulfate oral tablets, dextroamphetamine sulfate oral tablets. St Louis (MO): Mallinckrodt; 2007.
80. Product information: RITALIN oral tablets, methylphenidate hydrochloride oral tablets. East Hanover (NJ): Novartis; 2007.
81. Available at: https://www.fda.gov/ohrms/dockets/ac/06/briefing/2006-4202B1_07_FDA-Tab07.pdf. Accessed March 28, 2018.
82. Thorpy MJ. Modafinil/armodafinil in the treatment of narcolepsy. In: Goswami M, Thorpy MJ, Pandi-Perumal SR, editors. Narcolepsy. A clinical guide. Switzerland: Springer International Publishing; 2016. p. 331–9.
83. Ivanenko A, Tauman R, Gozal D. Modafinil in the treatment of excessive daytime sleepiness in children. Sleep Med 2003;4:579–82.
84. Harsh JR, Hayduk R, Rosenberg R, et al. The efficacy and safety of armodafinil as treatment for adults with excessive sleepiness associated with narcolepsy. Curr Med Res Opin 2006;22(4):761–74.
85. Dauvilliers Y, Bassetti C, Lammers GJ, et al. Pitolisant versus placebo or modafinil in patients with narcolepsy: a double-blind, randomised trial. Lancet Neurol 2013;12(11):1068–75.
86. Cak HT, Haliloglu G, Duzgun G, et al. Successful treatment of cataplexy in patients with Niemann Pick disease type C: use of tricyclic antidepressants. Eur J Paediatr Neurol 2014;18(6):811–5.
87. Morgenthaler TI, Kapur VK, Brown T, et al. Standards of practice committee of the AASM. Practice parameters for the treatment of narcolepsy and other hypersomnias of central origin. Sleep 2007;30(12):1705–11.
88. Lopez R, Dauvilliers Y. Pharmacotherapy options for cataplexy. Expert Opin Pharmacother 2013;14(7):895–903.
89. Lammers GJ, Arends J, Declerck AC, et al. Gammahydroxybutyrate and narcolepsy: a double-blind placebo-controlled study. Sleep 1993;16:216–20.

90. US Xyrem Multicenter Study Group. Sodium oxybate demonstrates long-term efficacy for the treatment of cataplexy in patients with narcolepsy. Sleep Med 2004;5:119–23.

91. Black J, Houghton WC. Sodium oxybate improves excessive daytime sleepiness in narcolepsy. Sleep 2006;29:939–46.

92. Van Schie MK, Werth E, Lammers GJ, et al. Improved vigilance after sodium oxybate treatment in narcolepsy: a comparison between in-field and in laboratory measures. J Sleep Res 2016;25(4):486–96.

93. Mansukhani M, Kotagal S. Sodium oxybate in the treatment of childhood narcolepsy-cataplexy: a retrospective study. Sleep Med 2012;13(6):606–10.

94. Lecendreux M, Poli F, Oudiette D, et al. Tolerance and efficacy of sodium oxybate in childhood narcolepsy with cataplexy: a retrospective study. Sleep 2012;35:709–11.

95. Rogers AE, Aldrich MS, Lin X. A comparison of three different sleep schedules for reducing daytime sleepiness in narcolepsy. Sleep 2001;24:385–91.

96. Picchietti DL, Bruni O, de Weerd A, et al. Pediatric restless legs syndrome diagnostic criteria: an update by the International Restless Legs Syndrome Study Group. Sleep Med 2013;14(12):1253–9.

97. Allen RP, Picchietti DL, Garcia-Borreguero D, et al. Restless legs syndrome/Willis-Ekbom disease diagnostic criteria: updated International Restless Legs Syndrome Study Group (IRLSSG) consensus criteria–history, rationale, description, and significance. Sleep Med 2014;15(8):860–73.

98. Picchietti MA, Picchietti DL. Restless legs syndrome and periodic limb movement disorder in children and adolescents. Semin Pediatr Neurol 2008;15(2):91–9.

99. Picchietti DL, Rajendran RR, Wilson MP, et al. Pediatric restless legs syndrome and periodic limb movement disorder: parent-child pairs. Sleep Med 2009;10(8):925–31.

100. Ohayon MM, O'Hara R, Vitiello MV. Epidemiology of restless legs syndrome: a synthesis of the literature. Sleep Med Rev 2012;16(4):283–95.

101. Picchietti D, Allen RP, Walters AS, et al. Restless legs syndrome: prevalence and impact in children and adolescents–the Peds REST study. Pediatrics 2007;120(2):253–66.

102. Zhang J, Lam SP, Li SX, et al. Restless legs symptoms in adolescents: epidemiology, heritability, and pubertal effects. J Psychosom Res 2014;76(2):158–64.

103. Allen RP. Restless leg syndrome/Willis-Ekbom disease pathophysiology. Sleep Med Clin 2015;10(3):207–14.

104. Rye DB. The molecular genetics of restless legs syndrome. Sleep Med Clin 2015 Sep;10(3):227–33.

105. Mindell JA, Emslie G, Blumer J, et al. Pharmacologic management of insomnia in children and adolescents: consensus statement. Pediatrics 2006;117(6):e1223–32.

106. Picchietti DL. Should oral iron be first-line therapy for pediatric restless legs syndrome and periodic limb movement disorder? Sleep Med 2017;32:220–1.

107. Dye TJ, Jain SV, Simakajornboon N. Outcomes of long-term iron supplementation in pediatric restless legs syndrome/periodic limb movement disorder (RLS/PLMD). Sleep Med 2017;32:213–9.

108. Picchietti DL, Stevens HE. Early manifestations of restless legs syndrome in childhood and adolescence. Sleep Med 2008;9(7):770–81.

109. Walters AS, Mandelbaum DE, Lewin DS. Dopaminergic therapy in children with restless legs/periodic limb movements in sleep and ADHD. Dopaminergic Therapy Study Group. Pediatr Neurol 2000;22(3):182–6.

Hypnotic Discontinuation in Chronic Insomnia

Jonathan P. Hintze, MD[a],*, Jack D. Edinger, PhD[b]

KEYWORDS

- Deprescribing • Discontinuation • Hypnotic • Benzodiazepines • Insomnia • Sleep disorder

KEY POINTS

- Patients with chronic insomnia are commonly prescribed hypnotic medications but discontinuation of these medications is difficult to achieve.
- A gradual taper is preferred over abrupt cessation to avoid rebound insomnia and withdrawal symptoms.
- Written information provided to the patient about medication discontinuation may be helpful.
- Cognitive behavioral therapy or behavioral therapies alone can improve hypnotic discontinuation outcomes.
- There is limited evidence for adjunct medications to assist in hypnotic cessation for insomnia.

INTRODUCTION

Insomnia disorder is common in adults and children. The estimated prevalence ranges from 9% to 15% in the general population, with higher prevalence in certain subpopulations.[1–6] Hypnotic medications are those that tend to produce sleep and are frequently used to treat insomnia.[7] Commonly used hypnotics in adults include benzodiazepines (BZDs), BZD receptor agonists (BzRAs), antihistamines, antidepressants, melatonin receptor agonists, orexin receptor antagonists, and antipsychotics. Although there are currently no medications for pediatric insomnia approved by the US Food and Drug Administration, commonly used medications include antihistamines, alpha agonists, antidepressants, BZDs, BzRAs, and antipsychotics.[8,9] The long-term health consequences of using hypnotics are not well described, and current guidelines recommend medication tapering and discontinuation when possible.[10] However, hypnotic discontinuation is difficult and often unsuccessful.[11] This article discusses strategies to discontinue hypnotics and evidence supporting their use.

HYPNOTIC TAPER STRATEGIES
Abrupt Hypnotic Cessation

Rapid drug cessation is an option for many medications. However, rebound insomnia and withdrawal symptoms may accompany abrupt hypnotic discontinuation. Rebound insomnia is generally defined as insomnia that is worse relative to baseline. This was first described with the discontinuation of triazolam[12] and has since been reported with several other BZDs[13,14]; sedating antidepressants, including amitriptyline[15] and trazodone[16]; and BzRAs, though with conflicting reports.[14,17–19] Additionally, withdrawal symptoms, largely defined as the emergence of previously absent symptoms, are frequently reported with abrupt discontinuation of BZDs.[20] Consequently, tapering hypnotics is generally preferred to abrupt cessation.

Disclosure Statement: J.P. Hintze has no potential conflicts of interest or funding sources. J.D. Edinger conflicts of interest or funding: grant support from Merck, Philips, Respironics, Inc.
a Division of Pediatric Sleep Medicine, University of South Carolina School of Medicine-Greenville, Greenville Health System, 200 Patewood Drive, Suite A330, Greenville, SC 29615, USA; b Department of Medicine, National Jewish Health, 1400 Jackson Street, Denver, CO 80206, USA
* Corresponding author.
E-mail address: jhintze@ghs.org

sleep.theclinics.com

Tapering Hypnotics

Reported tapering strategies vary widely, with no consensus on the optimal tapering protocol. A frequently described approach is a dose reduction of 25% every 1 to 2 weeks until discontinued completely.[21–25] Complete discontinuation rates ranged from 24% to 61% in these studies but there is variability in the frequency of office visits and the follow-up period in these reports. Withdrawal symptoms were commonly reported. A slightly slower wean was used by Lopez-Peig and colleagues.[26] Subjects all took BZDs, and were instructed to reduce their dose by 25% every 2 to 4 weeks. At the end of the taper period, 80.4% had successfully discontinued their BZD, and 64% remained BZD-free at 12 months. Another study weaned subjects from various BZDs by 10% to 25% every 2 to 3 weeks, with an approximately 40% hypnotic abstinence rate maintained at 36 months, without significant sleep dissatisfaction compared with a control group.[27] Drake[28] weaned subjects from temazepam by cutting doses roughly in half every 2 weeks, from 10 mg to 5 mg to 2 mg. Of the subjects, 59% successfully completed the taper, with 52% remaining hypnotic-free at follow-up 12 to 35 weeks later. Lemoine and colleagues[29] reported a similar taper with 2 BzRAs, zopiclone and zolpidem. In that study, subjects were weaned from zolpidem 10 mg to 5 mg for a week, followed by a placebo. Similarly, subjects were weaned from zopiclone 7.5 mg to 3.75 mg for a week, followed by a placebo. This regimen was associated with significantly higher withdrawal symptoms than the control group that was not weaned. In contrast, Raju and Meagher[30] used a more flexible taper protocol, in which subjects were able to control the rate of withdrawal. Given control over the weaning pace, some subjects rapidly discontinued hypnotic use (19 of 68), whereas others preferred a prolonged, yet complete, taper (13 of 68). The remainder did not completely discontinue medication use. To the authors' knowledge, there are no studies specifically comparing the success of different taper strategies. However, a clinical trial is currently underway that will compare different taper strategies among hypnotic-dependent subjects.[31]

Many practitioners find it helpful to switch from a short-acting to a long-acting BZD before initiating a taper.[27,32] This is done by switching to an equivalent dose of a long-acting BZD, commonly diazepam (**Table 1**). It is notable that a Cochrane Review published in 2006 noted higher dropout rates when tapering short half-life compounds compared with long-acting BZDs.[33] However,

Table 1
Approximate equivalent doses of benzodiazepines to 5 mg diazepam

BZD	Equivalent Dose (mg)
Alprazolam	0.25–0.5
Bromazepam	3–6
Lorazepam	0.5–1
Nitrazepam	5
Oxazepam	15
Temazepam	10
Triazolam	0.25

there was no difference in withdrawal symptoms between the groups, so switching from a short-acting to a long-acting BZD before a gradual taper was not supported. The authors are unaware of any studies specifically comparing the practice of switching to a long-acting BZD before gradual withdrawal versus a gradual withdrawal directly from a short-acting BZD.

ADJUNCT THERAPIES

Regardless of the taper strategy, several adjunct therapies have been studied to assist in hypnotic discontinuation. These include various degrees of patient education, psychological therapies, and medications.

Written Patient Education

There is some evidence that simply providing written information to patients can lead to hypnotic discontinuation. In 1 study, chronic BZD users were randomized to receive either routine care or advice during a single consultation supplemented by a self-help booklet.[34] The intervention resulted in a significant reduction in BDZ prescriptions compared with routine care alone (18% vs 5%). Several other studies used a letter sent to BZD users encouraging BZD reduction, with complete BZD cessation rates ranging from 14% to 27%.[23,24,35–37]

Psychological Therapies

Many studies have used psychological therapies to aid in medication discontinuation. A brief description of the different types of therapy is provided in **Table 2**.

Sleep hygiene education
Sleep hygiene education is routinely provided to patients with insomnia. However, there is insufficient evidence to recommend sleep hygiene as a

Table 2
Psychological therapies for insomnia

Therapy	Description
Sleep hygiene education	Guidelines about practices and habits that support or interfere with sleep (eg, obtaining regular exercise, avoid electronics before bed)
Relaxation therapy	Techniques used to reduce muscular tension and intrusive thought processes interfering with sleep
Stimulus control therapy	Reinforcing the association of the bed with sleep by getting out of bed when unable to fall asleep, only going to bed when sleepy, keeping a strict rise time, and avoiding napping
Sleep restriction therapy	Reducing the amount of time spent in bed to match actual sleep time, with periodic adjustments as necessary
Cognitive therapy	A method of challenging false beliefs about sleep that contribute to insomnia
Cognitive behavioral therapy	Combining cognitive therapy with another behavioral treatment (eg, sleep restriction or stimulus control)
Self-efficacy enhancement	Improving perceived coping capabilities by providing positive vicarious experiences, discussing obstacles from prior failed attempts, and social persuasion

stand-alone therapy regardless of the presence or absence of hypnotic use.[38] Additionally, the authors are unaware of any studies that used sleep hygiene alone as an intervention to assist in hypnotic discontinuation.

Relaxation therapy

Relaxation therapy is a technique used to reduce muscular tension and intrusive thought processes interfering with sleep, and involves tensing and relaxing major muscle groups. Giblin and Clift[39] studied the effects of relaxation therapy on hypnotic discontinuation in 20 subjects. Notably, their intervention also included a discussion about sleep and insomnia, hypnotics and their effects on sleep, and general advice about problem-solving and optimism. There was a significant decrease in the number of subjects who resumed nightly hypnotic use at 12 weeks in the treatment group (2 of 10) compared with the control group (8 of 10), without any significant difference between the groups in reported sleep onset latency and overall sleep quality.

Lichstein and Johnson[40] used relaxation therapy for hypnotic cessation, resulting in a substantial reduction (47%) in sleep medication use. Lichstein and colleagues[41] assessed the usefulness of progressive relaxation techniques in addition to a standard drug withdrawal program in a randomized trial. All subjects had a 79% reduction in hypnotic consumption, without any significant difference between the groups. However, those assigned to the relaxation group had fewer withdrawal symptoms, greater sleep efficiency, and higher reported quality of sleep.

Stimulus control therapy

Stimulus control therapy is a method pioneered by Bootzin[42] and is used to reestablish the association between the bed and sleep. Patients are encouraged to remove themselves from the bed when unable to fall asleep, and only go to bed when sleepy rather than at a designated bedtime. They are also encouraged to keep a strict rise time and to avoid napping. A study of 7 long-term hypnotic users found that most (6 of 7) were able to reduce or stop their medication when stimulus control therapy was used.[43] Riedel and colleagues[44] randomized 21 subjects to either a medication withdrawal program, or the withdrawal program and stimulus control therapy. Both groups had significant reductions in the amount of sleep medication use but the stimulus control group also had significant improvements in total sleep time, sleep efficiency, sleep quality, and daytime sleepiness. Several other studies included stimulus control therapy as part of their intervention (see later discussion).

Sleep restriction therapy

Sleep restriction therapy is used to curtail the amount of time spent awake in bed. This is done by determining the amount of sleep a patient is regularly getting and limiting the total allowable time in bed to the same amount. For example, if a patient is currently spending 10 hours in bed per night but only sleeps 6 hours, then the amount of time in bed per night would be limited to 6 to 6.5 hours, depending on the specific sleep restriction protocol used.

Although sleep restriction is a well-established therapy for insomnia in general,[45] Taylor and colleagues[46] performed the only known study examining the effectiveness of sleep restriction in the setting of hypnotic discontinuation. Forty-six subjects were assigned to either sleep hygiene education or sleep restriction with medication withdrawal. In the sleep restriction group, 52.6% completely discontinued hypnotic medication use, compared with 15.4% in the sleep hygiene group. Additionally, there was improvement in sleep-onset latency and sleep efficiency, which was maintained through a 12-month follow-up period.

Cognitive behavioral therapy
Cognitive therapy is the method of challenging a patient's current beliefs about sleep that contribute to insomnia. Cognitive behavioral therapy (CBT) combines behavioral therapy (eg, relaxation, stimulus control, sleep restriction) with cognitive therapy to form a multicomponent and omnibus intervention. Therefore, CBT is a combination therapy with variation depending on the specific methods used. CBT has long been used for insomnia and an early study demonstrated its usefulness in hypnotic discontinuation.[47] Several subsequent studies have been performed.

Many studies specifically evaluated BZD cessation. Baillargeon and colleagues[48] studied 65 subjects with chronic insomnia taking BZDs nightly, randomizing subjects to a gradual supervised taper alone or combined with 8 weeks of CBT. At treatment completion, more subjects had complete drug cessation in the combined group (77%) compared with the taper-alone group (38%), with similar results at a 12-month follow-up (70% vs 24%). Although several other studies reported no improvement in BZD discontinuation rates with CBT,[23,49,50] other measures of sleep quality were generally improved. Morin and colleagues[25] considered the differential effects of supervised BZD withdrawal and CBT in their randomized trial. Seventy-six subjects underwent supervised withdrawal, CBT, or both. Although all groups had a significant reduction in quantity (90%) and frequency (80%) of BZD use, the combined treatment group was the most successful at achieving complete drug cessation (85%), with supervised withdrawal and CBT alone producing less-successful results (48% and 54% respectively). Interestingly, the subjects in both groups that received CBT reported greater improvement in subjective sleep quality when compared with the group who only had supervised drug withdrawal. When a 24-month follow-up was conducted, 42.6% of subjects had resumed BZDs, with

greater relapse in the CBT-alone group (69.2%) when compared with the combined (33.3%) and supervised withdrawal (30.8%) groups.

BzRAs have also been studied. Zavesicka and colleagues[51] reported 15 zolpidem-dependent subjects who were successfully weaned while receiving CBT, with associated improved sleep efficiency and decreased wakefulness after sleep onset. An 8-week hypnotic taper program, including 53 subjects taking either BZDs or BzRAs, found that those randomized to receive CBT had improved sleep efficiency and decreased total wake time when compared with the control group.[52] However, both groups successfully reduced hypnotic use, with no significant additional reduction in the CBT group. In contrast, Morgan and colleagues[53] found that CBT greatly reduced hypnotic drug use while improving sleep efficiency and reducing sleep onset latency in a cohort of 209 chronic hypnotic users. Lichstein and colleagues[54] further validated the usefulness of CBT in hypnotic-dependent insomnia patients using BZDs, BzRAs, or sedating antidepressants by randomizing subjects to CBT with drug withdrawal, placebo biofeedback with drug withdrawal, or drug withdrawal alone. There were no significant differences between groups in medication reduction, which decreased by 84% posttreatment, and 66% at a 12-month follow-up. However, only the CBT group had significant improvement in sleep onset latency and subjective sleep measures.

Self-efficacy enhancement
In some analyses of factors leading to success in hypnotic cessation, an individual's perceived self-efficacy has been positively correlated with medication cessation.[50,55] To further pursue the effect of self-efficacy on patient outcomes, Yang and colleagues[56] randomized 48 long-term hypnotic users (BZDs or BzRAs) to a standard drug taper alone or a self-efficacy educational program followed by the same drug taper. Those in the treatment group had a higher percentage of dose reduction than those in the taper-alone group, suggesting that self-efficacy can be learned and can improve hypnotic cessation outcomes.

Pharmacologic Therapies
Several studies have evaluated the usefulness of medications to assist in BZD discontinuation, though generally in the setting of anxiety or other psychological disorders. These have included ondansetron,[57] imipramine,[58,59] buspirone,[58-60] paroxetine,[61] carbamazepine,[62] pregabalin,[63] progesterone,[64] antihistamines,[65] and propranolol.[66] Only a few have examined the usefulness of

medications to assist in BZDs cessation specifically for insomnia. There have also been some reports of other supplements to aid in hypnotic discontinuation.

Zopiclone

Withdrawal symptoms and rebound insomnia have been shown to be less severe with BzRAs compared with some BZDs.[18] Therefore, some investigators have proposed using a BzRA as a bridge to BZD discontinuation. Pat-Horenczyk and colleagues[67] studied 24 subjects taking flunitrazepam for insomnia. All underwent a 5-week withdrawal protocol and were followed with nightly actigraphy and serial polysomnograms during the withdrawal period. One group was transitioned to zopiclone and then weaned off, whereas the other was weaned off flunitrazepam directly. Both objective (polysomnogram and actigraphy) and subjective (sleep diaries) measures were improved in the zopiclone group compared with the flunitrazepam group. Similar positive findings were found in other reports.[68–70] Two studies indicated that abrupt medication substitution yielded better results than gradual substitution.[68,70]

Melatonin

Some have postulated that melatonin therapy could aid in the discontinuation of hypnotics. In a large retrospective study of prolonged-release melatonin, 31% discontinued hypnotic use (BZDs or BzRAs) after the melatonin was started.[71] Several randomized trials have also considered the usefulness of melatonin in hypnotic discontinuation, specifically BZDs. Although 2 of these trials showed some effectiveness,[72,73] most found that melatonin did not enhance BZD discontinuation.[74–78] A meta-analysis also concluded that melatonin supplementation did not affect rates of BZD discontinuation.[79]

Valerian

The evidence for the use of the herbal supplement valerian in insomnia to date has been inconclusive.[80] However, Poyares and colleagues[81] reported some positive outcomes with the use of valerian in BZD discontinuation. Subjects treated with valerian had better subjective sleep quality than the placebo group, with decreased wakefulness after sleep onset at a 2-week polysomnogram, though with a longer sleep onset latency.

SUMMARY

Discontinuation of hypnotic medications is often challenging. The current evidence suggests that a gradual taper is preferred over abrupt discontinuation owing to both rebound insomnia and withdrawal symptoms. However, an ideal taper schedule has not been well-established. A clinical trial is currently underway in an effort to improve understanding of the ideal wean schedule.[31] In addition to tapering hypnotics, providing patients with educational handouts may provide some benefit. Psychological therapies are also beneficial, with the most evidence supporting CBT in conjunction with a hypnotic taper. Some patients taking BZD hypnotics may benefit from bridging drug cessation with a BzRA. In those cases, an immediate switch to a BzRA was more beneficial than a gradual switch. Other medical therapies have not uniformly demonstrated benefit. Moreover, because most of the evidence for hypnotic discontinuation was done with BZDs, it is not clear that a similar approach can be made with sedating antidepressants, antihistamines, or other hypnotics. Furthermore, the discontinuation of hypnotics in the pediatric population is based only on the adult literature. Further research is needed to better establish optimal hypnotic discontinuation guidelines for both adults and children.

REFERENCES

1. Ohayon MM. Epidemiology of insomnia: what we know and what we still need to learn. Sleep Med Rev 2002;6(2):97–111.
2. Calhoun SL, Fernandez-Mendoza J, Vgontzas AN, et al. Prevalence of insomnia symptoms in a general population sample of young children and preadolescents: gender effects. Sleep Med 2014;15(1):91–5.
3. Chung KF, Yeung WF, Ho FY, et al. Cross-cultural and comparative epidemiology of insomnia: the Diagnostic and Statistical Manual (DSM), International Classification of Diseases (ICD) and International Classification of Sleep Disorders (ICSD). Sleep Med 2015;16(4):477–82.
4. Kronholm E, Partonen T, Härmä M, et al. Prevalence of insomnia-related symptoms continues to increase in the Finnish working-age population. J Sleep Res 2016;25(4):454–7.
5. Seow LS, Subramaniam M, Abdin E, et al. Sleep disturbance among people with major depressive disorders (MDD) in Singapore. J Ment Health 2016;25(6):492–9.
6. Kim KW, Kang SH, Yoon IY, et al. Prevalence and clinical characteristics of insomnia and its subtypes in the Korean elderly. Arch Gerontol Geriatr 2017;68: 68–75.
7. Walsh JK. Pharmacologic management of insomnia. J Clin Psychiatry 2004;65(Suppl 16):41–5.
8. Owens JA, Rosen CL, Mindell JA. Medication use in the treatment of pediatric insomnia: results of a survey of community-based pediatricians. Pediatrics 2003;111(5 Pt 1):e628–35.

9. Nguyen M, Tharani S, Rahmani M, et al. A review of the use of clonidine as a sleep aid in the child and adolescent population. Clin Pediatr (Phila) 2014; 53(3):211–6.

10. Schutte-Rodin S, Broch L, Buysse D, et al. Clinical guideline for the evaluation and management of chronic insomnia in adults. J Clin Sleep Med 2008; 4(5):487–504.

11. Ostini R, Jackson C, Hegney D, et al. How is medication prescribing ceased? A systematic review. Med Care 2011;49(1):24–36.

12. Kales A, Scharf MB, Kales JD. Rebound insomnia: a new clinical syndrome. Science 1978;201(4360): 1039–41.

13. Roehrs T. Rebound insomnia: its determinants and significance. Am J Med 1990;88(3A):39S–42S.

14. Soldatos CR, Dikeos DG, Whitehead A. Tolerance and rebound insomnia with rapidly eliminated hypnotics: a meta-analysis of sleep laboratory studies. Int Clin Psychopharmacol 1999;14(5): 287–303.

15. Staner L, Kerkhofs M, Detroux D, et al. Acute, subchronic and withdrawal sleep EEG changes during treatment with paroxetine and amitriptyline: a double-blind randomized trial in major depression. Sleep 1995;18(6):470–7.

16. Montgomery I, Oswald I, Morgan K, et al. Trazodone enhances sleep in subjective quality but not in objective duration. Br J Clin Pharmacol 1983;16(2): 139–44.

17. Monti JM, Attali P, Monti D, et al. Zolpidem and rebound insomnia–a double-blind, controlled polysomnographic study in chronic insomniac patients. Pharmacopsychiatry 1994;27(4):166–75.

18. Silvestri R, Ferrillo F, Murri L, et al. Rebound insomnia after abrupt discontinuation of hypnotic treatment: double-blind randomized comparison of zolpidem versus triazolam. Hum Psychopharmacol 1996;11(3):225–33.

19. Voshaar RC, van Balkom AJ, Zitman FG. Zolpidem is not superior to temazepam with respect to rebound insomnia: a controlled study. Eur Neuropsychopharmacol 2004;14(4):301–6.

20. Rickels K, Schweizer E, Case WG, et al. Long-term therapeutic use of benzodiazepines. I. Effects of abrupt discontinuation. Arch Gen Psychiatry 1990; 47(10):899–907.

21. Hopkins DR, Sethi KB, Mucklow JC. Benzodiazepine withdrawal in general practice. J R Coll Gen Pract 1982;32(245):758–62.

22. Murphy SM, Tyrer P. A double-blind comparison of the effects of gradual withdrawal of lorazepam, diazepam and bromazepam in benzodiazepine dependence. Br J Psychiatry 1991;158:511–6.

23. Voshaar RC, Gorgels WJ, Mol AJ, et al. Tapering off long-term benzodiazepine use with or without group cognitive-behavioural therapy: three-condition, randomised controlled trial. Br J Psychiatry 2003;182:498–504.

24. Gorgels WJ, Oude Voshaar RC, Mol AJ, et al. Discontinuation of long-term benzodiazepine use by sending a letter to users in family practice: a prospective controlled intervention study. Drug Alcohol Depend 2005;78(1):49–56.

25. Morin CM, Bastien CH, Guay B, et al. Randomized clinical trial of supervised tapering and cognitive-behavior therapy to facilitate benzodiazepine discontinuation in older adults with chronic insomnia. Am J Psychiatry 2004;161:332–42.

26. Lopez-Peig C, Mundet X, Casabella B, et al. Analysis of benzodiazepine withdrawal program managed by primary care nurses in Spain. BMC Res Notes 2012;5:684.

27. Vicens C, Sempere E, Bejarano F, et al. Efficacy of two interventions on the discontinuation of benzodiazepines in long-term users: 36-month follow-up of a cluster randomised trial in primary care. Br J Gen Pract 2016;66(643):e85–91.

28. Drake J. Temazepam 'Planpak': a multicentre general practice trial in planned benzodiazepine hypnotic withdrawal. Curr Med Res Opin 1991;12(6): 390–3.

29. Lemoine P, Allain H, Janus C, et al. Gradual withdrawal of zopiclone (7.5 mg) and zolpidem (10 mg) in insomniacs treated for at least 3 months. Eur Psychiatry 1995;10(Suppl 3):161s–5s.

30. Raju B, Meagher D. Patient-controlled benzodiazepine dose reduction in a community mental health service. Ir J Psychol Med 2005;22:42–5.

31. ClinicalTrials.gov. The role of tapering pace and selected traits on hypnotic discontinuation. Bethesda (MD): National Library of Medicine (US); 2016. Identifier NCT02831894, Available at: https://clinicaltrials.gov/ct2/show/NCT02831894. Accessed August 17, 2017.

32. Lader M, Tylee A, Donoghue J. Withdrawing benzodiazepines in primary care. CNS Drugs 2009;23(1): 19–34.

33. Denis C, Fatséas M, Lavie E, et al. Pharmacological interventions for benzodiazepine mono-dependence management in outpatient settings. Cochrane Database Syst Rev 2006;(3):CD005194.

34. Bashir K, King M, Ashworth M. Controlled evaluation of brief intervention by general practitioners to reduce chronic use of benzodiazepines. Br J Gen Pract 1994;44(386):408–12.

35. Cormack MA, Sweeney KG, Hughes-Jones H, et al. Evaluation of an easy, cost-effective strategy for cutting benzodiazepine use in general practice. Br J Gen Pract 1994;44(378):5–8.

36. Stewart R, Niessen WJ, Broer J, et al. General Practitioners reduced benzodiazepine prescriptions in an intervention study: a multilevel application. J Clin Epidemiol 2007;60(10):1076–84.

37. Tannenbaum C, Martin P, Tamblyn R, et al. Reduction of inappropriate benzodiazepine prescriptions among older adults through direct patient education: the EMPOWER cluster randomized trial. JAMA Intern Med 2014;174(6):890–8.

38. Morgenthaler T, Kramer M, Alessi C, et al, American Academy of Sleep Medicine. Practice parameters for the psychological and behavioral treatment of insomnia: an update. An american academy of sleep medicine report. Sleep 2006; 29(11):1415–9.

39. Giblin MJ, Clift AD. Sleep without drugs. J R Coll Gen Pract 1983;33(255):628–33.

40. Lichstein KL, Johnson RS. Relaxation for insomnia and hypnotic medication use in older women. Psychol Aging 1993;8(1):103–11.

41. Lichstein KL, Peterson BA, Riedel BW, et al. Relaxation to assist sleep medication withdrawal. Behav Modif 1999;23(3):379–402.

42. Bootzin RR. Stimulus control treatment for insomnia. Am Psychol Ass Proc 1972;7:395–6.

43. Baillargeon L, Demers M, Ladouceur R. Stimulus-control: nonpharmacologic treatment for insomnia. Can Fam Physician 1998;44:73–9.

44. Riedel B, Lichstein K, Peterson BA, et al. A comparison of the efficacy of stimulus control for medicated and nonmedicated insomniacs. Behav Modif 1998;22(1):3–28.

45. Morin CM, Bootzin RR, Buysse DJ, et al. Psychological and behavioral treatment of insomnia: update of the recent evidence (1998-2004). Sleep 2006; 29(11):1398–414.

46. Taylor DJ, Schmidt-Nowara W, Jessop CA, et al. Sleep restriction therapy and hypnotic withdrawal versus sleep hygiene education in hypnotic using patients with insomnia. J Clin Sleep Med 2010; 6(2):169–75.

47. Morin CM, Colecchi CA, Ling WD, et al. Cognitive behavior therapy to facilitate benzodiazepine discontinuation among hypnotic-dependent patients with insomnia. Behav Ther 1995;26(4):733–45.

48. Baillargeon L, Landreville P, Verreault R, et al. Discontinuation of benzodiazepines among older insomniac adults treated with cognitive-behavioural therapy combined with gradual tapering: a randomized trial. CMAJ 2003;169(10):1015–20.

49. Vorma H, Naukkarinen H, Sarna S, et al. Treatment of out-patients with complicated benzodiazepine dependence: comparison of two approaches. Addiction 2002;97(7):851–9.

50. O'Connor K, Marchand A, Brousseau L, et al. Cognitive-behavioural, pharmacological and psychosocial predictors of outcome during tapered discontinuation of benzodiazepine. Clin Psychol Psychother 2008;15(1):1–14.

51. Zavesicka L, Brunovsky M, Matousek M, et al. Discontinuation of hypnotics during cognitive behavioural therapy for insomnia. BMC psychiatry 2008;8(1):80.

52. Belleville G, Guay C, Guay B, et al. Hypnotic taper with or without self-help of insomnia: a randomized clinical trial. J Consult Clin Psychol 2007;75:325–35.

53. Morgan K, Dixon S, Mathers N, et al. Psychological treatment for insomnia in the management of long-term hypnotic drug use: a pragmatic randomised controlled trial. Br J Gen Pract 2003;53(497):923–8.

54. Lichstein KL, Nau SD, Wilson NM, et al. Psychological treatment of hypnotic-dependent insomnia in a primarily older adult sample. Behav Res Ther 2013;51(12):787–96.

55. Bélanger L, Morin CM, Bastien C, et al. Self-efficacy and compliance with benzodiazepine taper in older adults with chronic insomnia. Health Psychol 2005; 24(3):281–7.

56. Yang CM, Tseng CH, Lai YS, et al. Self-efficacy enhancement can facilitate hypnotic tapering in patients with primary insomnia. Sleep Biol Rhythms 2015;13(3):242–51.

57. Romach MK, Kaplan HL, Busto UE, et al. A controlled trial of ondansetron, a 5-HT3 antagonist, in benzodiazepine discontinuation. J Clin Psychopharmacol 1998;18(2):121–31.

58. Rickels K, DeMartinis N, García-España F, et al. Imipramine and buspirone in treatment of patients with generalized anxiety disorder who are discontinuing long-term benzodiazepine therapy. Am J Psychiatry 2000;157(12):1973–9.

59. Rynn M, García-España F, Greenblatt DJ, et al. Imipramine and buspirone in patients with panic disorder who are discontinuing long-term benzodiazepine therapy. J Clin Psychopharmacol 2003;23(5):505–8.

60. Ashton CH, Rawlins MD, Tyrer SP. A double-blind placebo-controlled study of buspirone in diazepam withdrawal in chronic benzodiazepine users. Br J Psychiatry 1990;157:232–8.

61. Nakao M, Takeuchi T, Nomura K, et al. Clinical application of paroxetine for tapering benzodiazepine use in non-major-depressive outpatients visiting an internal medicine clinic. Psychiatry Clin Neurosci 2006;60(5):605–10.

62. Schweizer E, Rickels K, Case WG, et al. Carbamazepine treatment in patients discontinuing long-term benzodiazepine therapy. Effects on withdrawal severity and outcome. Arch Gen Psychiatry 1991; 48(5):448–52.

63. Bobes J, Rubio G, Terán A, et al. Pregabalin for the discontinuation of long-term benzodiazepines use: an assessment of its effectiveness in daily clinical practice. Eur Psychiatry 2012;27(4):301–7.

64. Schweizer E, Case WG, Garcia-Espana F, et al. Progesterone co-administration in patients discontinuing long-term benzodiazepine therapy: effects on withdrawal severity and taper outcome. Psychopharmacology (Berl) 1995;117(4):424–9.

65. Gilhooly TC, Webster MG, Poole NW, et al. What happens when doctors stop prescribing temazepam? Use of alternative therapies. Br J Gen Pract 1998;48(434):1601–2.

66. Hallström C, Crouch G, Robson M, et al. The treatment of tranquilizer dependence by propranolol. Postgrad Med J 1988;64(Suppl 2):40–4.

67. Pat-Horenczyk R, Hacohen D, Herer P, et al. The effects of substituting zopiclone in withdrawal from chronic use of benzodiazepine hypnotics. Psychopharmacology (Berl) 1998;140(4):450–7.

68. Shapiro CM, MacFarlane JG, MacLean AW. Alleviating sleep-related discontinuance symptoms associated with benzodiazepine withdrawal: a new approach. J Psychosom Res 1993;37(Suppl 1):55–7.

69. Shapiro C, Sherman D, Peck D. Withdrawal from benzodiazepines by initially switching to zopiclone. Eur Psychiatry 1995;10(Suppl 3):145s–51s.

70. Lemoine P, Ohayon MM. Is hypnotic withdrawal facilitated by the transitory use of a substitute drug? Prog Neuropsychopharmacol Biol Psychiatry 1997; 21(1):111–24.

71. Kunz D, Bineau S, Maman K, et al. Benzodiazepine discontinuation with prolonged-release melatonin: hints from a German longitudinal prescription database. Expert Opin Pharmacother 2012;13(1):9–16.

72. Garfinkel D, Zisapel N, Wainstein J, et al. Facilitation of benzodiazepine discontinuation by melatonin: a new clinical approach. Arch Intern Med 1999; 159(20):2456–60.

73. Garzón C, Guerrero JM, Aramburu O, et al. Effect of melatonin administration on sleep, behavioral disorders and hypnotic drug discontinuation in the elderly: a randomized, double-blind, placebo-controlled study. Aging Clin Exp Res 2009;21(1): 38–42.

74. Cardinali DP, Gvozdenovich E, Kaplan MR, et al. A double blind-placebo controlled study on melatonin efficacy to reduce anxiolytic benzodiazepine use in the elderly. Neuroendocrinol Lett 2002; 23:55–60.

75. Peles E, Hetzroni T, Bar-Hamburger R, et al. Melatonin for perceived sleep disturbances associated with benzodiazepine withdrawal among patients in methadone maintenance treatment: a double-blind randomized clinical trial. Addiction 2007;102(12): 1947–53.

76. Vissers FH, Knipschild PG, Crebolder HF. Is melatonin helpful in stopping the long-term use of hypnotics? A discontinuation trial. Pharm World Sci 2007;29(6):641–6.

77. Lähteenmäki R, Puustinen J, Vahlberg T, et al. Melatonin for sedative withdrawal in older patients with primary insomnia: a randomized double-blind placebo-controlled trial. Br J Clin Pharmacol 2014; 77(6):975–85.

78. Baandrup L, Lindschou J, Winkel P, et al. Prolonged-release melatonin versus placebo for benzodiazepine discontinuation in patients with schizophrenia or bipolar disorder: a randomised, placebo-controlled, blinded trial. World J Biol Psychiatry 2016;17(7):514–24.

79. Wright A, Diebold J, Otal J, et al. The effect of melatonin on benzodiazepine discontinuation and sleep quality in adults attempting to discontinue benzodiazepines: a systematic review and meta-analysis. Drugs Aging 2015;32(12): 1009–18.

80. Fernández-San-Martín MI, Masa-Font R, Palacios-Soler L, et al. Effectiveness of Valerian on insomnia: a meta-analysis of randomized placebo-controlled trials. Sleep Med 2010;11(6):505–11.

81. Poyares DR, Guilleminault C, Ohayon MM, et al. Can valerian improve the sleep of insomniacs after benzodiazepine withdrawal? Prog Neuropsychopharmacol Biol Psychiatry 2002;26(3):539–45.

Effects of Chronic Opioid Use on Sleep and Wake

Michelle Cao, DO[a], Shahrokh Javaheri, MD[b,c],*

KEYWORDS

- Opiates • Daytime sleepiness • Depression • Poor sleep • Sleep-disordered breathing
- Central sleep apnea

KEY POINTS

- Chronic use of opioids has a multitude of negative effects on daytime function, including hypersomnolence, fatigue and depression, and sleep architecture and sleep-related breathing disorders, with resulting daytime consequences.
- Chronic opioid use is an established risk factor for sleep-disordered breathing, particularly for central sleep apnea.
- It is plausible to assume that patients on chronic opioid therapy may suffer from unrecognized sleep-disordered breathing and associated consequences, including respiratory depression and death.
- Sleep-disordered breathing associated with chronic opioid use is a diagnostic and therapeutic challenge.
- Although studies are limited, new-generation servo ventilators deserve further research and should be offered to patients with sleep-disordered breathing, including central sleep apnea, especially in those who do not respond to conventional modes of therapy, such as continuous positive airway pressure or bilevel positive airway pressure.

INTRODUCTION

Opioid medications are considered a significant component in the multidisciplinary management of chronic pain. In the past 2 decades, the use of opioid medications has dramatically risen in part due to an increased awareness by health care providers to treat chronic pain more effectively. In addition, patients themselves are encouraged to seek treatment. The release of a sentinel joint statement in 1997 by the American Academy of Pain Medicine and the American Pain Society in a national effort to increase awareness and support the treatment of chronic pain has undoubtedly contributed to the opioid crisis.[1] This effort and among others consequently led to an epidemic of opioid misuse (ie, without prescription or as directed by provider), abuse, and death related to overdose. A recent national large-scale survey reported that 91.8 million Americans used prescription opioids, 11.5 million misused them, and 1.9 million had opioid use disorder.[2] Cumulative data reported that increased use of opioids has resulted in increased morbidity and mortality, with more than 33,000 deaths due to opioid overdose in 2015.[3,4] Opioid-related deaths are most often from prescription opioid pain relievers and illicit use of synthetic compounds, including heroin and fentanyl.[4] With the support of the Secretary of Health and Human Services, President Donald Trump has declared the opioid crisis a national public health emergency.[4]

[a] Division of Sleep Medicine, Stanford University School of Medicine, 450 Broadway Street, Redwood City, CA 94063, USA; [b] Bethesda North Hospital, University of Cincinnati College of Medicine, 10535 Montgomery Road, Suite 200, Cincinnati, OH 45242, USA; [c] Division of Pulmonary, Critical Care and Sleep Medicine, The Ohio State University, 181 Taylor Avenue, Columbus, OH 43203, USA
* Corresponding author. 10535 Montgomery Road, Suite 200, Cincinnati, OH 45242.
E-mail address: shahrokhjavaheri@icloud.com

Sleep Med Clin 13 (2018) 271–281
https://doi.org/10.1016/j.jsmc.2018.02.002
1556-407X/18/© 2018 Elsevier Inc. All rights reserved.

The initial acceptance of opioid use for the relieve of chronic pain more than 20 years ago is now being challenged on efficacy and safety of these prescription practices. There is strong evidence to support short-term use of opioids for chronic pain, but support for long-term opioid use is lacking.[3] There are no studies of opioid therapy versus placebo, no opioid therapy, or nonopioid therapy for chronic pain evaluating long-term (≥1 year) outcomes related to pain, function, or quality of life. Most placebo-controlled randomized clinical trials were less than or equal to 6 weeks in duration.[5] Long-term use results in reduction or loss of analgesic efficacy due to pharmacologic tolerance or opioid-induced hyperalgesia (ie, worsening pain sensitivity). In the long run, among many other consequences, chronic use of opioids is associated with sleep dysfunction, leading to symptoms of excessive daytime sleepiness, daytime fatigue, depression, and notably, respiratory depression during sleep.

Daytime hypersomnolence, daytime fatigue, depression, copharmacy with benzodiazepines and/or antidepressants, and consequently poor general health quality are common in chronic opioid users. There may be a bidirectional relationship between poor sleep quality, sleep-disordered breathing (SDB), and daytime function. Chronic use of opioids is associated with disrupted sleep architecture and SDB, which encompasses a spectrum of ventilatory derangements, including hypoventilation, hypoxemia, obstructive and central apneas, periodic breathing, and ataxic or irregular breathing. The authors believe that a complex relationship exists between chronic pain, chronic use of opioids, sleep disorders, and daytime symptoms (**Fig. 1**).

OPIOIDS AND DAYTIME FUNCTION

Opioids have adverse effects on sleep and daytime function, effects that could be bidirectional. These effects could be modulated by the presence of chronic pain when present. Excessive daytime sleepiness, fatigue, depression, neurocognitive dysfunction, and poor general health are common in patients using opioids chronically. On the other hand, disrupted sleep architecture and SDB are frequently observed during polysomnography, together interacting in a complex manner (see **Fig. 1**).

In an early pilot study from Australia, Teichtahl and colleagues[6] assessed sleep and daytime function of 10 young patients (mean age 35 years) in a stable methadone maintenance program (MMP) with 9 control patients matched for age, gender, and body mass index. The methadone dose ranged between 50 mg per day and 120 mg per day. All patients were assessed by a psychologist and a physician. Compared with the control group, patients in the MMP were significantly more depressed based on the Beck

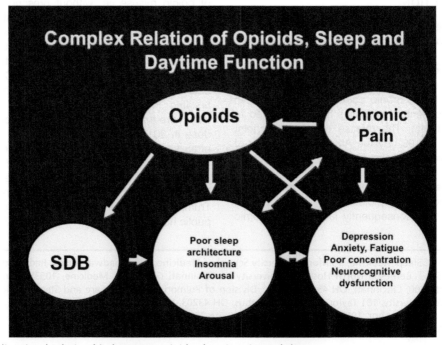

Fig. 1. Bidirectional relationship between opioids, chronic pain, and sleep.

Depression Inventory (BDI) scale, had more daytime sleepiness based on the Epworth Sleepiness Scale [ESS] (mean score of 11 for MMP group vs 3 for control group), and, not surprisingly, had significantly lower scores on general health quality. All MMP patients smoked tobacco cigarettes, and 8 admitted to regular cannabis use. Five MMP patients regularly used the benzodiazepine diazepam, with a daily dose of 20 mg to 30 mg.[6]

As discussed previously, poor sleep is common in patients on chronic opiates. In the study discussed previously,[6] polysomnograms on the MMP patients showed significantly lower sleep efficiency, lower percentage of stage N3 and rapid eye movement (REM) sleep, and higher percentage of stage N2 sleep compared with controls. Six patients had a central apnea index (CAI) greater than 5 events per hour (normal <5), 4 had a CAI greater than 10 events per hour, and 3 of these exhibited periodic breathing pattern during sleep (Fig. 2). Not surprisingly, the control group did not have central sleep apnea (CSA) because it is a rare occurrence in the general population.

In a larger and more comprehensive study, the same investigators reported on 50 subjects on methadone chronically and 20 control subjects, matched for age and body mass index.[7] All subjects underwent polysomnography and blood toxicology. In addition, all subjects completed several questionnaires, including the Epworth Sleepiness Scale (ESS), the Functional Outcome of Sleep Questionnaire (FOSQ), the BDI version 2 (BDI-II), and the Modified Mini-Mental State Examination (MMMSE). The FOSQ comprises 5 subscales evaluating general productivity, social outcome, activity level, vigilance, intimate relationship, and sexual activity.[8] BDI-II includes 4 items (agitation, worthlessness, concentration difficulty, and loss of energy) designed to assess for symptoms of depression. The MMMSE was designed to assess for neurocognitive impairment or organic mental disorders.[9] In this study, ESS, FOSQ, and BDI scores were significantly worse in patients on methadone compared with controls. The MMMSE showed a trend toward significance $(P = .09)$.[7]

From these studies, it cannot be determined conclusively if chronic opioid use was the cause of depression. Emerging epidemiologic evidence suggests, however, that chronic use of opioids is

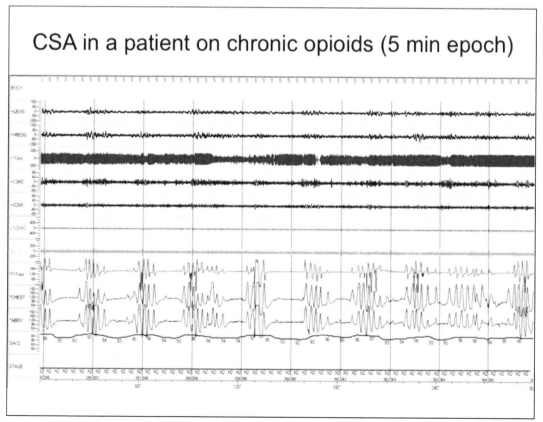

Fig. 2. An example of periodic breathing, central apneas, and ataxic breathing pattern in a patient on chronic opioids.

associated with incident depression and changes in neuronal mechanisms impacting relevant neurologic pathways.[10] Similarly, patients with remitted depression seemed at increased risk of relapse after exposure to chronic opioid analgesics.[11] These findings highlight the depressogenic effect of opioids and the importance of a careful assessment of past medical history of mood disturbances and depression as well as monitoring for the emergence of mood dysfunction before and during administration of opioids. The studies suggest that higher doses of opioids[12] and chronicity[13] are potential risk factors for depression. In a study by Merrill and colleagues,[12] more than 60% of patients receiving 120 mg or higher daily equivalent of morphine were clinically depressed, a 2.6-fold higher risk (95% CI, 1.5–4.4) than in patients on low-dose regimens (<20 mg daily). These data further highlight the importance of risk stratification before prescribing opioids for chronic use.

The daytime symptoms and presence of depression in association with chronic use of opioids are emphasized. In some of these studies, polysomnography was not performed, which might otherwise have discovered the presence of disrupted sleep architecture and SDB, both contributing to daytime impairment. Adverse effects of opioids on sleep and breathing are briefly reviewed.

OPIOIDS AND SLEEP

As depicted in **Fig. 1**, depression and anxiety may cause insomnia and poor sleep quantity and quality, and the latter could further contribute to a variety of daytime symptoms. Opioid use, although sedating, may actually interrupt sleep and impair sleep quality. To make matters more complicated, acute versus chronic opioid use (and withdrawal) have differing effects on sleep and daytime symptoms. Dimsdale and colleagues[14] evaluated the effects of 1 dose of sustained release morphine versus methadone on sleep architecture in healthy subjects. The investigators reported that both drugs significantly reduced percentage of time in slow-wave sleep (stage N3) and increased percentage of time in sleep stage N2, whereas neither drug had an effect on sleep efficiency, wake after sleep onset, or total sleep time. The latter findings perhaps were not surprising because control individuals were enrolled. Xiao and colleagues[15] compared sleep architecture of healthy controls and methadone-treated patients. Patients treated with chronic methadone had lower sleep efficiency, shorter total sleep time, more arousals, and a lower percentage of slow-wave sleep (stage N3). Correspondingly, the Pittsburgh Sleep Quality

Index and ESS scores were significantly higher than in control subjects. Although this study did not report a reduction in REM sleep, another study reported suppression of REM sleep with chronic opioid use.[6] Similar to SDB, the effects of opioids on sleep architecture seem dose dependent.[7,15]

The authors conclude that chronic use of opioids is associated with disturbed sleep architecture, low sleep efficiency, decreased slow-wave sleep and perhaps REM sleep, and daytime consequences.

OPIOIDS AND SLEEP-DISORDERED BREATHING

SDB associated with chronic opioid use is a complex form of sleep-related breathing disorder that combines elements of upper airway obstruction as well as suppression of the central nervous system pacemaker generating respiratory rhythm. Chronic opioid use as a risk factor for SDB is well established. The spectrum of SDB seen with chronic opioid use includes CSA, hypoventilation, hypoxemia, and ataxic or cluster breathing (see **Fig. 2**). Studies demonstrated that 30% to 90% of patients on chronic opioids have some form of SDB.[16–18] A recent review of 560 patients with chronic opioid use reported an overall CSA prevalence of 24%.[19] A morphine equivalent daily dose of 200 mg or more was strongly associated with severity of SDB, specifically CSA.[20]

Pathophysiology of Opioid-Induced Sleep-Disordered Breathing

Obstructive sleep apnea (OSA) and CSA induced by chronic use of opioid has been discussed in detail previously and is discussed briefly.[21] Experimental studies in neonatal rats have improved understanding of how respiration is controlled. Discovered in 1990s, there are 2 distinct respiratory rhythm generators located in the ventrolateral medullary portion of the neonatal rat brainstem, the pre-Bötzinger complex (pre-BotC) and the retrotrapezoid nucleus/parafacial respiratory group, which are normally coupled and generate normal respiratory rhythm.[22,23] In animal studies, the pre-BotC seems the dominant site for rhythm generation and contains the neurokinin-1 receptor (NK1R) and μ-opioid receptor.[24] In neonatal rodents, stimulation with μ-opioid agonists results in respiratory rate suppression.[25] Lesions in this area demonstrate apneas during sleep as well as an irregular breathing pattern during wakefulness and sleep.[26] A study in adult rats showed that accumulative loss of pre-BotC NK1R neurons led to progressive disturbances in sleep-related breathing initially in REM sleep, followed by

NREM sleep, with greater than 80% of neuronal loss in wakefulness. The abnormal breathing events were characterized by central hypopneas and central apneas and, when most severe, they were characterized as ataxic breathing.[27] In human polysomnographic studies, however, central apneas occur primarily in non-REM sleep.

Chronic opioid use contributes to an increased incidence and severity of SDB for several reasons: enhanced relaxation of upper airway musculature, alterations in hypercapnic and hypoxic ventilatory responses, and depression of respiratory rhythm generation. During sleep, activity of the dilator muscles of the upper airway is reduced[28] and in those who are prone to airway collapse (eg, anatomically small upper airway), opioids may further decrease the activity of these muscles and increase the likelihood of upper airway obstruction. The authors postulate that opioid-induced SDB is secondary to a combined effect of upper airway obstruction as well as suppression of the pacemaker generating breathing rhythm. There are no human studies on the pathophysiology of opioid-induced SDB.

Although large randomized studies have not been conducted, available data show that opioid-induced SDB may not respond to conventional positive airway pressure (PAP) devices and requires advanced PAP modes for effective treatment.[29–32]

MANAGEMENT GOALS

- Management of patients with opioid-related CSA is extremely challenging. The first and most important step is to assess ongoing need for opioids and, when possible, reduce dosage of opioid. This discussion should be made together with provider and patient within the first 4 weeks of initiating therapy and every 3 months or more frequently as part of the treatment plan. In an effort to minimize opioid overprescription and abuse, the Centers for Disease Control and Prevention recently published guidelines for prescribing opioids for chronic pain.[5] This guideline provides recommendations for clinicians who are prescribing opioids for chronic pain outside active cancer treatment, palliative care, and end-of-life care. The guideline addresses (1) when to initiate or continue opioids for chronic pain; (2) opioid selection, dosage, duration, follow-up, and discontinuation; and (3) assessing risk and addressing harms of opioid use.[5] The state prescription drug monitoring program data should be used to determine whether patients are receiving opioid dosages or dangerous combinations that put them at high risk for overdose.

- Consider nonopioid pharmacologic therapies when possible.
- If opioid is indicated, treatment should be initiated with immediate-release preparations rather than extended-release or long-acting preparations. The lowest effective dosage should be prescribed.
- Discontinue or taper opioid dosages if possible as clinically appropriate.
- For patients with underlying risk for respiratory depression or those with symptoms suggestive of SDB, diagnostic testing and treatment are indicated.

PHARMACOLOGIC STRATEGIES

When possible, supervised taper or withdrawal of opioids is recommended, but this is difficult to achieve. Unfortunately, pharmacologic interventions for SDB are limited. Discontinuation of opioids is the best option and studies have shown elimination of SDB by detoxification.[33,34] Importantly, these 2 studies[33,34] using polysomnography have unequivocally proved that opioids are a cause of SDB in humans.

Buprenorphine/Naloxone

Buprenorphine, a partial μ-opioid agonist, is widely used for the treatment of opioid dependency and chronic pain. Buprenorphine is a potent partial μ-agonist with a much higher receptor affinity than morphine and long dissociation half-life. The medication maintains an analgesic dose response across all levels without an increase in respiratory depression. In 2002, the US Food and Drug Administration approved buprenorphine monotherapy and a combination product of buprenorphine/naloxone for opioid detoxification therapy. Prescriptions for buprenorphine have exponentially risen due to its supposedly attractive safety profile regarding respiratory suppression compared with other full μ-agonists, such as methadone.

Farney and colleagues[35] reported that even at routine standard doses, buprenorphine showed significant respiratory impairment during sleep, with 63% showing evidence of mild SDB on polysomnography (an apnea-hypopnea index [AHI] >5 events/h), 17% of patients showing moderate to severe SDB (AHI >15 events/h), and 38% of patients had nocturnal hypoxemia (oxygen saturation as measured by pulse oximetry [Spo_2] <90% for 10% of total sleep time). The investigators concluded that clinically significant SDB occurred in many patients on buprenorphine/naloxone for opioid withdrawal therapy. Of significance, the respiratory disturbances consisted predominantly of central apneas and ataxic breathing, both of which are common respiratory events associated with opioids.

Acetazolamide

Opioids can cause continuous PAP (CPAP)-emergent CSA.[33] A case report described positive results with the use of acetazolamide, 250 mg, plus CPAP in the treatment of CSA secondary to chronic opioid use.[36] When the medication was discontinued after 5 months of treatment, central apneas reappeared while on CPAP.

Ampakines

Ampakines are a family of compounds that modulate the action of the excitatory neurotransmitter glutamate at the AMPA receptors by altering channel kinetics. Several studies using rat models demonstrated that ampakines, acting through glutamate-mediated neurotransmission via AMPA receptors, alleviate opiate-induced respiratory depression of central respiratory rhythmogenesis, which is hypothesized to originate from the pre-BotC.[37,38] Studies using adult rats showed that CX717, a synthetic ampakine compound, alleviates fentanyl-induced respiratory depression without inhibiting analgesia or sedation.[39–41]

Preliminary findings suggest that ampakines may be beneficial in counteracting opiate-induced respiratory depression, maintain upper airway patency, while preserving opioid's analgesic effect. In a study on 16 healthy human subjects, CX717 counteracted alfentanil-induced respiratory depression without affecting opiate-mediated analgesia.[42] Lorier and colleagues[43] showed that opiates induced upper airway obstruction by acting on the presynaptic inhibition of the hypoglossal (XII) motor neuron, affecting the tongue muscle involved in maintaining upper airway patency. Ampakines (CX 614 and CX717) successfully counteracted μ-opioid receptor mediated depression of hypoglossal (XII) motor-neuron inspiratory activity.[43] Dai and colleagues[44] demonstrated the use of a synthetic ampakine compound XD-8-17C to reverse opioid-induced acute respiratory depression without having an impact on the antinociceptive efficacy of morphine in rat model. Treatment with XD-8-17C reversed respiratory depression with restoration of arterial blood gas and lung function parameters to normal range. These findings show promise in novel therapeutic agents that protect against opioid-induced respiratory impairment without loss of analgesia.

Oxygen Therapy

The role of oxygen therapy for SDB secondary to chronic opioid use has not been established. To date, there are no studies evaluating the role of oxygen therapy as a single agent for the treatment of SDB due to chronic opioid use. Supplemental oxygen in combination with PAP therapy, however, has been reported and is discussed later. Given the understanding of the hypoxic and hypercapnic ventilatory responses, adding oxygen to patients with an already reduced hypercapnic ventilatory response may further worsen hypercapnia. Oxygen therapy may prolong hypoxemia or the duration of central apneas. On the other hand, in patients with elevated hypercapnic or hypoxic ventilatory responses (high loop gain), oxygen may stabilize respiration and abolish central apneas by reducing ventilatory chemoresponsiveness.

Chowdhuri and colleagues[45] used a protocol consisting of CPAP followed by CPAP + oxygen, then bilevel PAP [BPAP]+ oxygen, escalating in a stepwise titration to eliminate central apneas in veterans (N = 162) at an academic Veterans Affairs (VA) medical center; 47 patients were on opioid therapy for chronic pain, in whom CPAP, CPAP + oxygen, or BPAP + oxygen eliminated CSA in 54%, 28%, and 10% of the cases, respectively. The results showed that in individuals who fail initial CPAP therapy during a titration study, a majority of residual central apneas can be eliminated effectively by adding oxygen to PAP therapy. Obtaining oxygen using this protocol, however, may not be feasible in a non-VA setting given the current stringent oxygen criteria set forth by the Centers for Medicare and Medicaid Services.

POSITIVE AIRWAY PRESSURE THERAPY

See **Table 1** on studies using PAP therapy.

Continuous Positive Airway Pressure

Treatment of SDB secondary to chronic opioid use is challenging due to the presence of both OSA and CSA. In patients with OSA, the first treatment option is treatment with CPAP. As discussed later, however, CSA may emerge. CPAP does not treat central apneas associated with opioid use but rather increases the frequency of central apnea events.[29–31] Farney and colleagues[46] reported 1 of the earliest cases, of 3 patients who developed opioid-induced CSA that was unresponsive to CPAP. Allam and colleagues[32] undertook a retrospective study of 100 patients who failed conventional CPAP therapy for various types of CSA,

Table 1
Studies using positive airway pressure therapies for opioid-induced central sleep apnea

Study	Design	Intervention	Outcomes
Shapiro et al,[51] 2015	Prospective, randomized, crossover N = 34 First night titration then followed for 3 mo on ASV in the home setting	All subjects underwent CPAP, ASV without mandatory PS, ASV manual (PS min 6 cm H_2O) titration— then sent home with ASV with or without mandatory PS.	Significant reduction in AHI and CAI with ASV on initial titration, and at 3 mo compared with baseline diagnostic PSG and CPAP titration
Javaheri et al,[52] 2014	Prospective trial N = 20 acute 17 followed for a minimum of 9 mo up to 6 y	All subjects underwent CPAP titration with persistent CSA; 9 subjects underwent second CPAP titration with persistent CSA; all subjects underwent ASV titration.	Significant reductions in AHI and CAI and improvement in oxyhemoglobin saturation on ASV compared with diagnostic PSG and CPAP titration Mean adherence = 5.1 h $\pm$ 2.5 h
Cao et al,[50] 2014	Prospective, randomized crossover N = 18	All subjects underwent 1 night with bilevel ST titration, then crossover to 1 night with ASV titration.	ASV normalized AHI and CAI compared with bilevel ST (83.3% vs 33.3%, respectively)
Chowdhuri et al,[45] 2012	Retrospective, using protocol at a VA medical center N = 47 (opioid-induced CSA)	All subjects underwent a routine protocol, which consisted of CPAP titration, then CPAP + O_2, then bilevel + O_2 for persistent central apneas.	CPAP, CPAP + O_2, or BPAP + O_2 eliminated CSA in 54%, 28%, and 10% of cases, respectively. Using a protocol resulted in significant decline in AHI, CAI and an increase in Spo_2.
Ramar et al,[54] 2012	Retrospective N = 47	Comparative review on ASV titration for CSA due to opioids vs systolic heart failure	ASV was successful in 59.6% (28 of 47) in the opioid group (AHI <10 events/h).
Guilleminault et al,[29] 2010	Retrospective N = 44	All subjects underwent systematic protocol consisting of CPAP, bilevel S, and bilevel ST titration for persistent CSA.	Bilevel ST significantly reduced CAI (1.70 $\pm$ 0.58 events/h) compared with CPAP (13.81 $\pm$ 2.77 events/h) and bilevel S (11.52 $\pm$ 2.12 events/h).
Alattar & Scharf,[47] 2009	Retrospective case series N = 5	All 5 subjects underwent diagnostic PSG, then CPAP, then bilevel ST titration (4 subjects).	Three patients responded to bilevel ST with reduction of AHI from severe to mild.
Javaheri et al,[31] 2008	Retrospective case series N = 5	All underwent diagnostic PSG, followed by CPAP titration, then ASV titration due to an increase in central apneas on CPAP	CPAP titration resulted in increased CAI from 26 to 27 events/h. Mean CAI was 0 events/h on ASV compared with 37 events/h on CPAP.

(continued on next page)

Table 1
(continued)

Study	Design	Intervention	Outcomes
Farney et al,[30] 2008	Retrospective N = 22	All underwent diagnostic PSG, followed by CPAP titration, then ASV titration due to an increase in central apneas on CPAP.	ASV improved CAI compared with CPAP but did not reach significance, presumably due to an increase in obstructive events. Mean AHI was 66 events/h at baseline, 70 events/h on CPAP, and 54 events/h on ASV. Hypopnea index increased from 14.5 events/h to 35.7 events/h on ASV.
Allam et al,[32] 2007	Retrospective N = 100 (category of CSA included CompSA, idiopathic CSA, and CSA/CSR) 13 subjects used opioids chronically (within CompSA and CSA category).	All subjects underwent diagnostic PSG, followed by CPAP, bilevel S, bilevel ST, and ASV titration for persistently elevated CAI.	ASV significantly improved AHI to a mean of 5 events/h vs diagnostic PSG and CPAP titration night. Sixty-four patients responded to ASV with a mean AHI <10 events/h.[a]

Abbreviations: CompSA, complex sleep apnea; CSR, Cheyne-Stokes respiration; PSG, polysomnogram.
  [a] No specific data on those using opioids (lumped into complex sleep apnea and CSA success category).

including those due to opioids. These patients were successfully treated with an adaptive servo ventilator (ASV). In an early study,[30] Javaheri and colleagues[31] reported 5 patients with severe sleep apnea (overall AHI 70 ± 19, CAI 26 ± 27 events/h) who failed CPAP therapy (central apnea events increased on CPAP, CAI 37 ± 21 events/h). Farney and colleagues[30] performed a retrospective analysis of 22 patients with severe sleep apnea (AHI 66 ± 37 events/h), of whom 18 of 22 failed CPAP therapy (AHI on CPAP 70 ± 33 events/h). Guilleminault and colleagues[29] performed a case-control study evaluating 44 patients with severe OSA on chronic opioid therapy and observed CPAP-emergent CSA (diagnostic CAI = 0.6 ± 1 events/h, CPAP CAI = 14 ± 3 events/h).

Bilevel Positive Airway Pressure

Alattar and Scharf[47] reported 4 patients with opioid-induced CSA who failed CPAP as well as bilevel therapy; 3 of the 4 bilevel patients required supplemental oxygen due to persistent nocturnal hypoxemia.[47] Guilleminault and colleagues[29] attempted BPAP therapy on 44 patients with co-morbid OSA and CPAP-emergent CSA secondary to opioids. Although BPAP effectively treated obstructive respiratory events, central apneas present on CPAP persisted (bilevel CAI = 12 ± 2

events/h). Patients continued to complain of nocturnal awakenings and daytime hypersomno-lence on CPAP and BPAP.[29]

Bilevel Spontaneous Timed

BPAP with back-up respiratory rate (ie, bilevel spontaneous timed [ST]) has shown some success in treating CSA associated with chronic opioid use. Alattar and Scharf[47] reported 5 patients on methadone maintenance with central apneas (AHI ranged 28–106 events/h with >50% central apneas) that improved on BPAP therapy with back-up respiratory rate. A case-control study by Guilleminault and colleagues[29] in 44 chronic opioid users with OSA (mean AHI 44 ± 1 events/h) reported a high rate of central apneas on treatment with CPAP (CAI 14 ± 3 events/h) and BPAP (CAI 12 ± 2 events/h). Bilevel ST, however, effectively eliminated central apneas (CAI 1.7 ± 0.6 events/h) and OSAs and improved nocturnal oxyhemoglobin saturation and daytime hypersomnolence.

Adaptive Servo Ventilator

Recent literature supports the use of ASV over other modes of PAP therapy. New-generation pressure support (PS) servo ventilators use a breath-by-breath algorithm to analyze a patient's ventilatory status with real-time corresponding adjustments.[48] With this platform, dynamic anticyclic PS is applied during the "undershoot period" and a sloughing off of PS during the "overshoot period." This platform has been used with increasing popularity for other types of SDB, including treatment-emergent central apneas and complex sleep apneas, idiopathic CSAs, periodic breathing, and most recently, CSAs associated with chronic opioid use.[49] It has been shown to improve respiratory disturbances in patients with complex sleep apnea and mixed sleep apnea and is more effective than both CPAP and bilevel therapy.

Initial studies on ASV for CSA secondary to chronic opioid use were carried out by Farney and colleagues[30] and Javaheri and colleagues.[31] Farney and coworkers[30] conducted a retrospective study with ASV to treat comorbid OSA and CSA in chronic opioid users with somewhat disappointing results; 22 chronic opioid using patients referred for suspected SDB did not respond to CPAP and were subsequently placed on ASV. In this study, the end-expiratory pressure (EEP) was fixed at 5 cm H_2O (not titrated up for obstructive events), whereas the back-up respiratory rate was set at 15 breaths per minute. With EEP set at 5 cm H_2O, it is likely below the pressure required to maintain upper airway patency; therefore, obstructive events persisted. Around the same time, Javaheri and colleagues[31] evaluated 5 consecutive patients with SDB on chronic opioid therapy and found that the ASV effectively eliminated central apneas (AHI decreased from 70 events/h to 20 events/h, with a CAI of 0 events/h). In contrast to the study by Farney and colleagues[30] the EEP was titrated to effectively eliminate obstructive events. EEP titration with appropriate adjustment of both inspiratory and expiratory pressures is critical in treating comorbid OSA and CSA.

Cao and colleagues[50] randomized patients to bilevel ST versus new-generation ASV with a 1-night crossover design study. ASV with autotitrating expiratory PAP was superior to bilevel ST in normalizing respiratory events, including central apneas (83.3% vs 33.3% respectively). Two studies evaluated extended ASV use in the home setting. Shapiro and colleagues[51] performed a prospective interventional study comparing CPAP versus ASV on patients with CSA secondary to opioid use on initial titration study, then followed patients in the home setting for 3 months. All patients were using opioids prescribed at greater than 100 mg morphine equivalent. At 3 months of home ASV use, the AHI and CAI were significantly reduced compared with baseline diagnostic levels and CPAP treatment. Javaheri and colleagues[52] conducted a stepwise titration protocol on 20 patients with CSA secondary to chronic opioid therapy. CPAP titration was ineffective in reducing central apneas at initial titration and again 4 weeks later. The mean CAI was 32 events per hour at baseline, which was reduced to zero events per hour with ASV. Seventeen patients were followed for a period of 9 months up to 6 years, with persistently low CAI and a mean adherence of 5.1 ± 2.5 hours per night.[52]

A recent systematic review on current PAP therapies for opioid-induced CSA (n = 127 patients) showed conflicting results.[53] Opioid dosages ranged from 10 mg to 450 mg daily of morphine equivalent dose. CPAP was ineffective in reducing central apneic events. BPAP with and without supplemental oxygen achieved elimination of central apneas in 62% of patients. ASV yielded conflicting results with only 58% of participants achieving a CAI less than 10 events per hour. The investigators also found that the presence of ataxic breathing predicted a poor response to PAP therapy. Ramar and colleagues[54] also found a variable response to ASV. These data are in contrast to another study reporting good response, both acutely and chronically to ASV.[52] It must be emphasized that the complex algorithms of ASV devices and successful treatment of complex SDB require in-depth knowledge of these algorithms and the choice of appropriate pressure settings detailed elsewhere.[55,56]

SUMMARY

Chronic opioid use is an established risk factor for impaired sleep architecture and SDB, especially CSA. These sleep-related consequences result in daytime impairment, including daytime hypersomnolence, daytime fatigue, depression, and neurocognitive impairment. A careful medical history assessment and close follow-up are essential in patients using chronic opioids.

In addition, SDB associated with chronic opioid use is a diagnostic and therapeutic challenge for the clinician. There are no standard treatments for opioid-induced SDB. When possible, opiates should be tapered or discontinued. Optimal treatment modalities have not been extensively studied in long-term randomized trials as reflected by a paucity of the available literature. Although studies are limited, new-generation ASVs deserve further research and should be attempted in patients with SDB, including CSA induced by chronic opioid use, especially in those who do not respond to conventional modes of therapy, such as CPAP or BPAP. The overall impact of ASV on SDB induced by chronic opioid use on long-term morbidity and mortality is unknown.

REFERENCES

1. American Academy of Pain Medicine and the American Pain Society. The use of opioids for the treatment of chronic pain. A consensus statement from the American Academy of Pain Medicine and the American Pain Society. Clin J Pain 1997;13(1):6–8.
2. Han B, Compton WM, Blanco C, et al. Prescription opioid use, misuse, and use disorders in U.S. Adults: 2015 national survey on drug use and health. Ann Intern Med 2017;167:293–301.
3. Ballantyne JC. Opioid for the treatment of chronic pain: mistakes made, lessons learned, and future directions. Anesth Analg 2017;125:1769–78.
4. Rutkow J, Vernick JS. Emergency legal authority and the opioid crisis. N Engl J Med 2017;377(26): 2512–4.
5. Dowell D, Haegerich T, Chou R, et al. CDC guideline for prescribing opioids for chronic pain – United States, 2016. MMWR Recomm Rep 2016;65(1):1–49.
6. Teichtahl H, Prodromidis A, Miller B, et al. Sleep disordered breathing in stable methadone programme patients: a pilot study. Addiction 2001;96: 395–403.
7. Wang D, Teichtahl M, Drummer O, et al. Central sleep apnea in stable methadone maintenance treatment patients. Chest 2005;128:1348–56.
8. Weaver TE, Laizner AM, Evans LK, et al. An instrument to measure functional status outcomes for disorders of excessive sleepiness. Sleep 1997;20:835–43.
9. Patten SB, Fick GH. Clinical interpretation of the mini-mental state. Gen Hosp Psychiatry 1993;15: 254–9.
10. Fischer B, Murphy Y, Kurdyak P, et al. Depression - a major but neglected consequence contributing to the health toll from prescription opioids? Psychiatry Res 2016;243:331–4.
11. Scherrer JF, Salas J, Copeland LA, et al. Increased risk of depression recurrence after initiation of prescription opioids in non-cancer pain patients. J Pain 2016;17(4):473–82.
12. Merrill JO, Von Korff M, Banta-Green CJ, et al. Prescribed opioid difficulties, depression and opioid dose among chronic opioid therapy patients. Gen Hosp Psychiatry 2012;34(6):581–7.
13. Scherrer JF, Svrakic DM, Freedland KE, et al. Prescription opioid analgesics increase the risk of depression. J Gen Intern Med 2014;29(3):491–9.
14. Dimsdale JE, Norman D, DeJardin D, et al. The effect of opioids on sleep architecture. J Clin Sleep Med 2007;3(1):33–6.
15. Xiao L, Tang Y, Smith AK, et al. Nocturnal sleep architecture disturbances in early methadone treatment patients. Psychiatry Res 2010;179:91–5.
16. Mogri M, Desai H, Webster L, et al. Hypoxemia in patients on chronic opiate therapy with and without sleep apnea. Sleep Breath 2009;13(1):49–57.
17. Webster LR, Choi Y, Desai H, et al. Sleep-disordered breathing and chronic opioid therapy. Pain Med 2008;9(4):425–32.
18. Sharkey KM, Kurth ME, Anderson BJ, et al. Obstructive sleep apnea is more common than central sleep apnea in methadone maintenance patients with subjective sleep complaints. Drug Alcohol Depend 2010;108(1–2):77–83.
19. Correa D, Farney RJ, Chung F, et al. Chronic opioid use and central sleep apnea: a review of the prevalence, mechanisms, and perioperative considerations. Anesth Analg 2015;120:1273–85.
20. Walker JM, Farney RJ, Rhondeau SM, et al. Chronic opioid use is a risk factor for the development of central sleep apnea and ataxic breathing. J Clin Sleep Med 2007;3(5):455–61.
21. Chowdhuri S, Javaheri S. Sleep disordered breathing caused by chronic opioid use: diverse manifestations and their management. Sleep Med Clin 2017; 12(4):573–86.
22. Smith JC, Ellenberger HH, Ballanyi K, et al. Pre-Botzinger complex: a brainstem region that may generate respiratory rhythm in mammals. Science 1991;254(5032):726–9.
23. Feldman JL, Del Negro CA. Looking for inspiration: new perspectives on respiratory rhythm. Nat Rev Neurosci 2006;7(3):232–42.
24. Gray PA, Janczewski WA, Mellen N, et al. Normal breathing requires preBotzinger complex neurokinin-1 receptor-expressing neurons. Nat Neurosci 2001;4(9):927–30.
25. Gray PA, Rekling JC, Bocchiaro CM, et al. Modulation of respiratory frequency by peptidergic input to rhythmogenic neurons in the preBotzinger complex. Science 1999;286(5444):1566–8.
26. McKay LC, Janczewski WA, Feldman JL. Sleep-disordered breathing after targeted ablation of pre-Botzinger complex neurons. Nat Neurosci 2005; 8(9):1142–4.
27. McKay LC, Feldman JL. Unilateral ablation of pre-Botzinger complex disrupts breathing during sleep but not wakefulness. Am J Respir Crit Care Med 2008;178(1):89–95.
28. Edwards BA, White DP. Control of the pharyngeal musculature during wakefulness and sleep: implications in normal controls and sleep apnea. Head Neck 2011;33(Suppl 1):S37–45.
29. Guilleminault C, Cao M, Yue HJ, et al. Obstructive sleep apnea and chronic opioid use. Lung 2010; 188(6):459–68.
30. Farney RJ, Walker JM, Boyle KM, et al. Adaptive servoventilation (ASV) in patients with sleep disordered breathing associated with chronic opioid medications for non-malignant pain. J Clin Sleep Med 2008;4(4):311–9.
31. Javaheri S, Malik A, Smith J, et al. Adaptive pressure support servoventilation: a novel treatment for sleep

apnea associated with use of opioids. J Clin Sleep Med 2008;4(4):305–10.

32. Allam JS, Olson EJ, Gay PC, et al. Efficacy of adaptive servoventilation in treatment of complex and central sleep apnea syndromes. Chest 2007; 132(6):1839–46.

33. Javaheri S, Patel S. Opioids cause central and complex sleep apnea in humans and reversal with discontinuation: a plea for detoxification. J Clin Sleep Med 2017;13(6):829–33.

34. Davis MJ, Livingston M, Scharf SM. Reversal of central sleep apnea following discontinuation of opioids. J Clin Sleep Med 2012;8(5):579–80.

35. Farney RJ, McDonald AM, Boyle KM, et al. Sleep disordered breathing in patients receiving therapy with buprenorphine/naloxone. Eur Respir J 2013; 42:394–403.

36. Glidewell RN, Orr WC, Imes N. Acetazolamide as an adjunct to CPAP treatment: a case of complex sleep apnea in a patient on long-acting opioid therapy. J Clin Sleep Med 2009;5(1):63–4.

37. Ren J, Poon BY, Tang Y, et al. Ampakines alleviate respiratory depression in rats. Am J Respir Crit Care Med 2006;174(12):1384–91.

38. Ren J, Greer JJ. Modulation of perinatal respiratory rhythm by GABA(A)–and glycine receptor-mediated chloride conductances. Adv Exp Med Biol 2008;605:149–53.

39. Greer JJ, Ren J. Ampakine therapy to counter fentanyl-induced respiratory depression. Respir Physiol Neurobiol 2009;168(1–2):153–7.

40. Ren J, Ding X, Funk GD, et al. Ampakine CX717 protects against fentanyl-induced respiratory depression and lethal apnea in rats. Anesthesiology 2009; 110(6):1364–70.

41. Ren J, Lenal F, Yang M, et al. Coadministration of the AMPAKINE CX717 with propofol reduces respiratory depression and fatal apneas. Anesthesiology 2013; 118(6):1437–45.

42. Oertel BG, Felden L, Tran PV, et al. Selective antagonism of opioid-induced ventilatory depression by an ampakine molecule in humans without loss of opioid analgesia. Clin Pharmacol Ther 2010;87(2): 204–11.

43. Lorier AR, Funk GD, Greer JJ. Opiate-induced suppression of rat hypoglossal motoneuron activity and its reversal by ampakine therapy. PLoS One 2010; 5(1):e8766.

44. Dai W, Xiao D, Gao X, et al. A brain-targeted ampakine compound protects against opioid-induced respiratory depression. Eur J Pharmacol 2017;809: 122–9.

45. Chowdhuri S, Ghabsha A, Sinha P, et al. Treatment of central sleep apnea in US veterans. J Clin Sleep Med 2012;8(5):555–63.

46. Farney RJ, Walker JM, Cloward TV, et al. Sleep-disordered breathing associated with long-term opioid therapy. Chest 2003;123(2):632–9.

47. Alattar MA, Scharf SM. Opioid-associated central sleep apnea: a case series. Sleep Breath 2009; 13(1):201–6.

48. Javaheri S, Goetting MG, Khayat R, et al. The performance of two automatic servo-ventilation devices in the treatment of central sleep apnea. Sleep 2011; 34(12):1693–8.

49. Javaheri S. Positive airway pressure treatment of central sleep apnea with emphasis on heart failure, opioids, and complex sleep apnea. In: Berry RB, editor. Sleep medicine clinics. Philadelphia: WB Saunders; 2010. p. 407–17.

50. Cao M, Cardell C, Willes L, et al. A novel adaptive servoventilation (ASVauto) for the treatment of central sleep apnea associated with chronic use of opioids. J Clin Sleep Med 2014;10(8):855–61.

51. Shapiro CM, Chung SA, Wylie PE, et al. Home-use of servo-ventilation therapy in chronic pain patients with central sleep apnea: initial and 3-month follow up. Sleep Breath 2015;19:1285–92.

52. Javaheri S, Harris N, Howard J, et al. Adaptive servoventilation for treatment of opioid-associated central sleep apnea. J Clin Sleep Med 2014;10(6): 637–43.

53. Reddy R, Adamo D, Kufel T, et al. Treatment of opioid-related central sleep apnea with positive airway pressure: a systematic review. J Opioid Manag 2014;10(1):57–62.

54. Ramar K, Ramar P, Morgenthaler T. Adaptive servo-ventilation in patients with central or complex sleep apnea related to chronic opioid use and congestive heart failure. J Clin Sleep Med 2012;8(5):569–76.

55. Javaheri S, Brown L, Randerath W. Positive airway pressure therapy with adaptive servo-ventilation (Part 1: operational algorithms). Chest 2014;146: 514–23.

56. Javaheri S, Brown L, Randerath W. Positive airway pressure therapy with adaptive servo-ventilation (Part II: clinical Applications). Chest 2014;146: 855–68.

Moving?

Make sure your subscription moves with you!

To notify us of your new address, find your Clinics Account Number (located on your mailing label above your name), and contact customer service at:

Email: journalscustomerservice-usa@elsevier.com

800-654-2452 (subscribers in the U.S. & Canada)
314-447-8871 (subscribers outside of the U.S. & Canada)

Fax number: 314-447-8029

Elsevier Health Sciences Division
Subscription Customer Service
3251 Riverport Lane
Maryland Heights, MO 63043

To ensure uninterrupted delivery of your subscription, please notify us at least 4 weeks in advance of move.

Printed and bound by CPI Group (UK) Ltd, Croydon, CR0 4YY

03/10/2024

01040384-0008